Cardiovascular Mechanics

Cardiovascular Mechanics

Edited by
Michel R. Labrosse

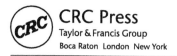

CRC Press
Taylor & Francis Group
Boca Raton London New York

CRC Press is an imprint of the
Taylor & Francis Group, an **informa** business

CRC Press
Taylor & Francis Group
6000 Broken Sound Parkway NW, Suite 300
Boca Raton, FL 33487-2742

First issued in paperback 2023

ISBN 13: 978-1-138-19723-7 (hbk)
ISBN 13: 978-1-03-265243-6 (pbk)
ISBN 13: 978-1-315-28029-5 (ebk)

DOI: 10.1201/b21917

Library of Congress Cataloging-in-Publication Data

Names: Labrosse, Michel (Michel R.), editor.
Title: Cardiovascular mechanics / [edited by] Michel Labrosse.
Description: Boca Raton, FL : CRC Press/Taylor & Francis Group, [2018] |
Includes bibliographical references.
Identifiers: LCCN 2018016353 (print) | LCCN 2018017115 (ebook) | ISBN
9781315280295 (Master eBook) | ISBN 9781315280288 (Pdf) | ISBN
9781315280271 (ePUB) | ISBN 9781315280264 (Mobipocket) | ISBN
9781138197237 (hardback)
Subjects: | MESH: Cardiovascular System | Biomechanical Phenomena
Classification: LCC QP101 (ebook) | LCC QP101 (print) | NLM WG 100 | DDC
612.1--dc23
LC record available at https://lccn.loc.gov/2018016353

Visit the Taylor & Francis Web site at
http://www.taylorandfrancis.com

and the CRC Press Web site at
http://www.crcpress.com

Contents

Contents

Preface

Decisions in cardiovascular surgery can be life-and-death decisions and often need to be made fast. This is the realm of evidence-based decision-making algorithms that are updated as practices evolve and new techniques are adopted. These algorithms originate from guidelines and recommendations elaborated after statistical treatment of data collected on whole cohorts of patients. While the decision to put knife to skin may be eminently binary, there are usually multiple ways to do so, and the amount of training of the surgeon and supporting team will heavily influence the patient outcome. Therefore, not only the initial decision needs to be adequate but also both the ensuing plan and implementation must be flawless. Surgical planning, as possibly aided by computer simulations to evaluate different scenarios, is one specific area in which biomedical engineers are increasingly involved, aside from their usual role in the development of new medical devices. Many surgeons have already shown an interest in such contributions.

Still, the questions addressed, along with the pace of investigation in biomedical engineering or basic science laboratories, are quite different from what clinicians may be familiar with. This is because experimental test methods need to be developed and mastered before producing consistent, meaningful data, and more often than not, simulation tools also need to be either developed from scratch or modified from existing computational tools. Computer models always need to be verified (i.e., do they solve the problem right? In other words, are the underlying mathematics and computer science correctly implemented?) Computer models also need to be validated (i.e., do they solve the right problem? In other words, does the idealized problem at hand include enough physical phenomena or is it oversimplified?) Both the verification and validation aspects of simulations are rather well established for biomedical engineering devices, thanks to regulatory compliance and certification procedures. However, they are still open-ended concepts, with no standards to speak of when it comes to cardiovascular modeling, because of, among other things, the complexity of their tissue mechanics.

It is hoped, through the present book, to make communication and understanding easier and more natural between clinicians, basic scientists, and biomedical engineers, by finding common language and letting them tell their side of the story. By taking stock of what is known and what has been achieved so far, one can also better appreciate what remains to be accomplished to further the standard of care.

Unraveling the detailed workings of the cardiovascular system and components is still a high priority in the twenty-first century, motivated not only by mankind's inquisitiveness but also by societal and clinical outlooks. According to the World Health Organization, each year, about a third of all deaths worldwide are due to cardiovascular disease. To put things in perspective, this represents the equivalent of 17 million people or half the population of a country like Canada vanishing each year because of cardiovascular disease. Aside from the obvious human loss the disease represents, its massive financial burden is also ballooning, owing to the aging of the population prevalent in many developing and developed countries.

The basic scientists, biomedical engineers, and clinicians engaged in the fight against cardiovascular disease have not been sitting idle. With recent developments such as fully integrated total artificial hearts and the bioprinting of coronary arteries, it is clear that innovative techniques and potential treatments are entering the fray at a rapid pace. In the last few decades, mechanobiology has emerged as a very promising and ever-expanding field, connecting mechanics to issues at the molecular, cellular, and tissue levels, with important ramifications for cardiovascular disease. With the apparent explosion, mosaic-like, of new highly specialized knowledge, it is timely to take a step back and piece together the larger picture of cardiovascular mechanics. There are multiple and excellent books that address one or a couple of specific topics (e.g., cardiovascular solid mechanics and mechanics of the circulation), but on review, it seemed that a book encompassing most major aspects of cardiovascular mechanics is yet to be written. Even if specialized scientific conferences and meetings strive to become increasingly inclusive, there are still significant divides between researchers in cardiovascular solids and fluids, between cellular biochemists and tissue engineers, and, regrettably, also between clinicians and biomedical engineers. The present book aims to provide the readers, irrespective of their backgrounds, with a comprehensive view that enables them to appraise the most recent developments and applications in cardiovascular mechanics through a presentation of the underlying principles and theories.

The first part of the book, comprising five chapters, introduces some fundamental concepts of modern cardiovascular mechanics. As such, Chapter 1 starts from the general anatomy and physiology of the cardiovascular system. Chapter 2 elaborates on the numerous cell and extracellular matrix interactions and, in so doing, underlines the importance of mechanobiological processes. Continuum mechanics, as it applies to the theoretical study of blood flow, is detailed in Chapter 3, whereas its applications to cardiovascular soft tissues are discussed in a brief ad hoc fashion in relevant chapters. For thorough presentations of continuum mechanics for soft tissues and related principles and mathematics, the reader is referred to the masters (Humphrey, 2013; Holzapfel, 2000; Taber, 2004). Next, Chapters 4 and 5 review the experimental and computational methods used in solid and fluid mechanics, providing a basis for discussion of the strengths and limitations of current experiments and computer simulations.

The second part of the book, in another seven chapters, focuses on specific areas of applications of cardiovascular mechanics. Aortic and arterial mechanics are discussed in detail in Chapter 6; atherosclerosis, the condition that develops when plaque builds up in the walls of the arteries and that underlies many problems related to cardiovascular disease, is reviewed in Chapter 7; blood and microcirculation mechanics are considered in Chapter 8; heart valve mechanics are covered in Chapters 9 and 10; and aging is discussed in Chapter 11. Finally, in Chapter 12, an overview of the native mechanobiology of the cardiovascular system is presented in the context of medical devices and drugs, followed by detailed reviews of specific devices that include both engineering and regulatory requirements.

I am deeply indebted to the contributors of this book. Their enthusiasm and support were second to none, and I simply cannot thank them enough! Lastly, although many eyes have reviewed the book's content, I take full responsibility for any error or omission and warmly welcome the readers' feedback.

Michel Labrosse

References

Holzapfel GA. *Nonlinear Solid Mechanics: A Continuum Approach for Engineering.* Chichester, UK: John Wiley & Sons; 2000.

Humphrey JD. *Cardiovascular Solid Mechanics: Cells, Tissues, and Organs.* New York: Springer Science & Business Media; 2013.

Taber LA. *Nonlinear Theory of Elasticity: Applications in Biomechanics.* River Edge, NJ: World Scientific; 2004.

Editor

Michel R. Labrosse is the founder of the Cardiovascular Mechanics Laboratory at the University of Ottawa, where he is a full professor in the Department of Mechanical Engineering. He has been an active researcher in academia in collaboration mainly with the University of Ottawa Heart Institute. He has authored or co-authored over 90 refereed documents, and supervised or co-supervised over 40 graduate students and post-docs.

Contributors

F. Auricchio
Department of Civil Engineering and
  Architecture
University of Pavia
Pavia, Italy

S. Avril
Mines Saint-Étienne
Université de Lyon
Saint-Étienne, France

M. Bender
Department of Experimental
  Biomedicine
University Hospital and Rudolf Virchow
  Center
Wuerzburg, Germany

M. Boodhwani
Division of Cardiac Surgery
University of Ottawa Heart Institute
Ottawa, Ontario, Canada

V. Chan
Department of Cardiac Surgery
University of Ottawa Heart Institute
Ottawa, Ontario, Canada

M. Conti
Department of Civil Engineering and
  Architecture
University of Pavia
Pavia, Italy

J. Dallard
Department of Mechanical Engineering
University of Ottawa
Ottawa, Ontario, Canada

M. Fenech
Department of Mechanical Engineering
University of Ottawa
Ottawa, Ontario, Canada

S. Gekle
Biofluid Simulation and Modeling,
  Physics Department
University of Bayreuth
Bayreuth, Germany

C. A. Gibbons Kroeker
Departments of Cardiac Science,
  Physiology, and Pharmacology
Faculties of Medicine and Kinesiology
University of Calgary
Calgary, Alberta, Canada

L. Haya
Department of Mechanical Engineering
University of Ottawa
Ottawa, Ontario, Canada

L. Horný
Department of Mechanics,
  Biomechanics and Mechatronics
Faculty of Mechanical Engineering
Czech Technical University in Prague
Prague, Czech Republic

L. Kadem
Department of Mechanical, Industrial
    and Aerospace Engineering
Concordia University
Montreal, Quebec, Canada

M. Kozakova
Department of Clinical and
    Experimental Medicine
University of Pisa
Pisa, Italy

M. R. Labrosse
Department of Mechanical Engineering
University of Ottawa
Ottawa, Ontario, Canada

A. Y. L. Lam
Institute of Biomaterials and Biomedical
    Engineering
Ted Rogers Centre for Heart Research
    Translational Biology and
    Engineering Program
University of Toronto
Toronto, Ontario, Canada

A. Lefieux
Division of Cardiology
Emory University
Atlanta, Georgia

K. May-Newman
Department of Mechanical Engineering
San Diego State University
San Diego, California

T. G. Mesana
Department of Cardiac Surgery
University of Ottawa Heart Institute
Ottawa, Ontario, Canada

S. Morganti
Department of Electrical, Computer,
    and Biomedical Engineering
University of Pavia
Pavia, Italy

C. Palombo
Department of Surgical, Medical and
    Molecular Pathology and Critical
    Care Medicine
University of Pisa
Pisa, Italy

A. Reali
Department of Civil Engineering and
    Architecture
University of Pavia
Pavia, Italy

G. Rozza
SISSA, International School for
    Advanced Studies
Mathematics Area, MathLab
Trieste, Italy

C. A. Simmons
Institute of Biomaterials and Biomedical
    Engineering
Ted Rogers Centre for Heart Research
    Translational Biology and
    Engineering Program
Department of Mechanical and
    Industrial Engineering
University of Toronto
Toronto, Ontario, Canada

A. Tran
Department of Surgery
University of Connecticut Health
    Center
Farmington, Connecticut

A. Veneziani
Department of Mathematics and
    Computer Science
Emory University
Atlanta, Georgia

and

School of Advanced Studies IUSS
    Pavia
Pavia, Italy

1

Cardiovascular System:
Anatomy and Physiology
C. A. Gibbons Kroeker

Contents

The cardiovascular system consists of three components: the heart, the blood, and the blood vessels. The heart behaves as a hydraulic pump, creating the driving force behind the pulsatile blood flow through the arterial system. The magnitude and behavior of this blood flow is dependent on the mechanical properties of the heart muscle and the blood vessel wall, as well as the fluid properties of the blood.

The human heart is roughly the size of a human fist, with an average mass of 275 g. It begins to beat within a few weeks of gestation, contracting approximately once per second through a lifetime (about 3 billion heart beats). The heart is a dual-pump system (Figure 1.1). The right side of the heart collects deoxygenated blood from the venous system to be sent to the pulmonary arteries and the lungs (the pulmonary circulation), while the left side collects oxygenated blood from the pulmonary veins to be sent out via the aorta to the body tissues (the systemic circulation). The pulmonary circulation has a lower pressure than the systemic circulation. It is a low-resistance system that moves 100% of the blood through the lungs, exchanging carbon dioxide for oxygen. In contrast, the systemic circulatory system acts as a parallel circuit, and the distribution of blood to each of the body organs varies, depending on the relative resistance of the arterioles and capillaries preceding the organ system. At rest, a large proportion of the total blood flow is directed to the digestive tract and the kidneys. With exercise, the arterioles to the muscle beds vasodilate, decreasing the resistance and redirecting more blood flow to this organ system, while decreasing the relative

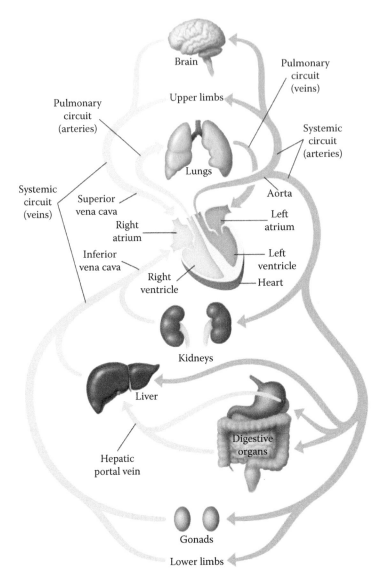

Figure 1.1 The circulatory system. While the pulmonary circuit receives 100% of the blood flow, the systemic system is arranged as a parallel circuit. Relative blood flow to each organ system will depend on the vascular tone of the vessel feeding the organ.

flow to the digestive tract and kidney. Although blood flow to many body organs may vary, blood flow to the brain remains constant.

1.1 The Heart

The heart is enclosed within the pericardium, a thin but tough connective tissue sheath. It provides protection and anchoring of the heart within the chest cavity, as well as acts as a constraint that prevents the overfilling of the heart chambers.

The fluid within the pericardial sac gives the heart some lubrication as it contracts and moves within the space. The heart muscle is supplied with blood and oxygen by the coronary circulation (the right, the left anterior descending, and the left circumflex coronary arteries). During systole (or contraction), the vessels are compressed by the muscle, so most of the coronary flow (roughly 70%) must occur during diastole (or relaxation). If nutrient supply is insufficient (e.g., by an occluded coronary artery in ischemia), damage to the heart muscle can occur.

The heart muscle is made up of cardiac muscle cells connected by intercalated discs. These discs consist of two cell junctions—a desmosome, which can withstand mechanical stress, and gap junctions, which allow for the movement of nerve impulses between cells. The muscle cells are arranged in a spiral pattern that results in ventricular torsion as the muscle contracts. It is believed that this "twisting" action aids in the ejection of blood, much like the effect seen when wringing out a wet cloth. In the isovolumic relaxation period, the muscle relaxes and the ventricular volume expands. This resulting drop in pressure may also aid in ventricular filling (known as the "diastolic suction" effect).

The heart is made up of four chambers—the left and right atria, which receive blood from the venous circulation, and the left and right ventricles, which eject blood into the arterial system (Figure 1.2). The blood enters the right atrium via the superior and inferior vena cavae (the great veins) and moves into the right ventricle, where it is ejected into the pulmonary arteries for circulation through the lungs. On return to the heart, via the pulmonary veins, it enters the left atrium and then the left ventricle, from where it is ejected into the aorta for circulation through the systemic arteries.

The atria are relatively small and thin-walled, reaching peak pressures of approximately 10 mmHg. They require only a minimal contraction to "top up" the ventricular volume, since most of the blood coming into the atria will directly flow into the ventricles during diastolic filling. The ventricles are divided by a muscular interventricular septum and contract simultaneously. The right ventricle will eject blood into the pulmonary circulation and develop peak pressures of approximately 30 mmHg. On the other hand, the left ventricle will eject blood into the higher-pressure, higher-resistance systemic circulation and will develop pressures of approximately 120 mmHg. To handle such high blood pressure, the muscle wall of the left ventricle is much thicker than that of the right ventricle.

The left ventricle ejects approximately 70 mL during each beat (this is known as the stroke volume) and about 5 L per minute (known as the cardiac output). Cardiac output is the product of stroke volume and heart rate. Stroke volume is dependent on the contractile ability of the heart muscle, as well as the amount of blood in the ventricles at the end of filling (the end-diastolic volume, or EDV). Commonly, the EDV in the left ventricle will be in the range of 110–120 mL. After contraction, the end-systolic volume (or ESV) ranges from 40 to 50 mL. The difference between the EDV and the ESV is the stroke volume. Clinically, the term ejection fraction is often used, which represents the stroke volume as a percentage of the EDV. Normal ejection fractions are approximately 66%–68%.

During exercise, when the sympathetic nervous system is stimulated and epinephrine is released, both the heart rate and the contractility of the heart increase. This results in large increases in both the stroke volume and the cardiac output and a decrease in the EDV. With aerobic training, the heart becomes larger and the wall

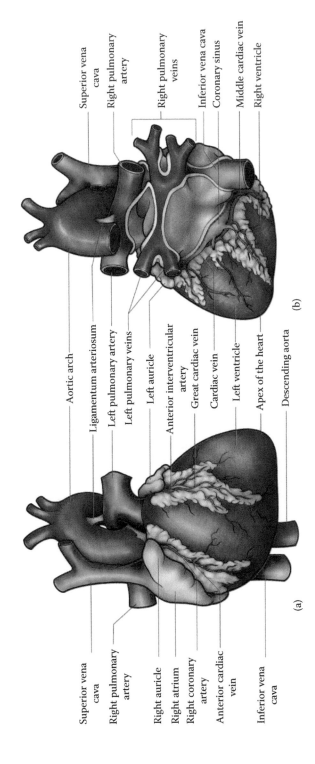

Figure 1.2 (a) The external anatomy of the heart, anterior view. (b) The external anatomy of the heart, posterior view.

thickness increases (eccentric hypertrophy). This allows for greater ventricular filling and a stronger contraction. Thus, a greater stroke volume can be achieved at rest. If cardiac demand is constant, then the resting heart rate can decrease and still maintain the required cardiac output.

1.2 The Heart Valves

To prevent the backflow of blood, the heart contains two sets of one-way valves (Figure 1.3)—the atrioventricular valves (A-V) and the aortic/pulmonary valves—which are supported by a connective tissue base called the fibrous skeleton. The valves may be open or closed, depending on the pressure difference on either side of the

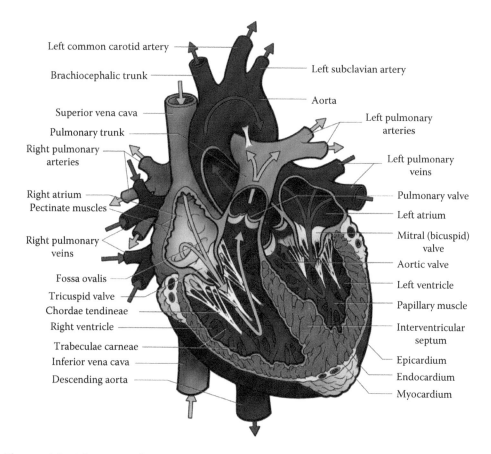

Figure 1.3 The internal anatomy of the heart, anterior view. Heart valves ensure unidirectional flow of blood through the heart. The atrio-ventricular (A-V) valves separate the atria from the ventricles, labeled as the Mitral valve on the left side and the tricuspid valve on the right. These are anchored by the chordae tendinae and the papillary muscle. The Pulmonary valve separates the right ventricle from the pulmonary artery, and the Aortic valve separates the aorta from the left ventricle.

valve. The A-V valves are situated between the atria and the ventricles. The right A-V valve has three cusps (or flaps) and is often referred to as the tricuspid valve. The left A-V valve has two cusps and is often referred to as the mitral valve or the bicuspid valve. When atrial pressure is higher than ventricular pressure during diastole (the relaxation phase), these valves are pushed open to allow for ventricular filling. When the ventricles begin to contract in systole, the increasing pressure in the ventricles pushes the valves closed, thus ensuring only forward blood flow. To prevent the A-V valves from everting, the valves are anchored by small tendon-like fibers called the chordae tendinae, which attach to the valve flaps and originate in the papillary muscle of the ventricles. As the ventricles contract, the papillary muscle also contracts, adding tension to the chordae tendinae and ensuring that the valve remains in a proper closed position. As the ventricles return to relaxation and the ventricular pressure drops below the atrial pressure, the valves open once again.

The aortic and pulmonary valves are found at the base of the heart, where the blood vessels attach. The pulmonary valve separates the right ventricle from the pulmonary artery, while the aortic valve separates the left ventricle from the aorta. During the diastole, the pressure in the blood vessels is higher than in the relaxed ventricles, and the back pressure shuts these valves. With systolic contraction, the pressure in the ventricles will rise. Once it exceeds the vessel pressure, it will push the aortic and pulmonary valves open, allowing for forward ejection of the blood. As diastole returns and the ventricle pressure once again drops below the vessel pressure, these valves will close due to the pressure differential. It is the closing of the valves that can be heard with a stethoscope. The first heart sound, "lub," is the closing of the A-V valves, while the second heart sound, "dup," is associated with the closure of the aortic and pulmonary valves.

The A-V valves and the aortic/pulmonary valves are never open at the same time. During diastolic filling, the A-V valves will be open and the aortic/pulmonary will be closed. During ejection, the aortic and pulmonary valves will be open but the A-V valves will be closed. There are two additional heart cycle phases—the isovolumic periods—when all four valves are shut. Because the atria are low-pressure chambers, the A-V valve shuts at the beginning of contraction and the pressure in the ventricle starts increasing. The A-V valve closure marks the beginning of systole. The aorta and the pulmonary arteries are relatively high-pressure systems, and the pressure in the ventricles must overcome this high pressure before they can push the valves open to eject blood. Thus, there is a period in contraction when the A-V valves have shut but the aortic/pulmonary valves are yet to open, and a similar period in relaxation, when the aortic/pulmonary valves have shut but the A-V valves are yet to open.

Heart murmurs are usually a result of a valve abnormality. A valve stenosis refers to a faulty opening of the valve and can be a result of stiff valve flaps or a narrowing of the valve annulus. This may be a congenital defect, caused by an illness such as rheumatic fever. With aging, calcification of the valve flaps also results in stenosis. A valve insufficiency (or regurgitation) refers to a faulty closure of the valve that allows for the backflow of blood. This "leak" can also be a result of a congenital condition, disease, or aging. Both conditions result in less forward blood flow and a drop in stroke volume and cardiac output, which can lead to heart failure. Defective valves may either be replaced with a valve prosthesis—a mechanical valve or a pig or cow valve—or be repaired. These aspects, along with the structure and function of the aortic and mitral valves, will be discussed in more detail in Chapters 9 and 10. Tissue engineering may soon allow for the development of valves from a patient's own cells.

There are no valves between the atria and the veins that deliver blood to these chambers. With the low pressures created in atrial contraction, the backflow into the veins is minimal.

1.3 Electrical Activity of the Heart

There are two types of cardiac muscle cells—the contractile cells, which create the muscle force, and the autorhythmic cells, which include the pacemaker cells and the conducting system (Figure 1.4). The heart requires no outside signal to contract. The action potential or nervous impulse is initiated in the pacemaker regions of the heart (the sinoatrial or the S-A node and the A-V node). It is then spread through the specialized conducting system (the bundle of His and the Purkinje fibers, which can also initiate action potentials). Each of these pacemaker regions depolarize themselves at different rates, with the S-A node exciting at a rate of 70 beats per minute, the A-V node exciting at a rate of 40 beats per minute, and the bundle of His and Purkinje fibers exciting at a rate of 20–30 beats per minute. Under normal circumstances, the action potential is initiated in the right atrium, by the S-A node, which has the fastest

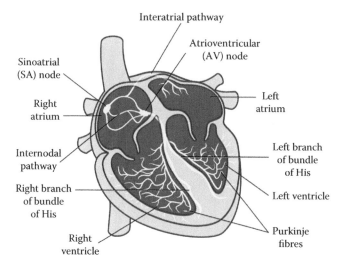

Figure 1.4 The conducting pathway of the heart. Electrical impulses are usually initiated in the pacemaker region called the sino-atrial (SA Node). It then spreads through the atria to initiate an atrial contraction. It also travels though the intermodal pathway to the Atrioventricular (AV) Node, to the Bundle of His, into the bundle branches and finally out to the Purkinje Fiber system, where the impulse initiates a ventricular contraction.

rate of pacemaker cycling (or action potential depolarization). As the impulse spreads to the other pacemaker regions, it causes them to excite before they have a chance to depolarize themselves. Thus, the heart rate (typically 70 beats per minute) is controlled by the S-A node. If this node stopped functioning, the A-V node (the next fastest depolarizing rate) would then control the heart rate (which would drop to about 40 beats per minute). At rest, the parasympathetic system is dominant and acts to suppress the heart rate (from an intrinsic rate of approximately 100 beats per minute, down to about 70 beats per minute). During exercise, when the sympathetic system is dominant, the heart rate increases and the conduction time is quickened.

Once the action potential is initiated in the S-A node, it spreads quickly across the atria via the intermodal pathway towards the A-V node and via the intra-atrial pathway and gap junctions to the left atrium (this takes about 30 ms). This ensures that all the atrial cells are depolarized at the same time and the resulting atrial contraction is unified. The impulse experiences a delay of approximately 100 ms at the A-V node. This delay ensures that the atria have fully contracted and ejected their blood into the ventricles before the ventricles begin their contraction. The impulse spreads from the A-V node through the bundle of His and into the left and right bundle branches before spreading out through the Purkinje fibers and gap junctions to depolarize the ventricles simultaneously (again, about 30 ms). The electrical activity can be recorded externally as an electrocardiogram (ECG) (Figure 1.5). There are typically three

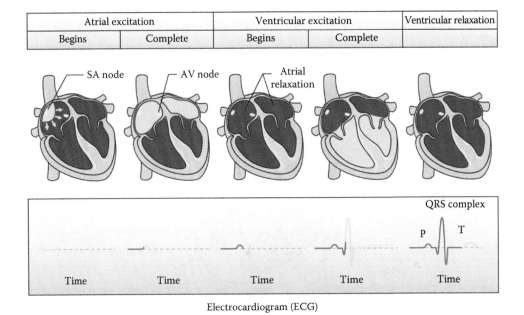

Electrocardiogram (ECG)

Figure 1.5 The electrocardiogram. The P-wave is the depolarization of the atria (initiated at the SA node) and is followed by an atrial contraction. The QRS complex represents the depolarization of the ventricles and is followed by ventricular contraction. The T-wave represents the repolarization of the ventricles, which starts at the apex of the heart and moves towards the base. It is followed by the relaxation of the ventricles.

waveforms recorded on an ECG—the P wave (which represents atrial depolarization and triggers atrial contraction), the QRS complex (which represents ventricular depolarization and triggers ventricular contraction), and the T wave (which represents ventricular repolarization and triggers ventricular relaxation). Abnormalities in the ECG waveforms can help diagnose arrhythmias such as heart block, atrial flutter, and atrial fibrillation, as well as myopathic conditions such as myocardial ischemia and infarction (commonly called a heart attack). If the coordination of the electrical impulses is lost and the myocardial cells are no longer contracting as a unit, the result is known as fibrillation. Ventricular fibrillation, which results in no significant ejection of blood, is life-threatening and requires electrical defibrillation for survival.

The contractile muscle fibers (which make up about 99% of the muscle cells) have a long recovery period (or refractory period) after they are depolarized. In this period, a second impulse or action potential is not possible. This ensures that the muscle repolarizes and relaxes (allowing for filling) before the next action potential and the contraction can occur.

1.4 The Cardiac Cycle

The cardiac cycle consists of diastole (or relaxation, which includes the isovolumic relaxation and the diastolic filling phases) and systole (or contraction, which includes the isovolumic contraction and ejection phases) (Figure 1.6). The cardiac cycle usually lasts about 800 ms, with most of that (about 500 ms) in the diastolic or relaxation phase. Systole (or contraction) usually lasts about 300 ms. With exercise, when heart rates increase, the diastolic phase is significantly shortened.

During diastolic filling, the atria and ventricles are relaxed. The atria receive blood from the venous system (the vena cava on the right side and the pulmonary veins on the left side), and the resulting pressure in the atria is enough to keep the A-V valves open. This allows the blood to move through the atria and directly in the ventricles. With the P wave and atrial depolarization, there is a contraction of the atria and a final ejection of blood into the ventricles. The next electrical event, the QRS complex, initiates ventricular contraction and the start of ventricular systole. As the pressure in the ventricles begins to rise, it quickly exceeds the pressure in the atria, and the A-V valves close. This is the start of the isovolumic contraction period. In this phase, there is no change in ventricular volume and no movement of blood (as all the valves are closed), but the pressure in the ventricles rises quickly. Once the pressure in the ventricles exceeds the pressures in the pulmonary artery and the aorta, the pulmonary and aortic valves open, beginning the ejection phase. As blood moves into the aorta and the pulmonary arteries, ventricular volume decreases but the pressure continues to increase until contraction ends. The T wave initiates ventricular relaxation, and at this point, ventricular pressure begins to fall. The pressure in the relaxing ventricles drops below the pressure in the aorta and pulmonary arteries (the latter pressure remains high because of the blood volume and the properties of the vessel) and the aortic and pulmonary valves close. This marks the beginning of

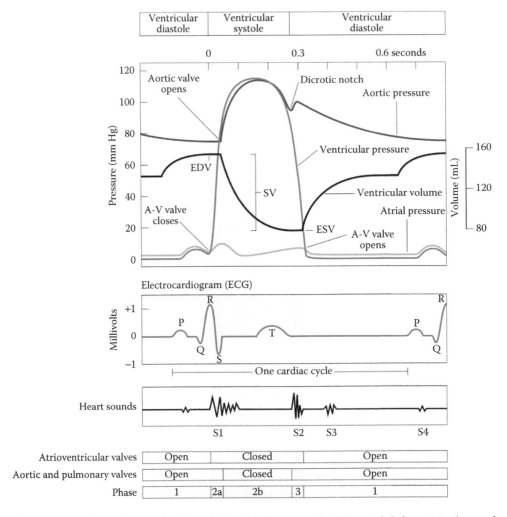

Figure 1.6 The cardiac cycle. The relationship between the left atrial, left ventricular, and aortic pressures, as well as left ventricular volume, during each period of the cardiac cycle. It also shows the relationship of these pressures to the ECG and to the valve openings and closures.

both ventricular diastole and of isovolumic relaxation. The pressure in the ventricles continues to decrease, but there is no movement of blood. Once the pressure in the fully relaxed ventricles drops below the atrial pressure, then the A-V valves are able to push open and diastolic filling begins again.

With high blood pressure (hypertension), the afterload effect is increased. The left ventricle must reach a higher pressure before it can push open the aortic valve against the higher aortic pressure. Thus, the isovolumic contraction period may be elongated, and there would be a shorter ejection period. This would result in a decrease in stroke volume that would have to be compensated for by a higher heart rate.

Over time, this can lead to heart failure. In response to hypertension, the ventricular muscle may sometimes thicken in an attempt to achieve higher pressures. Usually, this thickening comes at the expense of the lumen size (concentric hypertrophy), and stroke volumes may again be decreased. Heart failure can also develop with an aortic valve stenosis (decreased ejection) or after a myocardial infarction (weakened muscles and decreased ejection).

1.5 Blood Flow

After ejection from the left ventricle into the aorta, the blood enters the systemic arterial system, which carries blood away from the heart and into the tissues. Extensive branching takes place and the properties of the vessels change as they move from elastic arteries into muscular arteries and arterioles. At the level of the tissues, the capillaries allow for gas and nutrient exchange. On leaving the capillaries, the vessels converge into venules and veins and finally the vena cavae, before entering the heart at the right atrium.

Blood flow is directly dependent on the pressure gradient (ΔP) and inversely proportional to the vessels' resistance, which is primarily determined by the vessels' radius, r. The flow rate, Q, can be represented by Poiseuille's law:

$$Q = \frac{\pi \Delta P r^4}{8 \eta L}$$

where η represents blood viscosity and L represents vessel length (not a factor in situ). The blood pressure drops from the beginning of the vessel to the end of the vessel, and this difference, or gradient, is the determinant for flow, rather than the actual pressures within the vessel. As blood viscosity increases, as in dehydration, when blood plasma volume is decreased, the flow decreases proportionately. However, the resistance of a vessel increases to a far greater extent with a decrease in blood vessel radius (whose effect is to the fourth power). The blood flow properties will be discussed in more detail in Chapters 3 and 8.

1.6 Blood Vessel Properties

The blood vessel wall is made up of three layers: the tunica intima, the tunica media, and the tunica externa (Figure 1.7). The innermost layer, the tunica intima, is made up of a basement membrane and endothelium, which is in contact with the blood as the blood moves through the blood vessel lumen. The endothelial cells secrete chemicals such as endothelin and nitric oxide, which can trigger a local vasoconstriction or vasodilation. The endothelium also provides a smooth surface that minimizes the friction at the wall. The basement membrane and the internal elastic lamina make

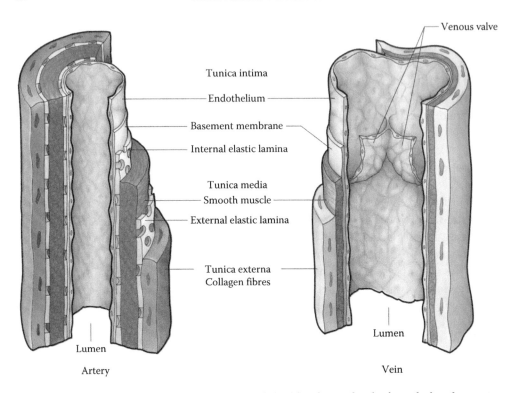

Venous valve

Tunica intima

Endothelium

Basement membrane

Internal elastic lamina

Tunica media
Smooth muscle

External elastic lamina

Tunica externa
Collagen fibres

Lumen

Lumen

Lumen

Artery

Vein

Figure 1.7 The layers making up the wall of the blood vessel, which includes the tunica intima (endothelium and elastic lamellae), the tunica media (containing smooth muscle), and the tunica externa.

up the rest of the tunica intima. The network of collagen fibers within the basement membrane and the layers of elastic fibers within the lamina provide tensile strength to the wall while also allowing for stretching and recoiling.

The tunica media is the middle layer of the vessel wall. It is made up of both smooth muscle and connective tissue and shows the greatest variation among the blood vessels of the circulatory system. When the smooth muscle contracts in vasoconstriction, there is a decrease in radius, an increase in resistance, and a resulting decrease in blood flow. The external elastic lamina forms the outer portion of the tunica media. The tunica externa (or adventitia) is made up of collagen and elastin fibers, which contribute to the mechanical properties of the blood vessels. It also helps anchor the vessels to the surrounding tissue. In the larger vessels, there are small blood vessels (the vasa vasorum) that supply the outer layers of the blood vessel wall with oxygen and nutrients. A weakened area of the wall with less connective tissue reinforcement may result in a region of expansion (a "bulge") known as an aneurysm. This could be a result of a genetic defect (such as Marfan's syndrome) or a disease state such as atherosclerosis and syphilis. If the wall becomes further stretched, it may result in rupture. Surgery is often done to repair this and prevent further rupture. This will be discussed further in Chapter 6.

1.7 The Arterial System

The arteries move blood away from the heart and, with the exception of the pulmonary artery, carry oxygenated blood. The elastic fibers within the arterial wall allow for high compliance or "expandability." The elastic arteries, or conducting arteries, include the aorta and its major branches. They range in diameter from 1 to 2.5 cm and contain a high proportion of elastin within the tunica layers. These arteries act as a pressure reservoir that expands as it receives blood from the left ventricle in systole and then recoils during diastole, helping to smooth out the pulsatile flow seen in these vessels. The thick wall and high percentage of elastic tissues help the vessel withstand the high and changing pressures. The peak arterial pressure (or systolic pressure) is seen during ventricular ejection, while the minimal arterial pressure (or diastolic pressure) occurs just before ejection begins. The difference in systolic and diastolic pressure is called the pulse pressure. It is dependent on the stroke volume ejected by the ventricle, as well as the vessel's elastic properties that determine arterial compliance. With aging, the arterial vessel walls can stiffen (arteriosclerosis) and result in a higher pulse pressure. This will be discussed in more detail in Chapters 6 and 11.

The properties of the blood vessels change as the blood moves from the elastic arteries into the muscular arteries. The muscular arteries have the thickest tunica media layer and contain relatively more smooth muscle and less elastic tissue than the elastic arteries. Thus, they are less distensible than the elastic arteries but are able to contribute to vasoconstriction. They range in size from 3 to 10 mm in diameter. The smallest arteries are called the arterioles, ranging in size from 10 μm to 0.3 mm. The larger arterioles contain all three tunicae, but as they decrease in size closer to the capillary bed, they become more like the capillary walls. Like the muscular arteries, they contain a high proportion of smooth muscle, which usually has some vascular tone (a condition of partial vasoconstriction). The diameter of the arterioles is a large determinant in the amount blood flow entering a connecting capillary bed. Vasoconstriction can be triggered by a change in sympathetic tone or by local effects such as a rise in O_2, decrease in CO_2, and cold. Conversely, vasodilation occurs when the smooth muscle relaxes, in response to local effectors such as high CO_2, high temperature, and histamine. As the blood leaves the arterioles, the pulsatile flow reduces to smooth flow.

1.8 The Microcirculation

The capillaries are thin-walled and form the site of gas exchange within the tissues. The average size of the capillaries is 8–10 μm in diameter, which ensures that the blood cells travel through the vessel in single file. The resistance is highest in the capillaries, making blood flow slow and allowing for maximal gas and nutrient exchange. Tissues that have high metabolic demands (such as muscle) have a high density of capillaries, while tissues such as tendons and ligaments have very few capillaries. Continuous capillaries are found in abundance in the muscle and the skin and are the least permeable. The wall is one-cell thick and has enough gaps to allow the movement of fluids and small particles. Fenestrated capillaries have larger pores and greater permeability. These are found in the kidney and the small intestine, where active filtration or absorption occurs. The sinusoid capillaries are the most "leaky," with pores large enough to allow blood cells to move through them. These are found in the liver and the spleen (where old red blood cells [RBCs] are removed from the circulation) and in the bone marrow (where new red cells are added to the circulation).

The capillary beds form the microcirculation through the tissues. The flow through the capillary bed is controlled by the vascular tone of the preceding arterioles as well as the precapillary sphincters. The smooth muscle that makes up the precapillary sphincters can contract to shut down some of the true capillaries within the bed if less gas exchange is required (e.g., at rest). The metarteriole or vascular channel remains open even when the sphincters are closed. If the tissue becomes active and requires more oxygen, the precapillary sphincters open and the entire capillary bed is perfused with blood, allowing an increase in gas and nutrient exchange.

Solutes such as glucose, oxygen, and carbon dioxide move between the capillary and the tissue by diffusion. Fluids are exchanged across the capillary wall by bulk flow (Figure 1.8). The fluid balance within the capillaries is dependent on the hydrostatic pressure differences as well as osmotic pressure gradients between the tissue and the capillary. If the blood pressure is higher in the capillary than in the tissues, the hydrostatic pressure difference encourages the movement of fluid from the capillaries and into the tissues. The plasma proteins that are too large to leave the capillaries

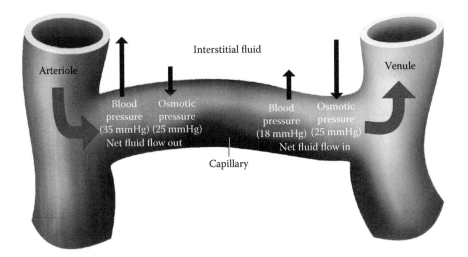

Figure 1.8 Capillary bulk flow. At the arteriolar end of the capillary bed where blood pressure is higher, the hydrostatic pressure dominates over the colloid osmotic pressure and fluid moves out of the capillary and into the tissue space. Closer to the venule end of the capillary bed where blood pressure is lower, the colloid osmotic pressure dominates over the hydrostatic pressure and draws fluid back into the capillary.

exert a colloid osmotic pressure that encourages the movement of fluid back into the vessel. At the arteriolar end of the capillary bed, the higher blood pressure means that the hydrostatic pressure effect is greater than that of the colloid osmotic gradient. Therefore, a net movement of fluid occurs from the capillary and into the tissues (on average, a volume of 20 L per day moving into the tissues). At the venous end of the capillary bed, where blood pressure is lower, the osmotic pressure gradient exceeds the hydrostatic pressure, and fluid moves back into the blood vessel at this end of the capillary bed (17 L per day on average). This reabsorption of fluids is dependent on the presence of plasma proteins. If the protein level within the blood is decreased, the osmotic pull is decreased, and more fluid remains in the tissues, resulting in edema or swelling. It should be noted that the tissue also exerts a hydrostatic pressure (although usually much smaller than the capillaries) as well as a colloid osmotic pressure. In the inflammation response, chemical messengers such as histamine are released, which cause the capillaries to dilate and flow to increase. It also changes the permeability of these vessels, allowing proteins, clotting factors, and blood cells to leave the blood and enter the tissue space. This increases the colloid osmotic pressure of the tissues and causes fluid to remain in the tissue space (causing swelling). With heart failure and poor ejection of the heart, the venous pressure increases. This causes a greater hydrostatic pressure within the capillary beds, particularly in the pulmonary circulation. This encourages more movement of fluid into the tissues, causing the systemic edema, seen with right-sided heart failure, and the pulmonary edema, seen with left-sided failure.

Despite the normal osmotic pull of the plasma proteins, there is an excess of fluids left in the tissues during bulk flow (approximately 3 L per day). This fluid is drained away by the lymphatic vessels—open-ended vessels that originate in the capillary beds and empty into the venous circulation. The lymph vessels have similar mechanical structure and properties as the veins. They are thin-walled, with low pressure. They contain valves in the vessels to aid the forward movement of flow. As the fluid moves toward the venous circulation, it moves through lymph nodes, which filter the fluid and remove pathogens that might be present from the tissue space.

1.9 The Venous System

The venules and veins move blood to the heart and, with the exception of the pulmonary vein, carry deoxygenated blood. Venules are the receiving vessels from the capillary beds and drain into the veins. Both the venules and veins are characterized by thin walls that are collapsible and have low pressures (10–15 mmHg). The postcapillary venules range in size from 10 to 50 μm, while the larger muscular venules are 50–200 μm in size. These venules are highly distensible and can act as blood reservoirs, with the ability to expand their blood volume by two to three times. When this blood is required by the circulation (e.g., during exercise), the smooth muscle in the muscular venules may contract and contribute to an increased venous return to the heart.

The veins range in size from 0.5-mm diameter near the venules to 3-cm diameter at the vena cava. The wall thickness is usually less than one-tenth of the vessel diameter. The veins are usually referred to as the capacitance vessels, because of their ability to expand and store blood. With an increase in blood volume on the arterial side, the arteries would be stretched and show recoil. On the venous side, the vessels would distend and show no recoil. The venous system contains the bulk of the blood volume (usually about 60%). Despite this storage ability, the blood in the venous system continues to move through the vessels and is encouraged to move forward in part by the driving force of the arterial system. Just as the water in a river would slow down if the river widens, the blood in the venous side slows down as it moves through the venous vessels. Veins have low amounts of smooth muscle and do not show the same vascular tone as is seen in the arterial system. There is a distinct difference between the arteries and the veins in terms of the effects of smooth muscle contraction. With vasoconstriction of the arterioles, there is an increase in resistance and a decrease in blood flow to the corresponding organs. With contraction of the venous smooth muscle (venoconstriction), there is a decreased compliance of the venous system, which encourages blood flow and creates a higher venous return to the heart.

Venous return (particularly against gravity) can be a challenge in the low-pressure, high-capacitance venous system. To help encourage venous return, the veins contain valves, which prevent backflow. If the valves begin to fail and allow backflow, the blood can pool in the veins, causing varicose veins. The stagnant blood in this condition increases the risk of blood clot formation.

The larger veins in the legs lie close to the skeletal muscle beds and can be compressed with skeletal muscle contraction. This compression pushes the venous blood forward toward the heart (and the valves prevent the backflow when the muscles relax). This is referred to as the skeletal muscle pump, and it is a factor in encouraging venous return. Other factors that aid in venous return include the respiratory suction (the negative pressure created on inspiration) and the diastolic suction (created during isovolumic relaxation); these help create a pressure gradient between the veins and the right atrium.

1.10 The Blood

The third component of the cardiovascular system is the blood that circulates through the vessels. The main components of the blood are the blood plasma (making up about 55% of the blood volume), the erythrocytes or RBCs (making up about 44% of the blood volume), the leukocytes (the while blood cells), and the platelets (together making up less than 1% of the blood volume).

The blood plasma is primarily water (90%) with dissolved nutrients, hormones, proteins, and electrolytes. The proteins can be classified as albumins, globulins, and fibrinogen (used for clotting). The proteins are a critical component for the bulk flow seen in the capillary beds, as their presence in the blood produces the colloid osmotic pressure that pulls fluid back into the capillary beds. With dehydration, the plasma volume is depleted, which can increase blood viscosity. This would increase the blood resistance and affect blood flow.

The primary function of the RBCs is to carry oxygen. They are formed in the red bone marrow, triggered by the hormone erythropoietin (or EPO). In the final stage of formation, the erythrocytes lose their nucleus and instead are filled with hemoglobin (the binding molecule for oxygen). Without a nucleus for cell repair, the erythrocytes can live for only about 120 days in circulation. The size of the RBCs (about 8 μm) is slightly bigger than some of the smallest capillaries, and the flexibility of the anucleated RBCs allows them to move through the vessels, in close contact with the capillary wall. This allows for maximal diffusion of nutrients and wastes within the microcirculation. As the RBC ages, it becomes less flexible and must be removed from circulation by the sinusoids of the spleen, rather than posing a risk of getting stuck within the small capillaries.

At higher elevations, as an adaptation to lower atmospheric oxygen, the body releases more erythropoietin, which increases the number of RBCs in circulation to improve the body's oxygen-carrying capacity (called secondary polycythemia). A reduced oxygen-carrying capacity is called anemia, and a common cause is an iron deficiency (a component needed for hemoglobin production).

The leukocytes, or white blood cells, are the cellular components of the body's immune system. There are five types of leukocytes: the neutrophils (circulating phagocytic cells), the lymphocytes (which activate antibody production and kill infected cells), the basophils (which produce histamine for the inflammation response), the monocytes (which are tissue macrophages), and the eosinophils (which become active in parasitic infections allergies).

The final components of the blood are the platelets or thrombocytes. They are not actual cells but cell fragments shed from megakaryocytes in the bone marrow. They are important in hemostasis—the stoppage of bleeding. When activated, the platelets can aggregate and form a platelet plug, which can seal off breaks in the blood vessel. The activated platelets are also an important cofactor in the coagulation pathways that form a more reinforcing blood clot.

The properties of the blood will be further discussed in Chapters 3 and 8.

Acknowledgment

Figure Artwork by Chaz Francis Comia.

2

Cell and Extracellular Matrix Interactions in a Dynamic Biomechanical Environment:
The Aortic Valve as an Illustrative Example

A. Y. L. Lam and C. A. Simmons

Contents

2.1 Introduction

As mentioned in Chapter 1, the cardiovascular system is made of various types of soft tissues, all of which, except blood, share the common feature that they are constituted of cells embedded in an extracellular matrix (ECM). Interactions between cells and the ECM play critical roles in supporting cell functions. The most basic function of the ECM is to provide a structural scaffold for cells. Cells begin secreting ECM components from the beginning of development, with ECM already being a part of mammalian embryos from the two-cell stage (Adams and Watt 1993). In healthy tissue, cells can maintain the ECM in a homeostatic state through carefully controlled secretion and degradation processes (Everts et al. 1996). However, in disease, this balance is disrupted, leading to maladaptive remodeling of the ECM by cells (Lu et al. 2011). In turn, the ECM can regulate a variety of cellular processes such as growth, migration, and differentiation (Schlie-Wolter et al. 2013, Gattazzo et al. 2014). Besides sensing the composition of the ECM structure through adhesion receptors, cells can also take cues from growth factors and cytokines that the ECM sequesters and the mechanical properties of the ECM. Thus, the relationship between cells and the ECM is dynamic and reciprocal, whereby cells sense cues from the surrounding ECM and can respond by modifying the ECM.

Dynamic cell–ECM interactions and their influence on cell and tissue function are exquisitely demonstrated in the aortic valve, a thin piece of tissue located between the aorta and the ventricle that serves to prevent backflow of the blood during diastole (see Chapter 1). The aortic valve opens and closes 40 million times a year for the duration of a person's life while experiencing strong hemodynamic shear, as well as tensile and bending forces. In this dynamic biomechanical environment, precise cell and ECM composition and organization are required to maintain proper valve function. Cell–ECM interactions will be explored in this chapter by using examples from the aortic valve as a model cardiovascular tissue, with a focus on the influence of mechanical forces. Readers specifically interested in cell–ECM interactions in the vasculature are directed to relevant reviews by Stegemann et al. (2005), Xu and Shi (2014), and Chistiakov et al. (2013).

2.2 The Aortic Valve

Normally, the aortic valve is composed of three leaflets that attach at their base in a semilunar manner to the aortic wall. The aortic valve is not muscularized and moves passively according to changes in blood flow and pressure. During diastole, left ventricular pressure is less than the pressure in the aorta, and the leaflets coapt at their tips to close the valve and prevent retrograde flow (Figure 2.1a). The leaflets must withstand substantial backpressure of 80 mmHg in normotensive individuals and more than 100 mmHg in hypertensive individuals, resulting in the leaflets stretching 10% in the circumferential direction and as much as 30% in the radial direction (Thubrikar 1990, Lo and Vesely 1995), with values of circumferential mechanical stress in the range of 300–600 kPa (Labrosse et al. 2010). During systole, the pressure gradient drops to zero (Thubrikar 1990) and the leaflets relax, allowing the valve to open (Figure 2.1b). Movement of the blood into the aorta creates high oscillatory shear stress varying between −5 and 7 Pa on the ventricular side of the leaflet (Yap et al. 2012), while the aortic side experiences lower shear stress peaking at 2 Pa (Yap et al. 2012), with flows that are generally thought to be more disturbed and complex (Balachandran et al. 2011). The complex mechanical environment of the aortic valve has resulted in the development of a highly optimized ECM.

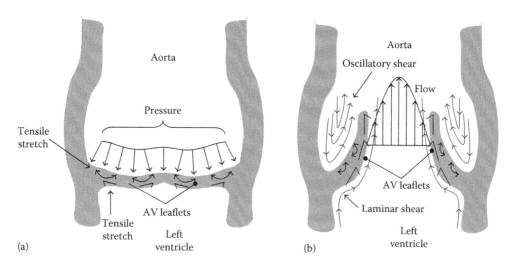

Figure 2.1 The aortic valve operates in a highly dynamic mechanical environment. (a) During peak diastole, the valve experiences significant back pressure from the blood and bends and stretches to keep the valve closed. (b) During peak systole, when the valve is open, the side facing the ventricle experiences high-magnitude laminar flow, while the side facing the aorta experiences low-magnitude oscillatory flow. (Adapted from Balachandran, K. et al., *Int. J. Inflam.*, 2011, 263870, 2011.)

2.2.1 Major Components of the Extracellular Matrix

The ECM comprises a wide variety of proteins, but around 300 proteins making up 1%–1.5% of the mammalian proteome are considered the "core matrisome" (Hynes and Naba 2012). Major categories in the matrisome include collagens, proteoglycans, and glycoproteins.

The aortic valve's ECM consists of about 55% collagen, 10% elastin, and 2% proteoglycan by dry weight (Naso et al. 2010), with each component performing a key mechanical function. Despite being only 1-mm thick (Sahasakul et al. 1988), the aortic valve is composed of three distinct layers (Figure 2.2): the fibrosa, which faces the aorta and is composed mainly of collagen; the ventricularis, which faces the ventricle and is composed mainly of elastin; and, in between, the spongiosa, which is composed mainly of proteoglycans and glycosaminoglycans (GAGs) (Latif et al. 2005a). The fibrosa and the ventricularis constitute 41% and 29%, respectively, of the valve thickness, with the spongiosa making up the remainder (Stella and Sacks 2007).

2.2.1.1 Collagen
Collagen is the most abundant protein in humans (Di Lullo et al. 2002) and is responsible for resisting tension and providing structural strength in tissue (Hynes and Naba 2012). This role is aided by a high rate of turnover, 5% per day in the heart, so

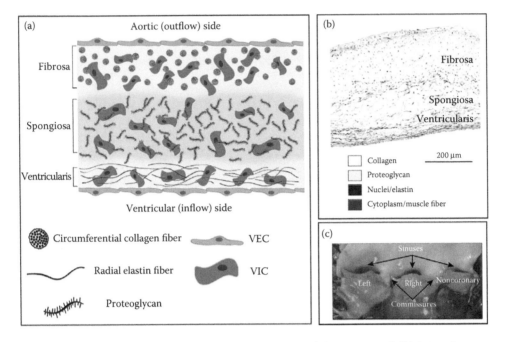

Figure 2.2 Structure of the aortic valve. (a) A detailed diagram, and (b) Movat's penta-chrome staining demonstrate the distinct ECM composition and alignment of the different layers of the valve, with the aorta-facing fibrosa composed of circumferentially oriented collagen fibers, the ventricle-facing ventricularis composed of radially oriented elastin fibers, and the spongiosa in between composed of proteoglycans. (c) Splayed view of the aortic valve displaying gross anatomy. (Reprinted from Blaser, M. C. et al., Implications for disease—Valvular fibrosis, in: Layton, B. (Ed.), *Molecular and Cellular Biomechanics*, Pan Stanford Publishing, Chicago, IL, 2015. With permission.)

that damaged collagen is quickly replaced (Laurent 1987). In total, 28 types of collagen have been identified, with type I fibrillar collagen being the most common.

Fibrillar collagen is formed hierarchically (Figure 2.3) (Mouw et al. 2014) and begins in the cell as α chains of repeating amino acid sequences in a Gly-X-Y pattern. Three α chains then form a homotrimer or a heterotrimer triple helix in the endoplasmic reticulum. This helix is about 300-nm long and about 2 nm in diameter. The collagen helices at this stage are called procollagen and are then excreted into the extracellular spaces, where they are further enzymatically modified by having their ends cleaved and are then packed side by side, 67-nm apart, to form fibrils (Kadler et al. 1996, Bailey et al. 1998). Fibrils are further bundled together to form collagen fibers, which can be 1–20 μm in diameter (Mouw et al. 2014). This extracellular assembly process is believed to be cell-mediated, where the cell membrane creates extracellular compartments that help guide collagen formation spatially and concentrate the release of required enzymes (Banos et al. 2008). Differences in assembly at each stage of the hierarchy, be it different amino acids making up the Gly-X-Y repeating sequence in the α chain, different α chains forming the triple helix, or differences in how the fibrils are formed, give rise to the different types of collagens with their unique mechanical characteristics.

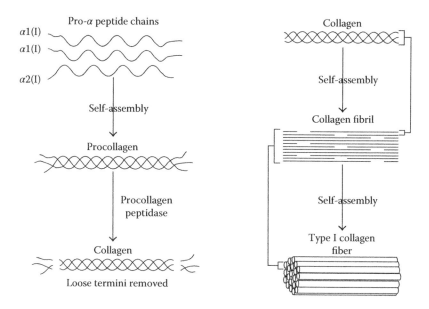

Figure 2.3 The hierarchical formation of collagen. Alpha chains of repeating Gly-X-Y sequences form triple helices and are excreted into the extracellular space as procollagen. Enzymatic cleavage of the ends of procollagen results in collagen that can be sequentially bundled into fibrils, followed by fibers. (Adapted from Kruger, T. E. et al., *Sci. World J.*, 2013, 1–6, 2013.)

The most common types of collagen in the aortic valve are type I, found mainly in the fibrosa, and type III, found throughout the leaflet (Latif et al. 2005a). Type I collagen is aligned circumferentially in the fibrosa (Figure 2.2a), corresponding to the direction of the highest tensile stress, as applied by backpressure during diastole (Thubrikar et al. 1986). Increased crosslinking of the circumferential collagen compared with the radial collagen also contributes to increased circumferential strength (Balguid et al. 2007). The collagen helps the valves maintain form and creates a tight seal during ventricular filling, preventing retrograde flow. The presence of collagen is estimated to reduce maximum stress on the leaflet by up to 60% (De Hart et al. 2004), and the alignment of the collagen in the circumferential direction is responsible for the circumferential stretch of the leaflet only being one-third of the radial stretch during diastole (Yap et al. 2010). Collagen fibers also play a role in systole to reduce the fluttering motion of the leaflets (De Hart et al. 2004). Collagen alignment not only causes an anisotropic effect on leaflet stretch but also results in the leaflet being stiffer circumferentially than radially (Vesely and Noseworthy 1992, Balguid et al. 2007).

Extra extensibility of the leaflet is also provided by excess length of the collagen and fibrosa. When the leaflet is relaxed, the collagen fibers are wavy and crimped and the fibrosa forms folds called corrugations in the radial direction. Under load, the unfolding of the collagen crimp and fibrosa corrugations allows the fibrosa to extend further radially, helping to ensure proper closure of the valve (Vesely and Noseworthy 1992).

2.2.1.2 Elastin

As the name suggests, elastic fibers easily stretch under load and recoil to their original dimensions when unloaded. Elastic fibers are extremely stable, with a half-life of 40 years (Arribas et al. 2006), helping tissues maintain proper form when healthy, but they have limited repair mechanisms if damaged or degraded. Elastic fibers are macromolecules formed around a core of insoluble elastin, which makes up 90% of the fiber (Sherratt 2009). The other 10% consists of glycoproteins, most commonly fibrillin, in the form of microfibrils that surround the elastin. Like collagen, elastin is also formed by a complex cell-mediated process, whereby cells release the soluble precursor tropoelastin into the extracellular space, where tropoelastin molecules aggregate into coacervate (Czirok et al. 2006). Cellular motion aides the coacervate in assembling, crosslinking, and extending into elastic fibers.

In the aortic valve, elastin is predominantly found in the ventricularis as radially aligned sheets of elastic fibers (Figure 2.2a) (Scott and Vesely 1996). This allows the ventricularis to stretch more radially than circumferentially (Vesely and Noseworthy 1992). The elastin in the ventricularis provides the valve with its elastic recoil, helping to open the valve during systole. Some circumferentially oriented elastin is also found in the fibrosa surrounding the circumferential collagen and is thought to help return the collagen to its crimped state on relaxation (Scott and Vesely 1996, Vesely 1998).

2.2.1.3 Proteoglycans and Glycosaminoglycans

Glycosaminoglycans and proteoglycans are important constituents of ECM, since they help bind and stabilize other ECM components, provide hydration and compressive stiffness, as well as retain growth factors and cytokines (Mouw et al. 2014). Glycosaminoglycans are long, linear chains of repeating disaccharides, with major types including chondroitin sulfate, dermatan sulfate, heparin sulfate, hyaluronic acid, and keratin sulfate (Lindahl et al. 2015). Glycosaminoglycans can be present in the ECM on their own, or they can attach covalently to a core protein to form proteoglycans. Hyaluronic acid is noteworthy because it lacks sulfate groups and does not bind covalently to form proteoglycans; however, it can interact with them noncovalently (Couchman and Pataki 2012).

Proteoglycans are named as families based on their core protein, such as aggrecan, biglycan, decorin, and versican, since the number, length, and arrangement of the attached GAG chains can vary, and their properties and function can be quite different (Lindahl et al. 2015). Aggrecan, for example, is composed of GAG chains with high negative charge that allows it to retain large amounts of water and resist compressive force, while decorin binds and regulates the formation of collagen fibers (Danielson et al. 1997, Couchman and Pataki 2012) (Figure 2.4).

In the aortic valve, proteoglycans and GAGs are present in all three layers but are most often found in the spongiosa (Figure 2.2a). The GAG hyaluronic acid on its own and the proteoglycan versican, which includes the GAG chondroitin sulfate, are most prominent in the spongiosa (Latif et al. 2005a, Stephens et al. 2008). Both these molecules are associated with hydration, which allows the spongiosa to link and lubricate the ventricularis and fibrosa layers as they shear relative to one another during leaflet flexure. The hydrated spongiosa can also provide compressibility to the overall valve leaflet.

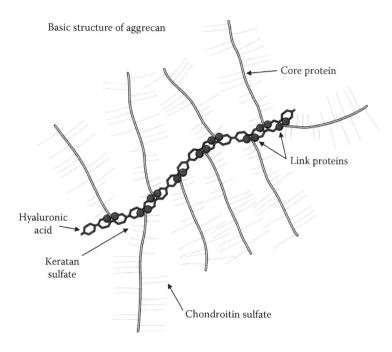

Figure 2.4 Proteoglycans (aggrecan shown here) are named after their core protein, which forms a backbone for the attachment of multiple GAG chains. The ends of proteoglycans can contain binding domains for other proteoglycans or glycoproteins. In this example, aggrecan can bind hyaluronic acid to assemble larger aggregates. (Reprinted from *Biochim. Biophys. Acta*, 1812, Oussoren, E. et al., Bone, joint and tooth development in mucopolysaccharidoses: Relevance to therapeutic options, 1542–1556, Copyright 2011, with permission from Elsevier.)

The proteoglycan biglycan, which has been found to bind elastin (Reinboth et al. 2002), is present in the ventricularis (Latif et al. 2005a, Stephens et al. 2008), where it may contribute to elastogenesis. Elastin retains its elastic properties only when hydrated and becomes brittle when dry (Lillie and Gosline 2002), so the presence of proteoglycans and GAGs in the elastin-rich ventricularis is likely important in maintaining the layer's mechanical properties. Decorin, which plays a role in collagen fibrillogenesis (Danielson et al. 1997), has been found in the collagen-rich fibrosa (Latif et al. 2005a, Stephens et al. 2008).

2.2.1.4 Matrix Metalloproteinases

In healthy tissues, matrix-degrading enzymes such as matrix metalloproteinases (MMPs) are involved in homeostatic renewal of the ECM as well as in degrading the ECM to facilitate cell migration and proliferation. More than 20 MMPs have been identified, which share three common domains: the prodomain, which is removed to activate the enzyme; the catalytic domain, which contains the active site that degrades the ECM target; and a hemopexin domain, which confers substrate specificity and can also bind inhibitors (Visse and Nagase 2003, Peng et al. 2012). Matrix metalloproteinases are grouped into families based on which ECM protein they can degrade; they include collagenases (MMP-1, MMP-8, MMP-13, and MMP-18), gelatinases (MMP-2 and MMP-9), and stromelysins (MMP-3, MMP-10, and MMP-11). Most MMPs are secreted into the ECM, but some types remain membrane-bound to the cell (Visse and Nagase 2003).

Activity of MMPs needs to be carefully regulated to avoid damaging the ECM. Key regulators of MMPs are matrix-degradation inhibitors such as tissue inhibitors of metalloproteinases (TIMPs). There are four TIMPs (TIMP-1 to TIMP-4) in mammals, but they are thought to have a common evolutionary origin, with TIMP-1 being the oldest (Murphy 2011). All TIMPs have some inhibitory activity against all MMPs, but binding affinities between individual pairs vary (Brew and Nagase 2010). Tissue inhibitors of metalloproteinases have two key domains: an N-terminal domain, which binds and inhibits the active site of the target MMP, and a C-terminal domain, which interacts with the hemopexin domain of MMPs to help stabilize the protein–protein interaction (Brew and Nagase 2010, Murphy 2011). Tissue inhibitors of metalloproteinases inhibit MMPs in a 1:1 ratio, and the balance between MMPs and TIMPs is an important determinant of the rate of ECM degradation (Visse and Nagase 2003, Peng et al. 2012). Besides their effect on MMPs, TIMPs can also serve as growth factors, promoting or inhibiting cell proliferation, depending on context (Stetler-Stevenson 2008). The following have been found in healthy aortic valves: MMP-1, MMP-2, MMP-9, TIMP-1, TIMP-2, and TIMP-3 (Dreger et al. 2002, Fondard et al. 2005).

2.2.1.5 Laminins and Fibronectin

Other important ECM components found in the aortic valve include laminins and fibronectin (Latif et al. 2005a). Laminins and fibronectin serve as specialized connector proteins that help bind the main structural proteins such as collagen and proteoglycans to each other to strengthen the ECM as well as link the structural proteins to cell surface receptors and bind growth factors (Halper and Kjaer 2014, Mouw et al. 2014). They, therefore, not only provide important structural functions in the ECM but are also important mediators of ECM–cell signaling.

Laminins are large heterotrimeric glycoproteins with α, β, and γ chains (Figure 2.5) (Domogatskaya et al. 2012). Five α chains, four β chains, and three γ chains have been identified, and their different combinations result in 16 laminin isoforms. Laminins are named as an abbreviation of their chain composition, so laminin-321 consists of $\alpha3\beta2\gamma1$ (Aumailley et al. 2005). Laminins have a cross- or T-shaped structure, with the triple helix forming the long arm and parts of each chain remaining exposed to form the two or three short arms. The α chain is the longest (~200–400 kDa), while the β and γ chains are shorter (~120–200 kDa) (Domogatskaya et al. 2012, Halper and Kjaer 2014), which means that when the chains form a triple helix, a part of the longer α chain remains exposed at the end of the long arm, which has important functional consequences, since it serves as an integrin-binding site (Domogatskaya et al. 2012, Mouw et al. 2014). Integrins, described in more detail in Section 2.2.3, are important cell surface receptors that connect cells to the ECM and have important cell signaling and force transmission functions. For example, the binding of laminin $\alpha4$ to integrin $\beta1$ induces Dll4, which reduces tip cell formation of endothelial cells and regulates angiogenesis

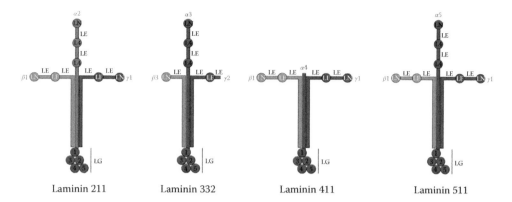

| Laminin 211 | Laminin 332 | Laminin 411 | Laminin 511 |

Figure 2.5   Sixteen laminin isoforms resulting from different combinations of α, β, and γ chains assembling in cross- or T-shaped heterotrimeric structures have been discovered. Laminins are named as an abbreviation of their chain composition, so laminin-211 consists of $\alpha2\beta1\gamma1$. Laminin serves important linking functions, with their end domains binding other ECM structural proteins and integrins. (Reprinted from *Trends Immunol.*, 38, Simon, T., and Bromberg, J. S., Regulation of the immune system by laminins, 858–871, Copyright 2017, with permission from Elsevier.)

(Stenzel et al. 2011). In turn, the short arms of laminins bind ECM components such as collagen and proteoglycans (Domogatskaya et al. 2012, Mouw et al. 2014).

Fibronectins are large glycoproteins formed with three types of repeating units called modules (Potts and Campbell 1994). Fibronectin is encoded by a single gene transcript, but alternative splicing results in 20 isoforms in humans (Singh et al. 2010, Halper and Kjaer 2014). Type I and II modules contain pairs of intramodule disulfide bonds, which stabilize the structure and prevent conformational changes (Potts and Campbell 1994, Schwarzbauer and DeSimone 2011). They contain binding sites for other ECM proteins such as collagen and fibrin (Potts and Campbell 1994). Type III modules do not contain disulfide bonds, can undergo conformational changes, and include binding sites for integrins and other fibronectins (Potts and Campbell 1994, Schwarzbauer and DeSimone 2011).

Fibronectin is secreted as a soluble dimer and assembles into an insoluble fibronectin fibril in the ECM with cellular assistance (Singh et al. 2010, Schwarzbauer and DeSimone 2011). Secreted fibronectin specifically binds to integrin $\alpha5\beta1$ at arginine-glycine-aspartate (RGD) and synergy sites (Huveneers et al. 2008), causing integrin clustering on the cell surface to create high local concentrations of soluble fibronectin (Singh et al. 2010, Schwarzbauer and DeSimone 2011). This is thought to promote the fibronectin–fibronectin interactions necessary to form fibrils. The fibronectin matrix needs to be constantly maintained, since it can degrade in as little as 6 hours if fibronectin polymerization is inhibited (Sottile and Hocking 2002).

Fibronectin is an important mediator in the assembly of other ECM proteins and is required for the formation of type I collagen (Sottile and Hocking 2002), for which fibronectin is thought to act as a scaffold (Singh et al. 2010). Fibronectin is also required for the formation of fibrillin (Sabatier et al. 2009), a key component in elastic fibers, and the incorporation into the ECM of transforming growth factor-β1 (TGF-β1) (Dallas et al. 2005), a key growth factor involved in myofibrogenesis and heart valve disease, discussed in more detail in Section 2.3.

2.2.2 Aortic Valve Cell Types

The resident cell types of the aortic valve include the valve endothelial cells (VECs), which form a monolayer around the outside of the leaflet, and the valve interstitial cells (VICs), which inhabit all three layers of the valve (Figure 2.2a).

The VECs form the blood-contacting surface of the leaflet and are thought to indirectly regulate ECM remodeling by controlling permeability (Tompkins et al. 1989), the adhesion of inflammatory cells (Muller et al. 2000), and paracrine signaling with VICs (Butcher and Nerem 2006). In vivo, VECs orient circumferentially in leaflets, following the alignment of collagen fibers, and perpendicular to flow (Deck 1986). In vitro, flow alone, without guidance from collagen fibers, has been reported to direct VECs to align perpendicular to flow. This makes the VECs distinct from aortic endothelial cells, which align parallel to flow (Butcher et al. 2004). The VECs and aortic endothelial cells also produce different gene transcription profiles in response to flow (Butcher et al. 2006). Distinct gene transcription profiles are also seen in VECs on different sides of the leaflet (Simmons et al. 2005), with inhibitors of calcification downregulated on the fibrosa side, indicating heterogeneity in the VEC population.

The VICs are embedded in the ECM and can directly remodel it. In vitro, the VICs have been found to express the mRNA for type I collagen, type III collagen, and elastin, necessary for matrix production (Dreger et al. 2006). The VICs have also been found to express MMP-1, MMP-2, MMP-8, MMP-13, MMP-14, TIMP-1, and TIMP-2 (Fondard et al. 2005, Dreger et al. 2006) and are thus able to degrade a variety of ECM components, including collagen, elastin, fibronectin, and proteoglycans. As such, VICs are responsible for maintenance and renewal of the valve ECM. This process is carefully controlled with, for example, valve tissue and VICs containing receptors to angiotensin II and bradykinin, which provide stimulatory and inhibitory signals, respectively, for collagen production (Weber et al. 1995). Renewal is also appropriately context-dependent, taking into account the mechanical forces experienced by the tissue, so that areas of the leaflet requiring the greatest strength see high structural protein synthesis, while the leaflet attachment region to the aortic wall, which needs flexibility, sees high GAG renewal, ensuring that proper valve function is maintained (Schneider and Deck 1981).

The VICs are a heterogenous population consisting mainly of fibroblasts and less than 5% myofibroblasts and smooth muscle cells (SMCs) in healthy adult valves (Cimini et al. 2003, Rabkin-Aikawa et al. 2004, Pho et al. 2008). The VICs have also been classified according to functionality, with fibroblasts being considered a quiescent VIC with a low rate of matrix synthesis and degradation (Liu et al. 2007). In contrast, myofibroblasts are considered activated VICs.

Myofibroblasts are traditionally identified as an intermediate cell type between fibroblasts and SMCs, with characteristic upregulated α-smooth muscle actin (αSMA).

They form stress fibers and vimentin, but lack the desmin, heavy-chain smooth muscle myosin, and smoothelin of SMCs (Darby et al. 2014). Myofibroblasts have been found to differentiate from a variety of cell types, most commonly fibroblasts, but also mesenchymal stem cells (MSCs), SMCs, and endothelial cells after endothelial-to-mesenchymal transition among others (Hinz et al. 2007, Barisic-Dujmovic et al. 2010). Transforming growth factor $\beta 1$ is a key regulator of myofibrogenesis by controlling αSMA expression (Desmouliere et al. 1993). Myofibroblasts have upregulated ECM synthesis, producing disorganized collagen and fibronectin in large amounts (Gabbiani et al. 1971, Torr et al. 2015), which when combined with upregulated MMP activity (Rabkin et al. 2001) means that myofibroblasts can remodel the ECM in a disruptive and disorganized manner. Myofibroblasts are also highly contractile due the presence of contractile bundles of actin and myosin (Hinz 2010). Upregulated ECM synthesis and contractility make myofibroblasts useful for wound healing, where they can rapidly close and stabilize the wound, but they are not capable of true regeneration, since original tissue function is not restored. On resolution of injury, recruited myofibroblasts should disappear via apoptosis (Desmouliere et al. 1995), while the continued presence of unregulated myofibroblasts leads to fibrosis. Similarly, the presence of low levels of myofibroblasts in the valve assists in valve homeostasis, but increased myofibrogenesis leads to valve disease (discussed in detail in Section 2.3).

Multiprogenitor VICs in humans have also been described but not directly proven (Liu et al. 2007). However, VICs from pigs grown in vitro have been found to have an MSC-like subpopulation, capable of osteogenesis, adipogenesis, chondrogenesis, and myofibrogenesis (Chen et al. 2009). These progenitor cells likely aid in tissue renewal and repair in healthy valves but are thought to become dysregulated and disruptive in disease.

2.2.3 Cellular Machinery

2.2.3.1 Integrins

Integrins are key transmembrane receptors. They are named so because of their role in integrating the ECM and the cell cytoskeleton (Tamkun et al. 1986), allowing the bidirectional transfer of mechanical forces and sensing of the structural protein composition of the surrounding ECM to regulate diverse cellular behaviors, including migration, differentiation, and survival (Gahmberg et al. 2009, Geiger et al. 2009, Harburger and Calderwood 2009, Barczyk et al. 2010). Integrins are heterodimers formed by noncovalent interaction between an α subunit and a β subunit, resulting in an extracellular globular head supported by two rod-like legs that pass through the cell membrane and extend briefly into the cytoplasm (Humphries et al. 2003). Eighteen α subunits and 8 β subunits have been identified, producing 24 different integrins (Figure 2.6) (Hynes 2002).

Ligand binding occurs at the globular head and involves a domain alternatively called an I domain or an A domain, which is homologous to von Willebrand factor A (Humphries et al. 2003, Barczyk et al. 2010). Nine of 18 α subunits contain an I domain referred to as an α-I domain, and all β subunits contain an analogous β-I domain.

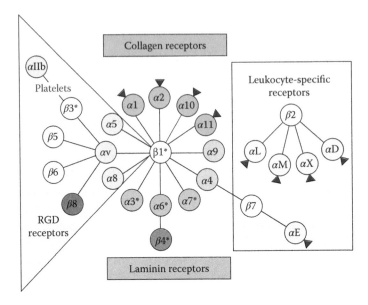

Figure 2.6   Integrins and their corresponding subunits and binding interactions. Eighteen α subunits and 8β subunits combine to form 24 integrins. The coloring of subunits indicates closely related subfamilies. Subunits with purple arrowheads contain I domains, and subunits with an asterisk have alternatively spliced isoforms. (Reprinted from Hynes, R. O., and Naba, A., *Cold Spring Harb. Perspect. Biol.*, 4, 1–16, 2012. With permission.)

For integrins that contain an α-I domain, ligand binding occurs at the α-I domain, otherwise the β-I domain is used (Barczyk et al. 2010). Cations are important mediators of ligand binding, and the I domain contains a "metal-ion-dependent adhesion site" (MIDAS) for a coordinating Mg^{2+} (Lee et al. 1995). Beta subunits are produced in excess, and the number of α subunits determines the number of integrins on the cell surface (Barczyk et al. 2010). The aortic valve and VICs have been found to contain mostly $\alpha1$, $\alpha2$, $\alpha3$, $\alpha5$, and $\beta1$ integrins (Latif et al. 2005b).

   Ligand-binding affinity to integrins can be modulated by the activation state of the integrin. When in an inactive, low-affinity state, the ligand-binding pocket is closed and is further obscured by the bending of the integrin legs, orienting the head and ligand-binding regions toward the cell membrane (Hynes 2002, Nishida et al. 2006, Gahmberg et al. 2009). Inactive integrins are considered in a low-affinity state because small ligands such as RGD peptides are still able to bind (Beer et al. 1992). An intermediate-affinity state can be achieved by a conformational change, extending the integrin legs to orient the integrin head toward the extracellular space while still keeping the ligand-binding pocket closed (Gahmberg et al. 2009). Finally, a high-affinity state occurs when the integrin is extended and the ligand-binding pocket is open (Hynes 2002, Gahmberg et al. 2009). A number of factors can regulate integrin activation state, including cations. The β-1 domain contains an adjacent-to-MIDAS (ADMIDAS) site, which inactivates integrin when Ca^{2+} is bound and activates integrin when Mn^{2++} is bound (Humphries et al. 2003). Inside-out signaling via molecules' binding to the integrin's cytoplasmic tail can also regulate activation, with talin binding promoting an active conformation (Tadokoro et al. 2003) and filamin binding inhibiting activation (Kiema et al. 2006). Both talin and filamin are linker molecules that join integrins to the actin cytoskeleton.

Integrins can bind a wide variety of ECM components, with major groupings including RGD receptors, glycine-phenylalanine-hydroxyproline-glycine-glutamate-arginine (GFOGER) receptors, leucine-aspartic acid-valine (LDV) receptors, and laminin receptors (Hynes 2002) (Humphries et al. 2006, Barczyk et al. 2010). The RGD sequence is most commonly associated with fibronectin and integrins, but it is also present in and allows integrin binding to vitronectin, fibrinogen, and the growth factor TGF-β1 through the latency-associated peptide (LAP) (Humphries et al. 2006). While denatured collagen I contains exposed RGD sequences (Davis 1992), intact fibrillar collagen uses a GFOGER sequence to bind to related integrins (Knight et al. 1998). The LDV sequence is related to RGD and is able to bind fibronectin, while variants of LDV bind vascular cell adhesion molecule 1 (VCAM-1), intercellular adhesion molecule 1 (ICAM-1), and other leukocyte adhesion proteins to mediate extravasation (Humphries et al. 2006). Some laminins contain exposed RGD sequences and can bind RGD integrins (Sasaki and Timpl 2001), but a number of specialized laminin-binding integrins that lack the α-I domain also exist (Humphries et al. 2006). Sequences such as RGD, GFOGER, and LDV represent the minimum recognition site for ligand receptor binding, and additional binding sites such as the synergy site of fibronectin are used to improve affinity (Mould et al. 1997, Huveneers et al. 2008). Although there is an overlap between what each integrin can bind to, every integrin appears to have a critical role, as knockout mouse models for each integrin result in distinct phenotypes (Hynes 2002).

2.2.3.2 Focal Adhesions

Ligand binding induces the clustering of integrins, which can lead to the formation of focal adhesions that provide a mechanical linkage between the cytoskeleton and the ECM, as well as a site for intracellular signaling by recruiting more than 50 different signaling molecules into the focal adhesion complex (Zamir and Geiger 2001, Romer et al. 2006, Geiger et al. 2009). This enables a variety of cell processes, including migration, proliferation, and differentiation. Formation of early focal adhesions, termed initial adhesions, is mediated by talin, which joins the initial clusters of integrins to F-actin (DePasquale and Izzard 1991, Jiang et al. 2003). Early signaling molecules recruited and activated include focal adhesion kinase (FAK), Src family kinases, and paxillin, which can interact with each other (Schaller et al. 1999, Hayashi et al. 2002) as well as with talin (Chen et al. 1995, Giannone et al. 2003) and integrins (Liu et al. 1999, Arias-Salgado et al. 2003). The multitude of interactions between these molecules ensures rapid formation of early focal adhesions called focal complexes. Focal adhesion kinase helps activate the small GTPase Rac (Chang et al. 2007), which in turn activates actin-related protein 2/3 (ARP2/3) (Miki et al. 2000) and helps in the recruitment of vinculin (DeMali et al. 2002) to promote actin assembly and organization. The small GTPase Rac promotes the formation of focal complexes, while activation of the small GTPase Rho enables the maturation of focal complexes into focal adhesions (Rottner et al. 1999). The stimuli of Rac and Rho are antagonistic to each other and help regulate the balance and turnover of focal complexes and focal

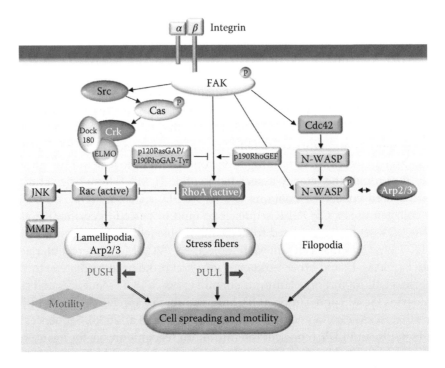

Figure 2.7 Cell migration is an integrin-mediated process involving a number of Rho GTPases, including Rac, RhoA, and Cdc42. As the cell moves forward, each ECM-engaged integrin drifts toward the back of the cell. Initially, filopodia extend on the cell's leading edge, facilitated by neural Wiskott–Aldrich syndrome protein (N-WASP) and actin polymerizing Arp2/3. Continued integrin engagement promotes integrin clustering and formation of focal complexes, along with the recruitment of key focal adhesion scaffolding and signaling proteins, including FAK, Src, p130CAS, Crk, Dock180, and engulfment and cell motility (ELMO), to drive Rac-stimulated promotion of Arp2/3 and lamellipodia extension. Focal complexes can mature into focal adhesions, with RhoA-mediated stress fiber formation enabling cellular contraction to retract the rear end of the cell. Cell movement in the ECM is assisted by JNK-mediated MMP activity. (With kind permission from Springer Science+Business Media: *Cell Tissue Res.*, Focal adhesion kinase (FAK) perspectives in mechanobiology: Implications for cell behavior, 357, 2014, 515–526, Tomakidi, P. et al.)

adhesions, allowing modulation of cell adhesiveness to the ECM, which is important for cell processes such as migration (Figure 2.7) (Rottner et al. 1999).

Mechanical forces, both intracellular and extracellular, play crucial roles in focal adhesion maturation. The application of internal or external force on initial adhesions stimulates their transition to focal complexes by recruiting vinculin to stabilize and strengthen the adhesion (Galbraith et al. 2002). Similarly, force generation induces the development of focal complexes into focal adhesions by activating Rho (Riveline et al. 2001). In focal adhesions, Rho regulates cellular contractility through two main mechanisms, which are mediated by two different integrin classes (Schiller et al. 2013). Engagement of αv-class integrins activates Rho and acts through mDia to promote actin stress fiber formation (Schiller et al. 2013). Actin stress fibers not only serve to provide a substrate for myosin to pull on but also serve to cluster integrins together to aid focal adhesion formation (Chrzanowska-Wodnicka and Burridge 1996). In contrast, engagement of $\alpha5\beta1$ integrins activates Rho and acts through Rho kinase (ROCK) to stimulate myosin II and force generation (Schiller et al. 2013). Cellular contractility is critical to focal adhesion formation, as inhibiting contractility leads to stress fiber and focal adhesion disassembly (Chrzanowska-Wodnicka and Burridge 1996).

The mechanical connection between the ECM and cell cytoskeleton through integrins means that mechanical force and properties between the two are closely linked. Cells sense and increase force generation proportionally with the stiffness of the surrounding matrix (Choquet et al. 1997, Wang et al. 2000), and correspondingly, increased ECM stiffness promotes the formation of larger, more stable actin stress fibers, and focal adhesions (Pelham and Wang 1997, Peyton and Putnam 2005). This leads to an increase the cell's own stiffness as the stiffness of its underlying substrate increases (Liu et al. 2013). Similarly, ECM stretch also enhances actin stress fiber and focal adhesion formation (Yoshigi et al. 2005).

More broadly, cells such as fibroblasts migrate preferentially toward stiffer substrates (Lo et al. 2000) and respond to stiffer substrates with increased cell spreading, increased DNA synthesis, and decreased apoptosis (Wang et al. 2000). Many cell types require adhesion for survival and undergo programmed cell death in the absence of any ECM interactions in a process called anoikis (Meredith et al. 1993). The importance of ECM stiffness in cell behavior is perhaps best illustrated by its effect on cell differentiation, where growing MSCs on different stiffness substrates is sufficient to direct differentiation, with soft brain-like stiffness-promoting neurogenesis, stiffer muscle-like stiffness-promoting myogenesis, and rigid bone-like stiffness-promoting osteogenesis (Engler et al. 2006).

2.2.3.3 Mechanosensors and Mechanosensitive Signaling Pathways

External mechanical forces are detected by cells through a number of mechanosensors, proteins that are directly modified by mechanical force to change conformation and/or enzymatic activity, which can then modulate intracellular signaling pathways to regulate cell behavior and gene transcription. A number of mechanosensors play key roles in the activation and assembly of focal adhesions, including integrins (Friedland et al. 2009, Chen et al. 2012), talin (del Rio et al. 2009), FAK (Zhou et al. 2015), and p130Crk-associated substrate (p130CAS) (Sawada et al. 2006). Integrin conformational change between inactive and active states is assisted by intracellular force through actin–myosin contraction (Friedland et al. 2009) as well as by extracellular force applied by the attached ECM ligand (Chen et al. 2012). Talin links integrins to actin and contains helical bundles in its structure. These bundles unfold when mechanically stretched to expose vinculin-binding domains, allowing vinculin recruitment to focal adhesions (del Rio et al. 2009). Vinculin mediates actin cytoskeleton reorganization and focal adhesion stability and also recruits other focal adhesion proteins such as Arp2/3 and paxillin in a force-dependent manner (Carisey and Ballestrem 2011, Carisey et al. 2013). Full activation of FAK requires recruitment and phosphorylation by Src, a key tyrosine kinase that phosphorylates many focal adhesion-associated proteins, at tyrosines 576 and 577 (Calalb et al. 1995). Initial recruitment of FAK to integrin and talin allows autophosphorylation of tyrosin 397, which opens a binding site for Src (Schaller et al. 1994) and is a process that in silico models predict to be mechanically assisted by pulling forces between FAK's attachment to the cell membrane and actin cytoskeleton (Zhou et al. 2015). Similar to talin, p130CAS also extends under applied force to expose its tyrosine phosphorylation site (Sawada et al. 2006). p130CAS is a substrate phosphorylated by Src (Ruest et al. 2001) and can enhance Src activity in reciprocity (Burnham et al. 2000). It is also an important scaffold for other proteins (Defilippi et al. 2006) and controls the activation of the Rac1 GTPase (Sharma and Mayer 2008).

Focal adhesion kinase is a key mediator of a number of important mechanosensitive signaling pathways, including mitogen-activated protein kinases (MAPK) (Figure 2.8) such as extracellular signal-regulated kinases 1/2 (ERK1/2) (Wang et al. 2001), p38 MAPK (Wang et al. 2001), and Jun N-terminal kinase (JNK) (Nadruz et al. 2005) and RhoA (Tomakidi et al. 2014). Extracellular signal-regulated kinases 1/2 regulates a number of cell processes, most notably migration, proliferation, and differentiation and can be activated by stimulation from growth factors such as fibroblast growth factor and vascular endothelial growth factor binding to their respective receptors, initiating a signaling cascade involving consecutive activation of the GTPase Ras, the GTPase Raf, mitogen-activated protein kinase (MEK), and ultimately ERK1/2 (Roskoski 2012). Focal adhesion kinase can activate Ras (Schlaepfer and Hunter 1997) through growth factor receptor-bound protein 2 (GRB2) (Schlaepfer et al. 1994) to trigger the Ras/Raf/MEK/ERK1/2 cascade, making Ras an important convergence point for mechanically mediated integrin and growth factor-related signaling. Ras (Li et al. 1996) and Rac (Sundberg et al. 2003) are able to activate the stress response pathway JNK to regulate cellular proliferation and apoptosis; however, JNK is more commonly activated by inflammatory cytokines, pathogens, and oxidative stress (Zeke et al. 2016). Jun N-terminal kinase also plays important roles in ECM remodeling by controlling expression of collagen (Kook et al. 2009) and MMPs (Hsia et al. 2003). Focal adhesion kinase activates p38 MAPK through p130CAS and Crk (Watanabe et al. 2009, Tomakidi et al. 2014) to direct cell proliferation (Watanabe et al. 2009) and apoptosis (Boosani et al. 2009). As FAK plays a role in the activation of all three MAPK pathways, other focal adhesion-associated proteins are likely responsible for the selective activation of individual MAPK pathways by different integrins (MacKenna et al. 1998).

Like other GTPases, Rho is inactive when bound to guanosine diphosphate (GDP) and is activated by guanine-nucleotide exchange factors (GEFs), which catalyze the exchange of GDP for GTP (Lessey et al. 2012). Rho's intrinsic GTPase activity can revert its active GTP-bound form to the inactive GDP-bound form, but this process can be catalyzed by GTPase-activating proteins (GAPs). Rho can be activated by a variety of mechanical forces, including shear stress, compression, and tension (Lessey et al. 2012). This process is mediated by GEFs and GAPs that associate with the cytoskeleton and focal adhesions (Schwartz 2004, Lessey et al. 2012). Notably, FAK

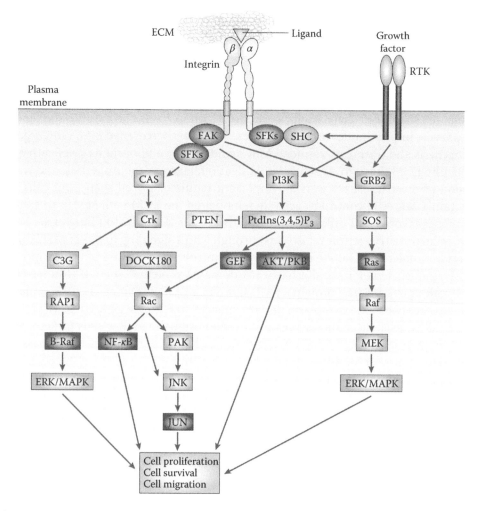

Figure 2.8 Along with more traditional control by growth factors and associated receptor tyrosine kinases (RTKs), mechanical forces can activate MAPKs by triggering mechanosensors such as integrin and FAK in order to control cell behaviors such as cell proliferation, survival, and migration. Mitogen-activated protein kinases are controlled by cascades with multiple levels of kinases. Focal adhesion kinase can stimulate GRB2 to activate the MAPK ERK through the Ras GTPase, Raf GTPase, and MAPK kinase (MEK) or, alternatively, with the help of additional focal adhesion-associated proteins such as SRK, CAS, and Crk, through the GEF C3G, RAP1 GTPase, and B-Raf GTPase. The MAPK JNK can be activated by FAK through recruitment of the GEF DOCK180 to trigger the Rac GTPase and eventually JNK, which regulates JUN transcription factors. Other important signaling pathways controlled by FAK include the inflammatory signaling pathways nuclear factor kappa-light-chain enhancer of activated B cells (NF-κB) and the phosphoinositide 3-kinase (PI3K)/protein kinase B (AKT) cell cycle/cell survival pathway. (Reprinted by permission from Macmillan Publishers Ltd. *Nat. Rev. Mol. Cell Biol.*, 5, 816–826, Guo, W., and Giancotti, F. G., 2004, copyright 2004.)

can activate Rho directly by binding and phosphorylating p190RhoGEF (Lim et al. 2008) and can inactivate Rho indirectly through Src to phosphorylate p190RhoGAP (Schober et al. 2007). RhoA's control of the actin–myosin machinery makes it an important signaling protein, mediating changes to cell structural behaviors such as cell shape response and migration in response to mechanical stimuli (Arthur and Burridge 2001, Peyton and Putnam 2005, Liu et al. 2014). While RhoA activity can change cell shape, cell shape itself can modulate RhoA levels and cytoskeletal tension and provide important developmental cues, with spread, flattened MSCs undergoing osteogenesis and unspread, rounded MSCs undergoing adipogenesis (McBeath et al. 2004). The ECM through structural organization, mechanical properties, and transmission of mechanical forces is an important regulator of cell shape, but cells can maintain a degree of control by actively remodeling the ECM with MMPs to assume cell shapes favorable to different differentiation fates (Figure 2.9) (Tang et al. 2013). Extracellular matrix stiffness also acts through RhoA signaling to direct MSC differentiation (Engler et al. 2006). RhoA activity controls the shuttling of transcriptional coactivators such as four and a half LIM domains protein 2 (FHL2) (Muller et al. 2002) and yes-associated protein (YAP)/tafazzin (TAZ) (Tang et al. 2013, Panciera et al. 2017) between the cytoplasm and the nucleus to regulate gene transcription.

In healthy cells, mechanosensing and mechanosignaling allow cells to detect and maintain their ideal mechanical environment, including preferred ECM stiffness and stress (Humphrey et al. 2014). They can do this through a variety of mechanisms, including exerting force on the ECM (Delvoye et al. 1991), remodeling the ECM by increasing ECM synthesis and degradation in response to increased mechanical loading (Gupta and Grande-Allen 2006), and reorienting the cytoskeleton to buffer the effects of externally applied forces on the cell (Webster et al. 2014). However, disease can result if the environment changes exceed the cells' homeostatic maintenance

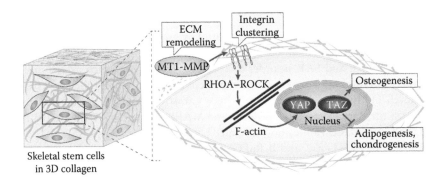

Figure 2.9 Stem cell differentiation is controlled by ECM properties, including stiffness and structure, which have an impact on cell shape. These mechanical cues are detected by RhoA, causing changes in actin cytoskeleton organization and intracellular tension and causing the nuclear translocation of YAP and TAZ to control the choice between osteogenesis and adipogenesis/chondrogenesis. Cells have a degree of control over their cell fate by remodeling the ECM by using MMPs such as MT1-MMP. (Reprinted by permission from Macmillan Publishers Ltd. *Nat. Rev. Mol. Cell Biol.*, 18, 758–770, Panciera, T. et al., 2017, copyright 2017.)

capability or if initially beneficial adaptive processes fail to stop. In the aortic valve, the development of calcific aortic valve disease helps illustrate some of these concepts.

2.3 Calcific Aortic Valve Disease

Calcific aortic valve disease (CAVD) encompasses a spectrum of diseases, from aortic valve sclerosis, where the valve begins to thicken and stiffen, to aortic valve stenosis, where the valve becomes calcified, no longer fully opens, and obstructs blood flow (Freeman and Otto 2005). It is the most common valvular disease (Benjamin et al. 2017) and is associated with age, where 25% of people over the age of 65 years have aortic valve sclerosis and 2% have aortic valve stenosis (Stewart et al. 1997). Besides age, other risk factors include male gender, smoking, hypertension, hypercholesterolemia, and having a congenital valve malformation such as a bicuspid valve (Stewart et al. 1997, Rabkin 2005, Roberts and Ko 2005). Although the milder aortic valve sclerosis does not impact valve function, it is associated with a 50% increased risk of death from cardiovascular events and myocardial infarction (Otto et al. 1999). There are currently no pharmaceutical treatments for CAVD, and patients with severe aortic stenosis require aortic valve replacement surgery (Hutcheson et al. 2014).

Calcific aortic valve disease was originally viewed as a degenerative wear-and-tear disorder, where mechanical stress combined with age results in passive calcification through damage to the valve (Freeman and Otto 2005). Observations that calcification occurs predominantly in areas that experience maximal mechanical stress in the valve were supportive of this view (Thubrikar et al. 1986). Calcific aortic valve disease is now understood as an active cell-mediated process involving complex cell–cell signaling, cell–matrix signaling, mechanical forces, and cellular differentiation (Chen and Simmons 2011, Merryman and Schoen 2013, Towler 2013, Yutzey et al. 2014).

Early lesions are found preferentially in the fibrosa (Otto et al. 1994, Sider et al. 2014) and are characterized by leaflet thickening and ECM disruption, most notably with the displacement, fragmentation, and reduplication of the elastic lamina and subendothelial basement membrane (Otto et al. 1994, Sider et al. 2014); fine extracellular mineralization (Otto et al. 1994); proteoglycan accumulation (Sider et al. 2014); lipid deposition (Otto et al. 1994, O'Brien et al. 1996); elevated osteochondral markers such as Sox9 and Msx2 (Sider et al. 2014); elevated osteogenic markers such as osteopontin, osteocalcin (OCN), Runx2, osterix, and Notch1 (Aikawa et al. 2007); elevated αSMA expression indicative of myofibroblasts (Otto et al. 1994); upregulated superoxide levels (Miller et al. 2008); downregulated antioxidant mechanisms (Miller et al. 2008); and the infiltration of inflammatory cells such as macrophages and T cells (Otto et al. 1994, Aikawa et al. 2007). These properties become more pronounced as disease progresses (Figure 2.10a). In addition, late-stage lesions develop extensive calcification with a study of patients undergoing aortic valve replacement surgery finding 83% have dystrophic calcification and 13% having osteogenic calcification with mature lamellar bone (Mohler et al. 2001).

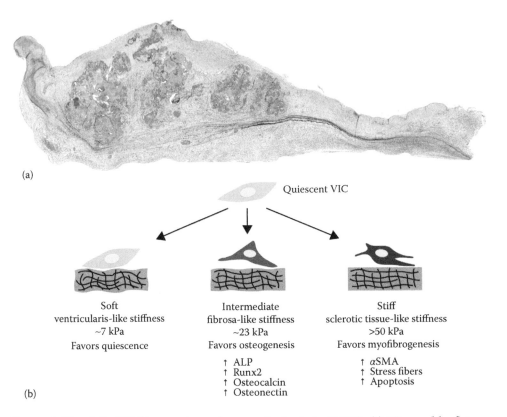

(a)

(b)

Figure 2.10 Cell–ECM interactions play a critical role in CAVD. (a) Diseased leaflets are characterized by the thickening and stiffening of the leaflet along with ECM disruption and the presence of calcific lesions that occur preferentially on the fibrosa side of the valve. The leaflet has been stained with Movat's pentachrome to show collagen (yellow), proteoglycan (blue), nuclei/elastin (purple/black), and cytoplasm/muscle fiber (red). (b) Mechanical forces are thought to play an important role in CAVD development. The healthy fibrosa contains uniquely stiff regions that may provide a permissive environment for the disease and contribute to preferential lesion formation in the fibrosa. In vitro, VICs preferentially undergo osteogenic differentiation, as shown by the osteogenic marker alkaline phosphatase (ALP), on the higher stiffness found in the fibrosa. Progressive stiffening of the valve with disease can promote myofibroblastic differentiation, which can lead to further ECM disruption and substrate stiffening in positive feedback. (Adapted from Chen, J.-H., and Simmons, C. A., *Circ. Res.*, 108, 1510–1524, 2011.)

Osteogenic calcification, on the one hand, refers to active bone formation (Rajamannan et al. 2003, Chen et al. 2009, Chen et al. 2015), and indeed, bone growth factors such as bone morphogenetic protein (BMP)-2 and -4 (Mohler et al. 2001), bone matrix components such as osteopontin (O'Brien et al. 1995, Rajamannan et al. 2003) and bone sialoprotein (BSP) (Rajamannan et al. 2003), bone transcription factors such as Runx2 (Rajamannan et al. 2003) (Alexopoulos et al. 2010) and osterix (Alexopoulos et al. 2010), and other bone markers such as alkaline phosphatase (ALP) (Rajamannan et al. 2003) and OCN (Rajamannan et al. 2003) are present in diseased valves. The primary source of these pro-osteogenic signals is believed to be VICs, which are multipotent and can differentiate into osteoblast-like cells in vitro when exposed to osteogenic media, forming nodules that demonstrate bone characteristics such as positive staining for calcium salts by von Kossa, ALP activity, and Runx2 expression (Chen et al. 2009, Yip et al. 2009). Circulating osteogenic precursor cells from the bone marrow that coexpress the bone marker collagen type I and hematopoietic marker CD45 have also been found in diseased valves and may contribute to osteogenic calcification (Egan et al. 2011).

Dystrophic calcification, on the other hand, is caused by cell death, a process involving myofibroblastic VICs (Jian et al. 2003, Yip et al. 2009, Chen et al. 2015). Diseased valves are enriched with TGF-β1, released in part by infiltrating lymphocytes, which in vitro promotes VICs to differentiate into a highly contractile myofibroblastic phenotype that aggregates into apoptotic nodules (Jian et al. 2003). Strikingly, a dramatic shift has been observed in the composition of the resident VIC population from one with low numbers of αSMA-positive myofibroblasts (1%–2%) in healthy valves to one with large numbers of αSMA-positive myofibroblasts (31%–36%) in diseased valves (Rabkin-Aikawa et al. 2004, Pho et al. 2008), which might explain the prevalence of dystrophic calcification. Temporary elevation in myofibroblast count is also seen in valve development, during adaption after valve transplant or in maturing tissue-engineered valves, but it eventually subsides. However, it persists in CAVD (Rabkin-Aikawa et al. 2004), suggesting that dysregulated repair and remodeling mechanisms contribute to the disease.

2.3.1 Changes to Extracellular Matrix Composition and Implications

Extracellular matrix disruption is a hallmark of CAVD (Otto et al. 1994, Hinton et al. 2006) interfering with the structural, mechanical, and chemical cues needed to maintain the health of the interior cell population and overall valve function. Notably, the stratification of the three layers of the valve, each with its distinct ECM composition and mechanical properties, is lost in advanced disease, as disorganized collagen and proteoglycan are deposited throughout the valve (Hinton et al. 2006).

In diseased valves, collagen fibers become disorganized due to upregulated MMP-1, MMP-2, MMP-3, and MMP-9 (Soini et al. 2001, Kaden et al. 2003, Fondard et al. 2005), along with TIMP-1 and TIMP-2 (Soini et al. 2001, Fondard et al. 2005). Infiltrating leukocytes are believed to play a role in this process by releasing the growth factor interleukin-1β to stimulate MMP activity in VICs (Kaden et al. 2003). Cathepsin K, a potent collagenase, is also upregulated in diseased valves (Helske et al. 2006). The result is a marked increase in collagen turnover, with collagen as a proportion of total protein in the valve dropping from 90% in healthy valves to 10% in calcified areas of diseased valves, despite a two- to three-fold increase in collagen synthesis (Eriksen et al. 2006). The development of calcific nodules also disrupts collagen organization (Fondard et al. 2005). As previously mentioned, while these collagen changes primarily affect the fibrosa, where collagen predominates, collagen is also dysregulated in the ventricularis and spongiosa in diseased valves (Fondard et al. 2005, Hinton et al. 2006).

Elastin content in diseased valves is reduced, becoming fragmented and disorganized (Fondard et al. 2005, Hinton et al. 2006), a process likely directed by the upregulated elastases MMP-2, MMP-9, cathepsin S, cathepsin K, and cathepsin V (Soini et al. 2001, Fondard et al. 2005, Helske et al. 2006). Elastin degradation reduces the extensibility and slightly increases the stiffness of the aortic valve (Lee et al. 2001).

Proteoglycan content increases in diseased valves and is present in all layers (Hinton et al. 2006). The proteoglycans biglycan and decorin colocalize with apolipoproteins (O'Brien 1995) and retain low-density lipoproteins through electrostatic interactions (Neufeld et al. 2014). Biglycan and decorin have a higher expression in early lesions than in mature lesions (Stephens et al. 2011), and it has been suggested that their lipid and growth factor retention properties help promote lesion progression (Grande-Allen et al. 2007). The proteoglycans biglycan and decorin are known to bind and regulate the availability of TGF-β1 (Macri et al. 2007). Supportive of that theory, a study of a porcine model of early disease suggests that the development of proteoglycan-rich onlays in the fibrosa between the endothelial layer and elastic lamina may be one of the earliest events in CAVD occurring before significant lipid accumulation, inflammatory cell infiltration, or myofibroblast activation (Sider et al. 2014).

While the increase in myofibroblastic VICs is in large part responsible for the upregulated ECM turnover (Rabkin-Aikawa et al. 2004), the ECM changes in turn regulate VIC behavior. Growing VICs on tissue culture polystyrene (TCPS) in vitro with or without TGF-β1 upregulates the myofibroblastic marker αSMA and the osteogenic markers ALP and Runx2, as well as promotes the formation of calcific nodules, but this VIC differentiation can be inhibited in a dose-dependent manner by coating the TCPS with collagen or fibronectin (Benton et al. 2008, Rodriguez and Masters 2009). In contrast, TCPS coated with laminin, heparin, or fibrin further enhanced VIC differentiation, with fibrin being particularly stimulatory (Benton et al. 2008, Rodriguez and Masters 2009). These results demonstrate the sensitivity of VICs to the composition of their surrounding ECM. In fact, ex vivo experiments growing excised porcine aortic valves in media have demonstrated that simply degrading collagen in the valve with collagenase is sufficient to induce VICs to express αSMA, ALP, OCN, and BSP and mineralize the leaflet compared with nondegraded control valves (Rodriguez et al. 2014), supporting the previous in vitro results. This may represent a positive-feedback mechanism toward disease, where falling collagen levels as a portion of total protein in diseased valves remove an inhibitory signal for VIC myofibrogenesis (Rodriguez and Masters 2009, Rodriguez et al. 2014), which in turn promotes additional collagen degradation.

Integrins mediate the differentiation signaling from structural ECM components, with the anticalcification signals from laminin and fibronectin being abrogated when their respective 67 kDa laminin receptors and α5β1 integrins are blocked (Gu and Masters 2010). Blocking α5β1 integrin, which is also a fibrin receptor, had no effect on fibrin's procalcific effect, and blocking α2β1 integrin, a collagen receptor, had no effect on collagen's anticalcific effect, indicating that they must use alternate integrins to signal cells (Gu and Masters 2010). Examining specific adhesion peptide sequences found that RGD is sufficient to replicate fibrin's procalcific effect while aspartic acid-glycine-glutamic acid-alanine (DGEA) and tyrosine-isoleucine-glycine-serine-arginine (YIGSR) found in collagen and laminin, respectively, are sufficient to replicate their anticalcific effect (Gu and Masters 2010). Blocking MEK or ERK1/2 downstream of MEK reduced nodule formation, ALP expression, TGF-β1 expression, and apoptosis of VICs grown on fibrin, suggesting that fibrin uses the MAPK/ERK pathway to promote calcification (Gu and Masters 2009).

Signaling from ECM structural components can also work in concert with growth factors present in the ECM to direct VIC differentiation. Fibronectin- and heparin-coated surfaces promote αSMA expression in VICs, which is thought to be due, in part, to be due to their TGF-β1-binding sites, which allow them to trap and present soluble TGF-β1 to VICs (Cushing et al. 2005). Detailed examination of heparin found that it not only aids in the adsorption of TGF-β1 but also promotes the production of TGF-β1 by VICs, making it a potent promoter of myofibrogenesis (Cushing et al. 2005). This effect can be further enhanced by adding soluble heparin to fibronectin-coated surfaces (Cushing et al. 2005). Experiments with elastin fragments and TGF-β1 in rat dermal fibroblasts have found that they also work synergistically to promote myofibrogenesis and osteogenesis (Simionescu et al. 2007). Alternatively, ECM structural components can induce growth factor release from VICs to control VIC differentiation. Biglycan has also been found to upregulate BMP-2 and TGF-β1 expression in VICs by signaling through Toll-like receptor-2 (Song et al. 2012) and -4 (Song et al. 2015), respectively, to promote ERK1/2 and nuclear factor (NF)κB signaling (Song et al. 2012). Biglycan is believed to promote osteogenesis in VICs, including increasing ALP expression and calcium deposition, indirectly through autocrine and paracrine BMP-2 and TGF-β1 releases, which work independently and synergistically through Smad1 and Smad3 signaling (Song et al. 2015). Oxidized low-density lipoprotein (oxLDL) found in diseased valves promotes VIC production of biglycan and collagen I (Cheng et al. 2017), which, combined with the previously described biglycan–VIC interactions, demonstrates the continuous, dynamic communication between the ECM and cells and how deleterious signals can propagate and magnify.

2.3.2 Influence of Mechanical Forces on Calcific Aortic Valve Disease

The aortic valve exists in a highly dynamic mechanical environment in which the cells and tissue experience shear stress and pressure from blood flow, bending and stretching forces from the valve opening and closing, and distinct stiffness properties in its three layers because of their different ECM compositions. As a result, mechanical forces play a central role in cell–matrix interactions in the valve, including during CAVD (Butcher et al. 2008, Balachandran et al. 2011, Chen and Simmons 2011, Merryman and Schoen 2013). A potent example of this is that simply preventing the valve from fully closing in an ex vivo bioreactor flow system causes differential regulation of 202 genes detected by microarray compared with the valves that can open and close normally (Maeda et al. 2016). Inflammatory genes saw the largest magnitude changes, while protein binding, developmental process, and stress response-related genes represent the groups with the most genes differentially regulated. Systemic forces such as increased blood pressure stimulate collagen and sulfated GAG production in the valve but not αSMA production (Xing et al. 2004), which may explain in part why hypertension is a risk factor for CAVD (Rabkin 2005).

A more local example of mechanical cell–matrix interaction is the release of TGF-β1 from the ECM through mechanical stress. Cells secrete TGF-β1 into the extracellular space, where it binds latency-associated proteins (LAPs) and latent-TGF-β-binding proteins (LTBP) to form large latent complexes (LLC) that attach to the ECM to store TGF-β1 (Annes, Munger, and Rifkin 2003). Contractile myofibroblasts can bind to the LAP by using integrins $\alpha_v\beta3$ and $\alpha_v\beta5$ and physically pull open the LAP by using mechanical stress to release the stored TGF-β1 (Wipff et al. 2007). This requires the presence of αSMA stress fibers in the cell to generate enough contractile force and a stiff-enough substrate (>5 kPa) to provide resistance to have the LLC open. Alternatively, myofibroblasts with appropriate stress fibers and integrin binding can provide the resistance that pulls open the LAP when the substrate is stretched. Released TGF-β1 binds to TGF-β1 receptor II, which phosphorylates and recruits TGF-β1 receptor I (Hinz 2007). This heterotrimeric receptor complex can then phosphorylate Smad2 and Smad3, inducing binding with Smad4 and translocation to the nucleus, where it can enhance transcription of myofibroblastic genes such as αSMA. This can quickly set up a positive-feedback loop, where TGF-β1 release by contractile myofibroblasts stimulates additional myofibrogenesis and contraction to release more TGF-β1, contributing to fibrosis.

Fibroblast growth factor 2 (FGF2) has also been found to play a role in TGF-β1 availability, since FGF2 and TGF-β1 appear to competitively bind to the proteoglycan betaglycan, so that increased FGF2 results in increased TGF-β1 availability (Han and Gotlieb 2012). As such, FGF2 increases VIC contractility seen in wound assays in a TGF-β1 pSmad2/3-dependent manner (Han and Gotlieb 2011). Interestingly, FGF2 has also been found to increase VIC contractility directly by signaling through Akt1 (Han and Gotlieb 2012), demonstrating the complex interplay of ECM structural components, growth factors, and cellular contractility.

Valve interstitial cells respond in vitro to TGF-β1 in a dose-dependent manner, with increasing αSMA expression and contractility (Walker et al. 2004). Increased mechanical tension in the underlying substrate enhances the effect of TGF-β1, and the activated VIC myofibroblasts remodel the ECM, which is thought to be the first step in CAVD initiation. Over time, VIC monolayers grown in vitro spontaneously contract into rounded nodules in a cellular contractility-mediated mechanism (Benton et al. 2009). Increasing αSMA through TGF-β1 or overexpression plasmid enhanced contractility and nodule formation, while αSMA knockdown inhibited the process. These types of nodules demonstrate not only the apoptosis expected of dystrophic calcification but also osteogenic markers, including upregulated ALP, Runx2, and OCN (Gu and Masters 2011). Nodule formation can also be regulated by Rho/ROCK contractile signaling, whose activation promotes nodule formation and promotes αSMA expression, while ROCK inhibition reduces the process (Gu and Masters 2011, Farrar et al. 2016).

In addition to tension between the cell and ECM promoting nodule formation, cell–cell tension mediated by Cadherin-11 is required for nodule formation in vitro (Hutcheson et al. 2013). Cadherin-11 is upregulated in human diseased valves (Hutcheson et al. 2013, Sung et al. 2016), and its overexpression in a mouse model promotes calcification (Sung et al. 2016). Dimensionality is also an important factor that directs VIC behavior, where, unlike two-dimensional (2D) culture, VICs grown in three-dimensional (3D) substrates maintain a more quiescent phenotype with lower expression of myofibroblast markers αSMA and vimentin (Hjortnaes et al. 2015).

Besides intracellularly generated forces, important mechanical signals in the aortic valve are provided by ECM stiffness and stretch, which will be discussed in Sections 2.3.2.1 and 2.3.2.2. The other key mechanical force on the aortic valve is shear stress from the blood, but as it does not directly relate to valve cell–matrix interactions, interested readers are directed to relevant reviews (Butcher et al. 2008, Balachandran et al. 2011, Arjunon et al. 2013).

2.3.2.1 Stiffness

The stiffness of the aortic valve naturally increases with age and varies with location, from 3.5 to 10.5 kPa in the belly from adolescence to adult and from 7.0 to 20.8 kPa in the commissure from adolescence to adult, as measured by low-strain biaxial testing (van Geemen et al. 2016). The different layers of the valve demonstrate many areas of similar stiffness, but on average, the fibrosa is stiffer than the ventricularis (Chen and Simmons 2011, Zhao et al. 2011). Calcific aortic valve disease lesions occur preferentially on the fibrosa side of the valve (Otto et al. 1994), and observations that the fibrosa contains regions with uniquely high stiffness have led to the theory that stiffness plays a role in the disease (Figure 2.10b) (Chen and Simmons 2011).

While valve stiffness is determined in large part by ECM composition (van Geemen et al. 2016), active regulation of valve stiffness is possible (El-Hamamsy et al. 2009, Warnock et al. 2010). Valve endothelial cell release of nitric oxide (NO) is thought to allow VIC relaxation and decrease valve stiffness (El-Hamamsy et al. 2009), while endothelin-1 (El-Hamamsy et al. 2009) and angiotensin II increase valve stiffness (Warnock et al. 2010).

Valve interstitial cells are able to sense and respond to increased substrate stiffness by increasing their own cellular stiffness, as measured by both micropipette aspiration (Merryman et al. 2006) and atomic force microscopy (Liu et al. 2013). Increased substrate stiffness promotes VIC activation to a myofibroblastic phenotype with increased αSMA expression (Merryman et al. 2006, Pho et al. 2008, Quinlan and Billiar 2012, Wang et al. 2013) and collagen production (Merryman et al. 2006, Wang et al. 2013). Cell density and cell area increase, and cells transition from a cuboid shape at low stiffness to an elongated shape at high stiffness (Quinlan and Billiar 2012). Valve interstitial cells require a stiffness less than 10 kPa to remain quiescent (Quinlan and Billiar 2012), which is most similar to the ventricularis (Chen and Simmons 2011) and may help explain why the ventricularis is less prone to disease. Valve interstitial cells are constantly probing their environment, and myofibrogenesis of VICs due to stiffness is reversible. Valve interstitial cells grown on photodegradable hydrogels of 32 kPa stiffness become myofibroblasts with increased αSMA expression but can return to a quiescent state with lowered αSMA levels after photodegrading the hydrogel to 7 kPa stiffness (Kloxin et al. 2010, Wang et al. 2012). The PI3K/Akt pathway helps direct stiffness-mediated VIC myofibrogenesis by activating at the gene and protein levels in response to increased stiffness (Wang et al. 2012). The inhibition of PI3K reduces myofibrogenesis on stiff substrates, and constitutive activation of PI3K promotes nodule formation on soft substrates. The inability of myofibroblasts to develop on soft substrates is due to an inability to form the mature focal adhesions that are required to anchor stress fibers and generate sufficient tension to recruit αSMA (Goffin et al. 2006).

The growth factor TGF-β1 can induce myofibroblast differentiation of VICs in a stiffness-dependent manner through β-catenin signaling (Chen et al. 2011). It also induces β-catenin nuclear translocation through TGF-β receptor I, which works alongside traditional TGF-β1 signaling through pSmad2/3 to promote αSMA expression. It induces very little VIC myofibrogenesis on substrates with a stiffness less than 22 kPa, moderate myofibrogenesis on substrates with a stiffness of 22–50 kPa, and large amounts of myofibrogenesis on substrate with a stiffness greater than 50 kPa. This TGF-β1 stiffness-dependent induction effect requires β-catenin, as β-catenin knockdown prevents myofibrogenesis on all stiffness.

The aortic valve is composed not only of ECM and VICs but also VECs, which provide important protective paracrine signals against myofibrogenesis in more physiologically relevant in vitro experiments. Coculture of VECs on the membrane of Transwell® inserts with VICs on hydrogels reduced αSMA expression in VICs on both 3 kPa and 27 kPa substrates (Gould et al. 2014). This protective effect is mediated by VEC NO release, as N^{ω}-Nitro-L-arginine methyl ester hydrochloride (L-NAME) inhibition of NO increased myofibroblast levels to that of VIC culture alone. Nitric oxide utilizes the cyclic guanosine monophosphate (cGMP) pathway in VICs to inhibit RhoA, and inhibiting soluble guanylyl cyclase or protein kinase G upstream of cGMP or activating RhoA directly overrides the protective effect of VEC.

Beyond just myofibrogenesis, substrate stiffness helps VICs decide between osteogenesis and myofibrogenesis and plays a role in calcific nodule formation (Yip et al. 2009). Long-term culture of VICs in osteogenic media on compliant 27 kPa collagen gels, a stiffness similar to early lesions, formed nodules that were osteogenic and preferentially expressed ALP, osteonectin, OCN, and Runx2, whereas VICs grown on stiff 113 kPa collagen gels, a stiffness similar to sclerotic valve tissue, formed nodules that were myofibroblastic and preferentially expressed filamentous αSMA. The nodules on stiff substrates were apoptotic and formed in part through a contractile process likely representing dystrophic calcification. Treatment with TGF-β1 enhanced nodule formation on stiff but not compliant gels (Yip et al. 2009), consistent with TGF-β1's difficulty in inducing myofibrogenesis at lower stiffness (Chen et al. 2011). This differential response may be due to lower detected TGF-β receptor I expression on compliant gels (Yip et al. 2009).

Valve interstitial cells grown in photocrosslinkable 3D hydrogels softer than the native valve, thought to mimic the soft proteoglycan-rich onlays formed in early disease (Sider et al. 2014, Duan et al. 2016), have also been found to promote osteogenesis (Duan et al. 2016). Runx2, OCN, and ALP are upregulated, and osteogenic differentiation stiffens the substrate by day 21, which accelerates the process in positive feedback. Dynamically stiffening the substrate with ultraviolet (UV) light after 7 days to physiological stiffness or inhibiting the stiffness sensing RhoA pathway with ROCK inhibitor reduced osteogenesis. Pathological differentiation of VICs on substrates both softer and stiffer than healthy aortic valves demonstrates how sensitive VICs are to stiffness and how any deviation from mechanical homeostasis can have dramatic effects.

2.3.2.2 Stretch

As will be discussed in detail in Chapter 15, the aorta stiffens with age (Haskett et al. 2010), and this is thought to contribute to increased mechanical strain on the valve (Fisher et al. 2013). Normal physiological stretch of the valve leaflets is 10% in the circumferential direction, while CAVD induces pathological stretch of 15% (Balachandran et al. 2009). Pathological 15% stretch on VICs in vitro (Ku et al. 2006) and on valves ex vivo (Balachandran et al. 2006, 2009) promotes ECM remodeling through increased collagen production (Balachandran et al. 2006, 2009, 2011, Ku et al. 2006), increased MMP-1, -2, -9 and the elastolytic proteases cathepsin S and K (Balachandran et al. 2009), and decreased TIMP-1 (Balachandran et al. 2009). Cell proliferation (Balachandran et al. 2009, 2011), apoptosis (Balachandran et al. 2009), and αSMA expression (Balachandran et al. 2006) also increase with pathological stretch. Valve endothelial cells undergoing pathological stretch present proinflammatory proteins such as VCAM-1 and ICAM-1 and have endothelial layer disruption (Metzler et al. 2008).

The effect of cyclic stretch is enhanced by 5-hydroxytryptamine (HT or serotonin) and is mediated by 5-HT receptor 2A, leading to increased cell proliferation, collagen production, and tissue stiffness (Balachandran et al. 2011, 2012). Cyclic stretch promotes expression of the gene for 5-HT receptor 2A, thereby increasing 5-HT responsiveness (Balachandran et al. 2011). The role of 5-HT and 5-HT receptors in the valve is an active area of research as an association between serotonin medications, and cardiac valvulopathy has been identified (Jick et al. 1998, Rothman et al. 2000).

Pathological cyclic stretch also works in concert with TGF-β1 to promote more collagen synthesis and αSMA expression than TGF-β1 or stretch alone (Merryman et al. 2007). Stretched VIC monolayers treated with TGF-β1 developed nodules that began as aggregates of apoptotic cells before developing into a necrotic core surrounded by apoptotic cells, mirroring dystrophic calcification (Fisher et al. 2013). Interestingly, cyclic stretch plays a key role in nodule growth by preventing cells from migrating out of the nodule. While Fisher proposed that the initiating event for apoptosis might be mechanical damage, cyclic stretch also promotes apoptotic cell signaling directly (Bouchareb et al. 2014). Pathological cyclic stretch increases ectonucleotide pyrophosphatase/phosphodiesterase 1 (ENPP1), an ectonucleotidase enzyme, which causes apoptosis in VICs in vitro through a process that includes the formation of spheroid microparticles rich in calcium and phosphorus. These microparticles have been found in diseased valves colocalized with high ENPP1. Mechanical control of ENPP1 transport to the cell surface, its site of action, is controlled by the Rho/ROCK pathway, where ROCK inhibition prevents ENPP1 localization and stretch-induced mineralization.

Osteogenic calcification of VICs is also cyclic stretch-dependent, acting through BMP (Balachandran et al. 2010). Pathological 15% stretch of aortic valves in osteogenic media supplemented with TGF-β1 induced calcification, as measured by alizarin red and von Kossa staining. Expressions of BMP-2, BMP-4, and Runx2 were present on the fibrosa and were stretch magnitude-dependent. Inhibiting BMP reduced calcium deposition and ALP activity induced by 15% strain toward that induced by physiological 10% strain.

While mechanical forces are usually studied individually to determine each one's contribution, the aortic valve experiences the combined forces simultaneously. Pathological 15% stretch alone promotes a contractile phenotype with increased myofibroblastic markers αSMA, vimentin, and caldesmon compared with physiological 10% stretch (Thayer et al. 2011). Interestingly, despite hypertension being a risk factor for CAVD, applying hypertensive pressure of 140/100 mmHg to aortic valves ex vivo in combination with 15% stretch reduces myofibroblastic activation to below that of physiological 10% stretch alone, demonstrating the complex relationship between mechanical forces and cell behavior in the valve.

2.4 Conclusion

Cell–ECM interactions occur in many forms, from cell-mediated assembly of ECM structural proteins, biophysical engagement between ECM structural proteins and integrins, growth factor secretion and sensing to the transfer of mechanical force. They represent a dynamic, interactive system where cells and the ECM influence each other. While cells normally seek to maintain ECM composition and mechanical properties in a homeostatic state, damage caused by aging and disease can exceed what cells can repair, and many cell–ECM interactions provide potent positive-feedback loops toward disruptive ECM remodeling and cell differentiation that accelerate tissue dysfunction. Understanding cell–matrix interactions, particularly which interactions promote a quiescent and homeostatic state and which interactions activate maladaptive behavior, is critical to understanding many diseases and also for tissue engineering applications.

References

Adams, J. C., and F. M. Watt. 1993. Regulation of development and differentiation by the extracellular matrix. *Development* 117 (4): 1183–1198.

Aikawa, E., M. Nahrendorf, D. Sosnovik, V. M. Lok, F. A. Jaffer, M. Aikawa, and R. Weissleder. 2007. Multimodality molecular imaging identifies proteolytic and osteogenic activities in early aortic valve disease. *Circulation* 115 (3): 377–386. doi:10.1161/CIRCULATIONAHA.106.654913.

Alexopoulos, A., V. Bravou, S. Peroukides, L. Kaklamanis, J. Varakis, D. Alexopoulos, and H. Papadaki. 2010. Bone regulatory factors NFATc1 and Osterix in human calcific aortic valves. *Int J Cardiol* 139 (2): 142–149. doi:10.1016/j.ijcard.2008.10.014.

Annes, J. P., J. S. Munger, and D. B. Rifkin. 2003. Making sense of latent TGFbeta activation. *J Cell Sci* 116 (Pt 2): 217–224.

Arias-Salgado, E. G., S. Lizano, S. Sarkar, J. S. Brugge, M. H. Ginsberg, and S. J. Shattil. 2003. Src kinase activation by direct interaction with the integrin beta cytoplasmic domain. *Proc Natl Acad Sci U S A* 100 (23): 13298–13302. doi:10.1073/pnas.2336149100.

Arjunon, S., S. Rathan, H. Jo, and A. P. Yoganathan. 2013. Aortic valve: Mechanical environment and mechanobiology. *Ann Biomed Eng* 41 (7): 1331–1346. doi:10.1007/s10439-013-0785-7.

Arribas, S. M., A. Hinek, and M. C. Gonzalez. 2006. Elastic fibres and vascular structure in hypertension. *Pharmacol Ther* 111 (3): 771–791. doi:10.1016/j.pharmthera.2005.12.003.

Arthur, W. T., and K. Burridge. 2001. RhoA inactivation by p190RhoGAP regulates cell spreading and migration by promoting membrane protrusion and polarity. *Mol Biol Cell* 12 (9): 2711–2720.

Aumailley, M., L. Bruckner-Tuderman, W. G. Carter, R. Deutzmann, D. Edgar, P. Ekblom, J. Engel et al. 2005. A simplified laminin nomenclature. *Matrix Biol* 24 (5): 326–332. doi:10.1016/j.matbio.2005.05.006.

Bailey, A. J., R. G. Paul, and L. Knott. 1998. Mechanisms of maturation and ageing of collagen. *Mech Ageing Dev* 106 (1–2): 1–56.

Balachandran, K., M. A. Bakay, J. M. Connolly, X. Zhang, A. P. Yoganathan, and R. J. Levy. 2011. Aortic valve cyclic stretch causes increased remodeling activity and enhanced serotonin receptor responsiveness. *Ann Thorac Surg* 92 (1): 147–153. doi:10.1016/j.athoracsur.2011.03.084.

Balachandran, K., S. Hussain, C. H. Yap, M. Padala, A. H. Chester, and A. P. Yoganathan. 2012. Elevated cyclic stretch and serotonin result in altered aortic valve remodeling via a mechanosensitive 5-HT(2A) receptor-dependent pathway. *Cardiovasc Pathol* 21 (3): 206–213. doi:10.1016/j.carpath.2011.07.005.

Balachandran, K., S. Konduri, P. Sucosky, H. Jo, and A. P. Yoganathan. 2006. An ex vivo study of the biological properties of porcine aortic valves in response to circumferential cyclic stretch. *Ann Biomed Eng* 34 (11): 1655–1665. doi:10.1007/s10439-006-9167-8.

Balachandran, K., P. Sucosky, H. Jo, and A. P. Yoganathan. 2009. Elevated cyclic stretch alters matrix remodeling in aortic valve cusps: implications for degenerative aortic valve disease. *Am J Physiol Heart Circ Physiol* 296 (3): H756–H764. doi:10.1152/ajpheart.00900.2008.

Balachandran, K., P. Sucosky, H. Jo, and A. P. Yoganathan. 2010. Elevated cyclic stretch induces aortic valve calcification in a bone morphogenic protein-dependent manner. *Am J Pathol* 177 (1): 49–57. doi:10.2353/ajpath.2010.090631.

Balachandran, K., P. Sucosky, and A. P. Yoganathan. 2011. Hemodynamics and mechanobiology of aortic valve inflammation and calcification. *Int J Inflam* 2011: 263870. doi:10.4061/2011/263870.

Balguid, A., M. P. Rubbens, A. Mol, R. A. Bank, A. J. Bogers, J. P. van Kats, B. A. de Mol, F. P. Baaijens, and C. V. Bouten. 2007. The role of collagen cross-links in biomechanical behavior of human aortic heart valve leaflets–relevance for tissue engineering. *Tissue Eng* 13 (7): 1501–1511. doi:10.1089/ten.2006.0279.

Banos, C. C., A. H. Thomas, and C. K. Kuo. 2008. Collagen fibrillogenesis in tendon development: Current models and regulation of fibril assembly. *Birth Defects Res C Embryo Today* 84 (3): 228–244. doi:10.1002/bdrc.20130.

Barczyk, M., S. Carracedo, and D. Gullberg. 2010. Integrins. *Cell Tissue Res* 339 (1): 269–280. doi:10.1007/s00441-009-0834-6.

Barisic-Dujmovic, T., I. Boban, and S. H. Clark. 2010. Fibroblasts/myofibroblasts that participate in cutaneous wound healing are not derived from circulating progenitor cells. *J Cell Physiol* 222 (3): 703–712. doi:10.1002/jcp.21997.

Beer, J. H., K. T. Springer, and B. S. Coller. 1992. Immobilized Arg-Gly-Asp (RGD) peptides of varying lengths as structural probes of the platelet glycoprotein IIb/IIIa receptor. *Blood* 79 (1): 117–128.

Benjamin, E. J., M. J. Blaha, S. E. Chiuve, M. Cushman, S. R. Das, R. Deo, S. D. de Ferranti et al. 2017. Heart disease and stroke statistics-2017 update: A report from the American Heart Association. *Circulation* 135 (10): e146–e603. doi:10.1161/CIR.0000000000000485.

Benton, J. A., H. B. Kern, and K. S. Anseth. 2008. Substrate properties influence calcification in valvular interstitial cell culture. *J Heart Valve Dis* 17 (6): 689–699.

Benton, J. A., H. B. Kern, L. A. Leinwand, P. D. Mariner, and K. S. Anseth. 2009. Statins block calcific nodule formation of valvular interstitial cells by inhibiting alpha-smooth muscle actin expression. *Arterioscler Thromb Vasc Biol* 29 (11): 1950–1957. doi:10.1161/ATVBAHA.109.195271.

Blaser, M. C. et al., Implications for disease—Valvular fibrosis. In: B. Layton (Ed.), *Molecular and Cellular Biomechanics*. Chicago, IL: Pan Stanford Publishing, 2015.

Boosani, C. S., N. Nalabothula, V. Munugalavadla, D. Cosgrove, V. G. Keshamoun, N. Sheibani, and A. Sudhakar. 2009. FAK and p38-MAP kinase-dependent activation of apoptosis and caspase-3 in retinal endothelial cells by alpha1(IV)NC1. *Invest Ophthalmol Vis Sci* 50 (10): 4567–4575. doi:10.1167/iovs.09-3473.

Bouchareb, R., M. C. Boulanger, D. Fournier, P. Pibarot, Y. Messaddeq, and P. Mathieu. 2014. Mechanical strain induces the production of spheroid mineralized microparticles in the aortic valve through a RhoA/ROCK-dependent mechanism. *J Mol Cell Cardiol* 67: 49–59. doi:10.1016/j.yjmcc.2013.12.009.

Brew, K., and H. Nagase. 2010. The tissue inhibitors of metalloproteinases (TIMPs): An ancient family with structural and functional diversity. *Biochim Biophys Acta* 1803 (1): 55–71. doi:10.1016/j.bbamcr.2010.01.003.

Burnham, M. R., P. J. Bruce-Staskal, M. T. Harte, C. L. Weidow, A. Ma, S. A. Weed, and A. H. Bouton. 2000. Regulation of c-SRC activity and function by the adapter protein CAS. *Mol Cell Biol* 20 (16): 5865–5878.

Butcher, J. T., and R. M. Nerem. 2006. Valvular endothelial cells regulate the phenotype of interstitial cells in co-culture: Effects of steady shear stress. *Tissue Eng* 12 (4): 905–915. doi:10.1089/ten.2006.12.905.

Butcher, J. T., A. M. Penrod, A. J. Garcia, and R. M. Nerem. 2004. Unique morphology and focal adhesion development of valvular endothelial cells in static and fluid flow environments. *Arterioscler Thromb Vasc Biol* 24 (8): 1429–1434. doi:10.1161/01.ATV.0000130462.50769.5a.

Butcher, J. T., C. A. Simmons, and J. N. Warnock. 2008. Mechanobiology of the aortic heart valve. *J Heart Valve Dis* 17 (1): 62–73.

Butcher, J. T., S. Tressel, T. Johnson, D. Turner, G. Sorescu, H. Jo, and R. M. Nerem. 2006. Transcriptional profiles of valvular and vascular endothelial cells reveal phenotypic differences: Influence of shear stress. *Arterioscler Thromb Vasc Biol* 26 (1): 69–77. doi:10.1161/01.ATV.0000196624.70507.0d.

Calalb, M. B., T. R. Polte, and S. K. Hanks. 1995. Tyrosine phosphorylation of focal adhesion kinase at sites in the catalytic domain regulates kinase activity: A role for Src family kinases. *Mol Cell Biol* 15 (2): 954–963.

Carisey, A., and C. Ballestrem. 2011. Vinculin, an adapter protein in control of cell adhesion signalling. *Eur J Cell Biol* 90 (2–3): 157–163. doi:10.1016/j.ejcb.2010.06.007.

Carisey, A., R. Tsang, A. M. Greiner, N. Nijenhuis, N. Heath, A. Nazgiewicz, R. Kemkemer, B. Derby, J. Spatz, and C. Ballestrem. 2013. Vinculin regulates the recruitment and release of core focal adhesion proteins in a force-dependent manner. *Curr Biol* 23 (4): 271–281. doi:10.1016/j.cub.2013.01.009.

Chang, F., C. A. Lemmon, D. Park, and L. H. Romer. 2007. FAK potentiates Rac1 activation and localization to matrix adhesion sites: A role for betaPIX. *Mol Biol Cell* 18 (1): 253–264. doi:10.1091/mbc.E06-03-0207.

Chen, H. C., P. A. Appeddu, J. T. Parsons, J. D. Hildebrand, M. D. Schaller, and J. L. Guan. 1995. Interaction of focal adhesion kinase with cytoskeletal protein talin. *J Biol Chem* 270 (28): 16995–16999.

Chen, J., J. R. Peacock, J. Branch, and W. David Merryman. 2015. Biophysical analysis of dystrophic and osteogenic models of valvular calcification. *J Biomech Eng* 137 (2): 020903. doi:10.1115/1.4029115.

Chen, J. H., W. L. Chen, K. L. Sider, C. Y. Yip, and C. A. Simmons. 2011. beta-catenin mediates mechanically regulated, transforming growth factor-beta1-induced myofibroblast differentiation of aortic valve interstitial cells. *Arterioscler Thromb Vasc Biol* 31 (3): 590–597. doi:10.1161/ATVBAHA.110.220061.

Chen, J. H., and C. A. Simmons. 2011. Cell-matrix interactions in the pathobiology of calcific aortic valve disease: Critical roles for matricellular, matricrine, and matrix mechanics cues. *Circ Res* 108 (12): 1510–1524. doi:10.1161/CIRCRESAHA.110.234237.

Chen, J. H., C. Y. Yip, E. D. Sone, and C. A. Simmons. 2009. Identification and characterization of aortic valve mesenchymal progenitor cells with robust osteogenic calcification potential. *Am J Pathol* 174 (3): 1109–1119. doi:10.2353/ajpath.2009.080750.

Chen, W., J. Lou, E. A. Evans, and C. Zhu. 2012. Observing force-regulated conformational changes and ligand dissociation from a single integrin on cells. *J Cell Biol* 199 (3): 497–512. doi:10.1083/jcb.201201091.

Cheng, H., Q. Yao, R. Song, Y. Zhai, W. Wang, D. A. Fullerton, and X. Meng. 2017. Lysophosphatidylcholine activates the Akt pathway to upregulate extracellular matrix protein production in human aortic valve cells. *J Surg Res* 213: 243–250. doi:10.1016/j.jss.2017.02.028.

Chistiakov, D. A., I. A. Sobenin, and A. N. Orekhov. 2013. Vascular extracellular matrix in atherosclerosis. *Cardiol Rev* 21 (6): 270–288. doi:10.1097/CRD.0b013e31828c5ced.

Choquet, D., D. P. Felsenfeld, and M. P. Sheetz. 1997. Extracellular matrix rigidity causes strengthening of integrin-cytoskeleton linkages. *Cell* 88 (1): 39–48.

Chrzanowska-Wodnicka, M., and K. Burridge. 1996. Rho-stimulated contractility drives the formation of stress fibers and focal adhesions. *J Cell Biol* 133 (6): 1403–1415.

Cimini, M., K. A. Rogers, and D. R. Boughner. 2003. Smoothelin-positive cells in human and porcine semilunar valves. *Histochem Cell Biol* 120 (4): 307–317. doi:10.1007/s00418-003-0570-z.

Couchman, J. R., and C. A. Pataki. 2012. An introduction to proteoglycans and their localization. *J Histochemi Cytochem* 60 (12): 885–897. doi:10.1369/0022155412464638.

Cushing, M. C., J. T. Liao, and K. S. Anseth. 2005. Activation of valvular interstitial cells is mediated by transforming growth factor-beta1 interactions with matrix molecules. *Matrix Biol* 24 (6): 428–437. doi:10.1016/j.matbio.2005.06.007.

Czirok, A., J. Zach, B. A. Kozel, R. P. Mecham, E. C. Davis, and B. J. Rongish. 2006. Elastic fiber macro-assembly is a hierarchical, cell motion-mediated process. *J Cell Physiol* 207 (1): 97–106. doi:10.1002/jcp.20573.

Dallas, S. L., P. Sivakumar, C. J. Jones, Q. Chen, D. M. Peters, D. F. Mosher, M. J. Humphries, and C. M. Kielty. 2005. Fibronectin regulates latent transforming growth factor-beta (TGF beta) by controlling matrix assembly of latent TGF beta-binding protein-1. *J Biol Chem* 280 (19): 18871–18880. doi:10.1074/jbc.M410762200.

Danielson, K. G., H. Baribault, D. F. Holmes, H. Graham, K. E. Kadler, and R. V. Iozzo. 1997. Targeted disruption of decorin leads to abnormal collagen fibril morphology and skin fragility. *J Cell Biol* 136 (3): 729–743.

Darby, I. A., B. Laverdet, F. Bonte, and A. Desmouliere. 2014. Fibroblasts and myofibroblasts in wound healing. *Clin Cosmet Investig Dermatol* 7: 301–311. doi:10.2147/CCID.S50046.

Davis, G. E. 1992. Affinity of integrins for damaged extracellular matrix: Alpha v beta 3 binds to denatured collagen type I through RGD sites. *Biochem Biophys Res Commun* 182 (3): 1025–1031.

De Hart, J., G. W. Peters, P. J. Schreurs, and F. P. Baaijens. 2004. Collagen fibers reduce stresses and stabilize motion of aortic valve leaflets during systole. *J Biomech* 37 (3): 303–311.

Deck, J. D. 1986. Endothelial cell orientation on aortic valve leaflets. *Cardiovasc Res* 20 (10): 760–767.

Defilippi, P., P. Di Stefano, and S. Cabodi. 2006. p130Cas: A versatile scaffold in signaling networks. *Trends Cell Biol* 16 (5): 257–263. doi:10.1016/j.tcb.2006.03.003.

del Rio, A., R. Perez-Jimenez, R. Liu, P. Roca-Cusachs, J. M. Fernandez, and M. P. Sheetz. 2009. Stretching single talin rod molecules activates vinculin binding. *Science* 323 (5914): 638–641. doi:10.1126/science.1162912.

Delvoye, P., P. Wiliquet, J. L. Leveque, B. V. Nusgens, and C. M. Lapiere. 1991. Measurement of mechanical forces generated by skin fibroblasts embedded in a three-dimensional collagen gel. *J Invest Dermatol* 97 (5): 898–902.

DeMali, K. A., C. A. Barlow, and K. Burridge. 2002. Recruitment of the Arp2/3 complex to vinculin: Coupling membrane protrusion to matrix adhesion. *J Cell Biol* 159 (5): 881–891. doi:10.1083/jcb.200206043.

DePasquale, J. A., and C. S. Izzard. 1991. Accumulation of talin in nodes at the edge of the lamellipodium and separate incorporation into adhesion plaques at focal contacts in fibroblasts. *J Cell Biol* 113 (6): 1351–1359.

Desmouliere, A., A. Geinoz, F. Gabbiani, and G. Gabbiani. 1993. Transforming growth factor-beta 1 induces alpha-smooth muscle actin expression in granulation tissue myofibroblasts and in quiescent and growing cultured fibroblasts. *J Cell Biol* 122 (1): 103–111.

Desmouliere, A., M. Redard, I. Darby, and G. Gabbiani. 1995. Apoptosis mediates the decrease in cellularity during the transition between granulation tissue and scar. *Am J Pathol* 146 (1): 56–66.

Di Lullo, G. A., S. M. Sweeney, J. Korkko, L. Ala-Kokko, and J. D. San Antonio. 2002. Mapping the ligand-binding sites and disease-associated mutations on the most abundant protein in the human, type I collagen. *J Biol Chem* 277 (6): 4223–4231. doi:10.1074/jbc.M110709200.

Domogatskaya, A., S. Rodin, and K. Tryggvason. 2012. Functional diversity of laminins. *Annu Rev Cell Dev Biol* 28: 523–553. doi:10.1146/annurev-cellbio-101011-155750.

Dreger, S. A., P. M. Taylor, S. P. Allen, and M. H. Yacoub. 2002. Profile and localization of matrix metalloproteinases (MMPs) and their tissue inhibitors (TIMPs) in human heart valves. *J Heart Valve Dis* 11 (6): 875–880; discussion 880.

Dreger, S. A., P. Thomas, E. Sachlos, A. H. Chester, J. T. Czernuszka, P. M. Taylor, and M. H. Yacoub. 2006. Potential for synthesis and degradation of extracellular matrix proteins by valve interstitial cells seeded onto collagen scaffolds. *Tissue Eng* 12 (9): 2533–2540. doi:10.1089/ten.2006.12.2533.

Duan, B., Z. Yin, L. Hockaday Kang, R. L. Magin, and J. T. Butcher. 2016. Active tissue stiffness modulation controls valve interstitial cell phenotype and osteogenic potential in 3D culture. *Acta Biomater* 36: 42–54. doi:10.1016/j.actbio.2016.03.007.

Egan, K. P., J. H. Kim, E. R. Mohler, 3rd, and R. J. Pignolo. 2011. Role for circulating osteogenic precursor cells in aortic valvular disease. *Arterioscler Thromb Vasc Biol* 31 (12): 2965–2971. doi:10.1161/ATVBAHA.111.234724.

El-Hamamsy, I., K. Balachandran, M. H. Yacoub, L. M. Stevens, P. Sarathchandra, P. M. Taylor, A. P. Yoganathan, and A. H. Chester. 2009. Endothelium-dependent regulation of the mechanical properties of aortic valve cusps. *J Am Coll Cardiol* 53 (16): 1448–1455. doi:10.1016/j.jacc.2008.11.056.

Engler, A. J., S. Sen, H. L. Sweeney, and D. E. Discher. 2006. Matrix elasticity directs stem cell lineage specification. *Cell* 126 (4): 677–689. doi:10.1016/j.cell.2006.06.044.

Eriksen, H. A., J. Satta, J. Risteli, M. Veijola, P. Vare, and Y. Soini. 2006. Type I and type III collagen synthesis and composition in the valve matrix in aortic valve stenosis. *Atherosclerosis* 189 (1): 91–98. doi:10.1016/j.atherosclerosis.2005.11.034.

Everts, V., E. van der Zee, L. Creemers, and W. Beertsen. 1996. Phagocytosis and intracellular digestion of collagen, its role in turnover and remodelling. *Histochem J* 28 (4): 229–245.

Farrar, E. J., V. Pramil, J. M. Richards, C. Z. Mosher, and J. T. Butcher. 2016. Valve interstitial cell tensional homeostasis directs calcification and extracellular matrix remodeling processes via RhoA signaling. *Biomaterials* 105: 25–37. doi:10.1016/j.biomaterials.2016.07.034.

Fisher, C. I., J. Chen, and W. D. Merryman. 2013. Calcific nodule morphogenesis by heart valve interstitial cells is strain dependent. *Biomech Model Mechanobiol* 12 (1): 5–17. doi:10.1007/s10237-012-0377-8.

Fondard, O., D. Detaint, B. Iung, C. Choqueux, H. Adle-Biassette, M. Jarraya, U. Hvass et al. 2005. Extracellular matrix remodelling in human aortic valve disease: The role of matrix metalloproteinases and their tissue inhibitors. *Eur Heart J* 26 (13): 1333–1341. doi:10.1093/eurheartj/ehi248.

Freeman, R. V., and C. M. Otto. 2005. Spectrum of calcific aortic valve disease: Pathogenesis, disease progression, and treatment strategies. *Circulation* 111 (24): 3316–3326. doi:10.1161/CIRCULATIONAHA.104.486738.

Friedland, J. C., M. H. Lee, and D. Boettiger. 2009. Mechanically activated integrin switch controls alpha5beta1 function. *Science* 323 (5914): 642–644. doi:10.1126/science.1168441.

Gabbiani, G., G. B. Ryan, and G. Majne. 1971. Presence of modified fibroblasts in granulation tissue and their possible role in wound contraction. *Experientia* 27 (5): 549–550.

Gahmberg, C. G., S. C. Fagerholm, S. M. Nurmi, T. Chavakis, S. Marchesan, and M. Gronholm. 2009. Regulation of integrin activity and signalling. *Biochim Biophys Acta* 1790 (6): 431–444. doi:10.1016/j.bbagen.2009.03.007.

Galbraith, C. G., K. M. Yamada, and M. P. Sheetz. 2002. The relationship between force and focal complex development. *J Cell Biol* 159 (4): 695–705. doi:10.1083/jcb.200204153.

Gattazzo, F., A. Urciuolo, and P. Bonaldo. 2014. Extracellular matrix: A dynamic microenvironment for stem cell niche. *Biochim Biophys Acta* 1840 (8): 2506–2519. doi:10.1016/j.bbagen.2014.01.010.

Geiger, B., J. P. Spatz, and A. D. Bershadsky. 2009. Environmental sensing through focal adhesions. *Nat Rev Mol Cell Biol* 10 (1): 21–33. doi:10.1038/nrm2593.

Giannone, G., G. Jiang, D. H. Sutton, D. R. Critchley, and M. P. Sheetz. 2003. Talin1 is critical for force-dependent reinforcement of initial integrin-cytoskeleton bonds but not tyrosine kinase activation. *J Cell Biol* 163 (2): 409–419. doi:10.1083/jcb.200302001.

Goffin, J. M., P. Pittet, G. Csucs, J. W. Lussi, J. J. Meister, and B. Hinz. 2006. Focal adhesion size controls tension-dependent recruitment of alpha-smooth muscle actin to stress fibers. *J Cell Biol* 172 (2): 259–268. doi:10.1083/jcb.200506179.

Gould, S. T., E. E. Matherly, J. N. Smith, D. D. Heistad, and K. S. Anseth. 2014. The role of valvular endothelial cell paracrine signaling and matrix elasticity on valvular interstitial cell activation. *Biomaterials* 35 (11): 3596–3606. doi:10.1016/j.biomaterials.2014.01.005.

Grande-Allen, K. J., N. Osman, M. L. Ballinger, H. Dadlani, S. Marasco, and P. J. Little. 2007. Glycosaminoglycan synthesis and structure as targets for the prevention of calcific aortic valve disease. *Cardiovasc Res* 76 (1): 19–28. doi:10.1016/j.cardiores.2007.05.014.

Gu, X., and K. S. Masters. 2009. Role of the MAPK/ERK pathway in valvular interstitial cell calcification. *Am J Physiol Heart Circ Physiol* 296 (6): H1748–H1757. doi:10.1152/ajpheart.00099.2009.

Gu, X., and K. S. Masters. 2010. Regulation of valvular interstitial cell calcification by adhesive peptide sequences. *J Biomed Mater Res A* 93 (4): 1620–1630. doi:10.1002/jbm.a.32660.

Gu, X., and K. S. Masters. 2011. Role of the Rho pathway in regulating valvular interstitial cell phenotype and nodule formation. *Am J Physiol Heart Circ Physiol* 300 (2): H448–H458. doi:10.1152/ajpheart.01178.2009.

Guo, W., and F. G. Giancotti. 2004. Integrin signalling during tumour progression. *Nat Rev Mol Cell Biol* 5: 816–826.

Gupta, V., and K. J. Grande-Allen. 2006. Effects of static and cyclic loading in regulating extracellular matrix synthesis by cardiovascular cells. *Cardiovasc Res* 72 (3): 375–383. doi:10.1016/j.cardiores.2006.08.017.

Halper, J., and M. Kjaer. 2014. Basic components of connective tissues and extracellular matrix: Elastin, fibrillin, fibulins, fibrinogen, fibronectin, laminin, tenascins and thrombospondins. *Adv Exp Med Biol* 802: 31–47. doi:10.1007/978-94-007-7893-1_3.

Han, L., and A. I. Gotlieb. 2011. Fibroblast growth factor-2 promotes in vitro mitral valve interstitial cell repair through transforming growth factor-beta/Smad signaling. *Am J Pathol* 178 (1): 119–127. doi:10.1016/j.ajpath.2010.11.038.

Han, L., and A. I. Gotlieb. 2012. Fibroblast growth factor-2 promotes in vitro heart valve interstitial cell repair through the Akt1 pathway. *Cardiovasc Pathol* 21 (5): 382–389. doi:10.1016/j.carpath.2011.12.001.

Harburger, D. S., and D. A. Calderwood. 2009. Integrin signalling at a glance. *J Cell Sci* 122 (Pt 2): 159–163. doi:10.1242/jcs.018093.

Haskett, D., G. Johnson, A. Zhou, U. Utzinger, and J. Vande Geest. 2010. Microstructural and biomechanical alterations of the human aorta as a function of age and location. *Biomech Model Mechanobiol* 9 (6): 725–736. doi:10.1007/s10237-010-0209-7.

Hayashi, I., K. Vuori, and R. C. Liddington. 2002. The focal adhesion targeting (FAT) region of focal adhesion kinase is a four-helix bundle that binds paxillin. *Nat Struct Biol* 9 (2): 101–106. doi:10.1038/nsb755.

Helske, S., S. Syvaranta, K. A. Lindstedt, J. Lappalainen, K. Oorni, M. I. Mayranpaa, J. Lommi et al. 2006. Increased expression of elastolytic cathepsins S, K, and V and their inhibitor cystatin C in stenotic aortic valves. *Arterioscler Thromb Vasc Biol* 26 (8): 1791–1798. doi:10.1161/01.ATV.0000228824.01604.63.

Hinton, R. B., Jr., J. Lincoln, G. H. Deutsch, H. Osinska, P. B. Manning, D. W. Benson, and K. E. Yutzey. 2006. Extracellular matrix remodeling and organization in developing and diseased aortic valves. *Circ Res* 98 (11): 1431–1438. doi:10.1161/01.RES.0000224114.65109.4e.

Hinz, B. 2007. Formation and function of the myofibroblast during tissue repair. *J Invest Dermatol* 127 (3): 526–537. doi:10.1038/sj.jid.5700613.

Hinz, B. 2010. The myofibroblast: Paradigm for a mechanically active cell. *J Biomech* 43 (1): 146–155. doi:10.1016/j.jbiomech.2009.09.020.

Hinz, B., S. H. Phan, V. J. Thannickal, A. Galli, M. L. Bochaton-Piallat, and G. Gabbiani. 2007. The myofibroblast: One function, multiple origins. *Am J Pathol* 170 (6): 1807–1816. doi:10.2353/ajpath.2007.070112.

Hjortnaes, J., G. Camci-Unal, J. D. Hutcheson, S. M. Jung, F. J. Schoen, J. Kluin, E. Aikawa, and A. Khademhosseini. 2015. Directing valvular interstitial cell myofibroblast-like differentiation in a hybrid hydrogel platform. *Adv Healthc Mater* 4 (1): 121–130. doi:10.1002/adhm.201400029.

Hsia, D. A., S. K. Mitra, C. R. Hauck, D. N. Streblow, J. A. Nelson, D. Ilic, S. Huang et al. 2003. Differential regulation of cell motility and invasion by FAK. *J Cell Biol* 160 (5): 753–767. doi:10.1083/jcb.200212114.

Humphrey, J. D., E. R. Dufresne, and M. A. Schwartz. 2014. Mechanotransduction and extracellular matrix homeostasis. *Nat Rev Mol Cell Biol* 15 (12): 802–812. doi:10.1038/nrm3896.

Humphries, J. D., A. Byron, and M. J. Humphries. 2006. Integrin ligands at a glance. *J Cell Sci* 119 (Pt 19): 3901–3903. doi:10.1242/jcs.03098.

Humphries, M. J., P. A. McEwan, S. J. Barton, P. A. Buckley, J. Bella, and A. P. Mould. 2003. Integrin structure: Heady advances in ligand binding, but activation still makes the knees wobble. *Trends Biochem Sci* 28 (6): 313–320.

Humphries, M. J., E. J. Symonds, and A. P. Mould. 2003. Mapping functional residues onto integrin crystal structures. *Curr Opin Struct Biol* 13 (2): 236–243.

Hutcheson, J. D., E. Aikawa, and W. D. Merryman. 2014. Potential drug targets for calcific aortic valve disease. *Nat Rev Cardiol* 11 (4): 218–231. doi:10.1038/nrcardio.2014.1.

Hutcheson, J. D., J. Chen, M. K. Sewell-Loftin, L. M. Ryzhova, C. I. Fisher, Y. R. Su, and W. D. Merryman. 2013. Cadherin-11 regulates cell-cell tension necessary for calcific nodule formation by valvular myofibroblasts. *Arterioscler Thromb Vasc Biol* 33 (1): 114–120. doi:10.1161/ATVBAHA.112.300278.

Huveneers, S., H. Truong, R. Fassler, A. Sonnenberg, and E. H. Danen. 2008. Binding of soluble fibronectin to integrin alpha5 beta1—Link to focal adhesion redistribution and contractile shape. *J Cell Sci* 121 (Pt 15): 2452–2462. doi:10.1242/jcs.033001.

Hynes, R. O. 2002. Integrins: Bidirectional, allosteric signaling machines. *Cell* 110 (6): 673–687.

Hynes, R. O., and A. Naba. 2012. Overview of the matrisome—An inventory of extracellular matrix constituents and functions. *Cold Spring Harb Perspect Biol* 4 (1): a004903. doi:10.1101/cshperspect.a004903.

Jian, B., N. Narula, Q. Y. Li, E. R. Mohler, 3rd, and R. J. Levy. 2003. Progression of aortic valve stenosis: TGF-beta1 is present in calcified aortic valve cusps and promotes aortic valve interstitial cell calcification via apoptosis. *Ann Thorac Surg* 75 (2): 457–465; discussion 465–466.

Jiang, G., G. Giannone, D. R. Critchley, E. Fukumoto, and M. P. Sheetz. 2003. Two-piconewton slip bond between fibronectin and the cytoskeleton depends on talin. *Nature* 424 (6946): 334–337. doi:10.1038/nature01805.

Jick, H., C. Vasilakis, L. A. Weinrauch, C. R. Meier, S. S. Jick, and L. E. Derby. 1998. A population-based study of appetite-suppressant drugs and the risk of cardiac-valve regurgitation. *N Engl J Med* 339 (11): 719–724. doi:10.1056/NEJM199809103391102.

Kaden, J. J., C. E. Dempfle, R. Grobholz, H. T. Tran, R. Kilic, A. Sarikoc, M. Brueckmann et al. 2003. Interleukin-1 beta promotes matrix metalloproteinase expression and cell proliferation in calcific aortic valve stenosis. *Atherosclerosis* 170 (2): 205–211.

Kadler, K. E., D. F. Holmes, J. A. Trotter, and J. A. Chapman. 1996. Collagen fibril formation. *Biochem J* 316 (Pt 1): 1–11.

Kiema, T., Y. Lad, P. Jiang, C. L. Oxley, M. Baldassarre, K. L. Wegener, I. D. Campbell, J. Ylanne, and D. A. Calderwood. 2006. The molecular basis of filamin binding to integrins and competition with talin. *Mol Cell* 21 (3): 337–347. doi:10.1016/j.molcel.2006.01.011.

Kloxin, A. M., J. A. Benton, and K. S. Anseth. 2010. In situ elasticity modulation with dynamic substrates to direct cell phenotype. *Biomaterials* 31 (1): 1–8. doi:10.1016/j.biomaterials.2009.09.025.

Knight, C. G., L. F. Morton, D. J. Onley, A. R. Peachey, A. J. Messent, P. A. Smethurst, D. S. Tuckwell, R. W. Farndale, and M. J. Barnes. 1998. Identification in collagen type I of an integrin alpha2 beta1-binding site containing an essential GER sequence. *J Biol Chem* 273 (50): 33287–33294.

Kook, S. H., J. M. Hwang, J. S. Park, E. M. Kim, J. S. Heo, Y. M. Jeon, and J. C. Lee. 2009. Mechanical force induces type I collagen expression in human periodontal ligament fibroblasts through activation of ERK/JNK and AP-1. *J Cell Biochem* 106 (6): 1060–1067. doi:10.1002/jcb.22085.

Kruger, T. E., A. H. Miller, and J. Wang. 2013. Collagen scaffolds in bone sialoprotein-mediated bone regeneration. *Sci World J* 2013: 1–6.

Ku, C. H., P. H. Johnson, P. Batten, P. Sarathchandra, R. C. Chambers, P. M. Taylor, M. H. Yacoub, and A. H. Chester. 2006. Collagen synthesis by mesenchymal stem cells and aortic valve interstitial cells in response to mechanical stretch. *Cardiovasc Res* 71 (3): 548–556. doi:10.1016/j.cardiores.2006.03.022.

Latif, N., P. Sarathchandra, P. M. Taylor, J. Antoniw, and M. H. Yacoub. 2005a. Localization and pattern of expression of extracellular matrix components in human heart valves. *J Heart Valve Dis* 14 (2): 218–227.

Latif, N., P. Sarathchandra, P. M. Taylor, J. Antoniw, and M. H. Yacoub. 2005b. Molecules mediating cell-ECM and cell-cell communication in human heart valves. *Cell Biochem Biophys* 43 (2): 275–287. doi:10.1385/CBB:43:2:275.

Labrosse, M. R., K. Lobo, and C. J. Beller. 2010. Structural analysis of the natural aortic valve in dynamics: From unpressurized to physiologically loaded. *J Biomech* 43 (10): 1916–1922.

Laurent, G. J. 1987. Dynamic state of collagen: Pathways of collagen degradation in vivo and their possible role in regulation of collagen mass. *Am J Physiol* 252 (1 Pt 1): C1–C9.

Lee, J. O., P. Rieu, M. A. Arnaout, and R. Liddington. 1995. Crystal structure of the A domain from the alpha subunit of integrin CR3 (CD11b/CD18). *Cell* 80 (4): 631–638.

Lee, T. C., R. J. Midura, V. C. Hascall, and I. Vesely. 2001. The effect of elastin damage on the mechanics of the aortic valve. *J Biomech* 34 (2): 203–210.

Lessey, E. C., C. Guilluy, and K. Burridge. 2012. From mechanical force to RhoA activation. *Biochemistry* 51 (38): 7420–7432. doi:10.1021/bi300758e.

Li, Y. S., J. Y. Shyy, S. Li, J. Lee, B. Su, M. Karin, and S. Chien. 1996. The Ras-JNK pathway is involved in shear-induced gene expression. *Mol Cell Biol* 16 (11): 5947–5954.

Lillie, M. A., and J. M. Gosline. 2002. The viscoelastic basis for the tensile strength of elastin. *Int J Biol Macromol* 30 (2): 119–127.

Lim, Y., S. T. Lim, A. Tomar, M. Gardel, J. A. Bernard-Trifilo, X. L. Chen, S. A. Uryu et al. 2008. PyK2 and FAK connections to p190Rho guanine nucleotide exchange factor regulate RhoA activity, focal adhesion formation, and cell motility. *J Cell Biol* 180 (1): 187–203. doi:10.1083/jcb.200708194.

Lindahl, U., J. Couchman, K. Kimata, and J. D. Esko. 2015. Proteoglycans and Sulfated Glycosaminoglycans. In *Essentials of Glycobiology*, edited by A. Varki, R. D. Cummings,

J. D. Esko, P. Stanley, G. W. Hart, M. Aebi, A. G. Darvill et al. Cold Spring Harbor, NY: Cold Spring Harbor Laboratory Press.

Liu, A. C., V. R. Joag, and A. I. Gotlieb. 2007. The emerging role of valve interstitial cell phenotypes in regulating heart valve pathobiology. *Am J Pathol* 171 (5): 1407–1418. doi:10.2353/ajpath.2007.070251.

Liu, B., S. Lu, Y. L. Hu, X. Liao, M. Ouyang, and Y. Wang. 2014. RhoA and membrane fluidity mediates the spatially polarized Src/FAK activation in response to shear stress. *Sci Rep* 4: 7008. doi:10.1038/srep07008.

Liu, H., Y. Sun, and C. A. Simmons. 2013. Determination of local and global elastic moduli of valve interstitial cells cultured on soft substrates. *J Biomech* 46 (11): 1967–1971. doi:10.1016/j.jbiomech.2013.05.001.

Liu, S., S. M. Thomas, D. G. Woodside, D. M. Rose, W. B. Kiosses, M. Pfaff, and M. H. Ginsberg. 1999. Binding of paxillin to alpha4 integrins modifies integrin-dependent biological responses. *Nature* 402 (6762): 676–681. doi:10.1038/45264.

Lo, C. M., H. B. Wang, M. Dembo, and Y. L. Wang. 2000. Cell movement is guided by the rigidity of the substrate. *Biophys J* 79 (1): 144–152. doi:10.1016/S0006-3495(00)76279-5.

Lo, D., and I. Vesely. 1995. Biaxial strain analysis of the porcine aortic valve. *Ann Thorac Surg* 60 (2 Suppl): S374–S378.

Lu, P., K. Takai, V. M. Weaver, and Z. Werb. 2011. Extracellular matrix degradation and remodeling in development and disease. *Cold Spring Harb Perspect Biol* 3 (12). doi:10.1101/cshperspect.a005058.

MacKenna, D. A., F. Dolfi, K. Vuori, and E. Ruoslahti. 1998. Extracellular signal-regulated kinase and c-Jun NH2-terminal kinase activation by mechanical stretch is integrin-dependent and matrix-specific in rat cardiac fibroblasts. *J Clin Invest* 101 (2): 301–310. doi:10.1172/JCI1026.

Macri, L., D. Silverstein, and R. A. Clark. 2007. Growth factor binding to the pericellular matrix and its importance in tissue engineering. *Adv Drug Deliv Rev* 59 (13): 1366–1381. doi:10.1016/j.addr.2007.08.015.

Maeda, K., X. Ma, F. L. Hanley, and R. K. Riemer. 2016. Critical role of coaptive strain in aortic valve leaflet homeostasis: Use of a novel flow culture bioreactor to explore heart valve mechanobiology. *J Am Heart Assoc* 5 (8). doi:10.1161/JAHA.116.003506.

McBeath, R., D. M. Pirone, C. M. Nelson, K. Bhadriraju, and C. S. Chen. 2004. Cell shape, cytoskeletal tension, and RhoA regulate stem cell lineage commitment. *Dev Cell* 6 (4): 483–495.

Meredith, J. E., Jr., B. Fazeli, and M. A. Schwartz. 1993. The extracellular matrix as a cell survival factor. *Mol Biol Cell* 4 (9): 953–961.

Merryman, W. D., H. D. Lukoff, R. A. Long, G. C. Engelmayr, Jr., R. A. Hopkins, and M. S. Sacks. 2007. Synergistic effects of cyclic tension and transforming growth factor-beta1 on the aortic valve myofibroblast. *Cardiovasc Pathol* 16 (5): 268–276. doi:10.1016/j.carpath.2007.03.006.

Merryman, W. D., and F. J. Schoen. 2013. Mechanisms of calcification in aortic valve disease: Role of mechanokinetics and mechanodynamics. *Curr Cardiol Rep* 15 (5): 355. doi:10.1007/s11886-013-0355-5.

Merryman, W. D., I. Youn, H. D. Lukoff, P. M. Krueger, F. Guilak, R. A. Hopkins, and M. S. Sacks. 2006. Correlation between heart valve interstitial cell stiffness and transvalvular pressure: Implications for collagen biosynthesis. *Am J Physiol Heart Circ Physiol* 290 (1): H224–H231. doi:10.1152/ajpheart.00521.2005.

Metzler, S. A., C. A. Pregonero, J. T. Butcher, S. C. Burgess, and J. N. Warnock. 2008. Cyclic strain regulates pro-inflammatory protein expression in porcine aortic valve endothelial cells. *J Heart Valve Dis* 17 (5): 571–577; discussion 578.

Miki, H., H. Yamaguchi, S. Suetsugu, and T. Takenawa. 2000. IRSp53 is an essential inter-
    mediate between Rac and WAVE in the regulation of membrane ruffling. *Nature*
    408 (6813): 732–735. doi:10.1038/35047107.
Miller, J. D., Y. Chu, R. M. Brooks, W. E. Richenbacher, R. Pena-Silva, and D. D. Heistad.
    2008. Dysregulation of antioxidant mechanisms contributes to increased oxidative
    stress in calcific aortic valvular stenosis in humans. *J Am Coll Cardiol* 52 (10): 843–850.
    doi:10.1016/j.jacc.2008.05.043.
Mohler, E. R., 3rd, F. Gannon, C. Reynolds, R. Zimmerman, M. G. Keane, and F. S. Kaplan.
    2001. Bone formation and inflammation in cardiac valves. *Circulation* 103 (11):
    1522–1528.
Mould, A. P., J. A. Askari, Si Aota, K. M. Yamada, A. Irie, Y. Takada, H. J. Mardon, and
    M. J. Humphries. 1997. Defining the topology of integrin alpha5beta1-fibronectin inter-
    actions using inhibitory anti-alpha5 and anti-beta1 monoclonal antibodies. Evidence
    that the synergy sequence of fibronectin is recognized by the amino-terminal repeats of
    the alpha5 subunit. *J Biol Chem* 272 (28): 17283–17292.
Mouw, J. K., G. Ou, and V. M. Weaver. 2014. Extracellular matrix assembly: A multiscale
    deconstruction. *Nat Rev Mol Cell Biol* 15 (12): 771–785. doi:10.1038/nrm3902.
Muller, A. M., C. Cronen, L. I. Kupferwasser, H. Oelert, K. M. Muller, and C. J. Kirkpatrick.
    2000. Expression of endothelial cell adhesion molecules on heart valves: Up-regulation
    in degeneration as well as acute endocarditis. *J Pathol* 191 (1): 54–60. doi:10.1002/
    (SICI)1096-9896(200005)191:1<54::AID-PATH568>3.0.CO;2-Y.
Muller, J. M., E. Metzger, H. Greschik, A. K. Bosserhoff, L. Mercep, R. Buettner, and R. Schule.
    2002. The transcriptional coactivator FHL2 transmits Rho signals from the cell mem-
    brane into the nucleus. *EMBO J* 21 (4): 736–748.
Murphy, G. 2011. Tissue inhibitors of metalloproteinases. *Genome Biol* 12 (11): 233.
    doi:10.1186/gb-2011-12-11-233.
Nadruz, W., Jr., M. A. Corat, T. M. Marin, G. A. Guimaraes Pereira, and K. G. Franchini.
    2005. Focal adhesion kinase mediates MEF2 and c-Jun activation by stretch: Role in the
    activation of the cardiac hypertrophic genetic program. *Cardiovasc Res* 68 (1): 87–97.
    doi:10.1016/j.cardiores.2005.05.011.
Naso, F., A. Gandaglia, M. Formato, A. Cigliano, A. J. Lepedda, G. Gerosa, and M. Spina.
    2010. Differential distribution of structural components and hydration in aortic and
    pulmonary heart valve conduits: Impact of detergent-based cell removal. *Acta Biomater*
    6 (12): 4675–4588. doi:10.1016/j.actbio.2010.06.037.
Neufeld, E. B., L. M. Zadrozny, D. Phillips, A. Aponte, Z. X. Yu, and R. S. Balaban. 2014. Decorin
    and biglycan retain LDL in disease-prone valvular and aortic subendothelial intimal
    matrix. *Atherosclerosis* 233 (1): 113–121. doi:10.1016/j.atherosclerosis.2013.12.038.
Nishida, N., C. Xie, M. Shimaoka, Y. Cheng, T. Walz, and T. A. Springer. 2006. Activation
    of leukocyte beta2 integrins by conversion from bent to extended conformations.
    Immunity 25 (4): 583–594. doi:10.1016/j.immuni.2006.07.016.
O'Brien, K. D., J. Kuusisto, D. D. Reichenbach, M. Ferguson, C. Giachelli, C. E. Alpers, and
    C. M. Otto. 1995. Osteopontin is expressed in human aortic valvular lesions. *Circulation*
    92 (8): 2163–2168.
O'Brien, K. D., C. M. Otto, D. D. Reichenbach, C. E. Alpers, and T. N. Wight. 1995. Regional
    accumulation of proteoglycans in lesions of degenerative valvular aortic stenosis and
    their relationship to apolipoproteins. *Circulation* 92: 612.
O'Brien, K. D., D. D. Reichenbach, S. M. Marcovina, J. Kuusisto, C. E. Alpers, and C. M. Otto.
    1996. Apolipoproteins B, (a), and E accumulate in the morphologically early lesion of
    'degenerative' valvular aortic stenosis. *Arterioscler Thromb Vasc Biol* 16 (4): 523–532.

Otto, C. M., J. Kuusisto, D. D. Reichenbach, A. M. Gown, and K. D. O'Brien. 1994. Characterization of the early lesion of 'degenerative' valvular aortic stenosis. Histological and immunohistochemical studies. *Circulation* 90 (2): 844–853.

Otto, C. M., B. K. Lind, D. W. Kitzman, B. J. Gersh, and D. S. Siscovick. 1999. Association of aortic-valve sclerosis with cardiovascular mortality and morbidity in the elderly. *N Engl J Med* 341 (3): 142–147. doi:10.1056/NEJM199907153410302.

Oussoren, E., M. M. M. G. Brands, G. J. G. Ruijter, A. T. van der Ploeg, and A. J. J. Reuser. 2011. Bone, joint and tooth development in mucopolysaccharidoses: Relevance to therapeutic options. *Biochim. Biophys. Acta* 1812: 1542–1556.

Panciera, T., L. Azzolin, M. Cordenonsi, and S. Piccolo. 2017. Mechanobiology of YAP and TAZ in physiology and disease. *Nat Rev Mol Cell Biol* 18 (12): 758–770. doi:10.1038/nrm.2017.87.

Pelham, R. J., Jr., and Yl Wang. 1997. Cell locomotion and focal adhesions are regulated by substrate flexibility. *Proc Natl Acad Sci U S A* 94 (25): 13661–13665.

Peng, W. J., J. W. Yan, Y. N. Wan, B. X. Wang, J. H. Tao, G. J. Yang, H. F. Pan, and J. Wang. 2012. Matrix metalloproteinases: A review of their structure and role in systemic sclerosis. *J Clin Immunol* 32 (6): 1409–1414. doi:10.1007/s10875-012-9735-7.

Peyton, S. R., and A. J. Putnam. 2005. Extracellular matrix rigidity governs smooth muscle cell motility in a biphasic fashion. *J Cell Physiol* 204 (1): 198–209. doi:10.1002/jcp.20274.

Pho, M., W. Lee, D. R. Watt, C. Laschinger, C. A. Simmons, and C. A. McCulloch. 2008. Cofilin is a marker of myofibroblast differentiation in cells from porcine aortic cardiac valves. *Am J Physiol Heart Circ Physiol* 294 (4): H1767–H1778. doi:10.1152/ajpheart.01305.2007.

Potts, J. R., and I. D. Campbell. 1994. Fibronectin structure and assembly. *Curr Opin Cell Biol* 6 (5): 648–655.

Quinlan, A. M., and K. L. Billiar. 2012. Investigating the role of substrate stiffness in the persistence of valvular interstitial cell activation. *J Biomed Mater Res A* 100 (9): 2474–2482. doi:10.1002/jbm.a.34162.

Rabkin, E., M. Aikawa, J. R. Stone, Y. Fukumoto, P. Libby, and F. J. Schoen. 2001. Activated interstitial myofibroblasts express catabolic enzymes and mediate matrix remodeling in myxomatous heart valves. *Circulation* 104 (21): 2525–2532.

Rabkin, S. W. 2005. The association of hypertension and aortic valve sclerosis. *Blood Press* 14 (5): 264–272. doi:10.1080/08037050500233320.

Rabkin-Aikawa, E., M. Farber, M. Aikawa, and F. J. Schoen. 2004. Dynamic and reversible changes of interstitial cell phenotype during remodeling of cardiac valves. *J Heart Valve Dis* 13 (5): 841–847.

Rajamannan, N. M., M. Subramaniam, D. Rickard, S. R. Stock, J. Donovan, M. Springett, T. Orszulak et al. 2003. Human aortic valve calcification is associated with an osteoblast phenotype. *Circulation* 107 (17): 2181–2184. doi:10.1161/01.CIR.0000070591.21548.69.

Reinboth, B., E. Hanssen, E. G. Cleary, and M. A. Gibson. 2002. Molecular interactions of biglycan and decorin with elastic fiber components: Biglycan forms a ternary complex with tropoelastin and microfibril-associated glycoprotein 1. *J Biol Chem* 277 (6): 3950–3957. doi:10.1074/jbc. M109540200.

Riveline, D., E. Zamir, N. Q. Balaban, U. S. Schwarz, T. Ishizaki, S. Narumiya, Z. Kam, B. Geiger, and A. D. Bershadsky. 2001. Focal contacts as mechanosensors: Externally applied local mechanical force induces growth of focal contacts by an mDia1-dependent and ROCK-independent mechanism. *J Cell Biol* 153 (6): 1175–1186.

Roberts, W. C., and J. M. Ko. 2005. Frequency by decades of unicuspid, bicuspid, and tricuspid aortic valves in adults having isolated aortic valve replacement for aortic stenosis, with or without associated aortic regurgitation. *Circulation* 111 (7): 920–925. doi:10.1161/01. CIR.0000155623.48408.C5.

Rodriguez, K. J., and K. S. Masters. 2009. Regulation of valvular interstitial cell calcification by components of the extracellular matrix. *J Biomed Mater Res A* 90 (4): 1043–1053. doi:10.1002/jbm.a.32187.

Rodriguez, K. J., L. M. Piechura, A. M. Porras, and K. S. Masters. 2014. Manipulation of valve composition to elucidate the role of collagen in aortic valve calcification. *BMC Cardiovasc Disord* 14: 29. doi:10.1186/1471-2261-14-29.

Romer, L. H., K. G. Birukov, and J. G. Garcia. 2006. Focal adhesions: Paradigm for a signaling nexus. *Circ Res* 98 (5): 606–616. doi:10.1161/01.RES.0000207408.31270.db.

Roskoski, R., Jr. 2012. ERK1/2 MAP kinases: Structure, function, and regulation. *Pharmacol Res* 66 (2): 105–143. doi:10.1016/j.phrs.2012.04.005.

Rothman, R. B., M. H. Baumann, J. E. Savage, L. Rauser, A. McBride, S. J. Hufeisen, and B. L. Roth. 2000. Evidence for possible involvement of 5-HT(2B) receptors in the cardiac valvulopathy associated with fenfluramine and other serotonergic medications. *Circulation* 102 (23): 2836–2841.

Rottner, K., A. Hall, and J. V. Small. 1999. Interplay between Rac and Rho in the control of substrate contact dynamics. *Curr Biol* 9 (12): 640–648.

Ruest, P. J., N. Y. Shin, T. R. Polte, X. Zhang, and S. K. Hanks. 2001. Mechanisms of CAS substrate domain tyrosine phosphorylation by FAK and Src. *Mol Cell Biol* 21 (22): 7641–7652. doi:10.1128/MCB.21.22.7641-7652.2001.

Sabatier, L., D. Chen, C. Fagotto-Kaufmann, D. Hubmacher, M. D. McKee, D. S. Annis, D. F. Mosher, and D. P. Reinhardt. 2009. Fibrillin assembly requires fibronectin. *Mol Biol Cell* 20 (3): 846–858. doi:10.1091/mbc.E08-08-0830.

Sahasakul, Y., W. D. Edwards, J. M. Naessens, and A. J. Tajik. 1988. Age-related changes in aortic and mitral valve thickness: Implications for two-dimensional echocardiography based on an autopsy study of 200 normal human hearts. *Am J Cardiol* 62 (7): 424–430.

Sasaki, T., and R. Timpl. 2001. Domain IVa of laminin alpha5 chain is cell-adhesive and binds beta1 and alphaVbeta3 integrins through Arg-Gly-Asp. *FEBS Lett* 509 (2): 181–185.

Sawada, Y., M. Tamada, B. J. Dubin-Thaler, O. Cherniavskaya, R. Sakai, S. Tanaka, and M. P. Sheetz. 2006. Force sensing by mechanical extension of the Src family kinase substrate p130Cas. *Cell* 127 (5): 1015–1026. doi:10.1016/j.cell.2006.09.044.

Schaller, M. D., J. D. Hildebrand, and J. T. Parsons. 1999. Complex formation with focal adhesion kinase: A mechanism to regulate activity and subcellular localization of Src kinases. *Mol Biol Cell* 10 (10): 3489–3505.

Schaller, M. D., J. D. Hildebrand, J. D. Shannon, J. W. Fox, R. R. Vines, and J. T. Parsons. 1994. Autophosphorylation of the focal adhesion kinase, pp125FAK, directs SH2-dependent binding of pp60src. *Mol Cell Biol* 14 (3): 1680–1688.

Schiller, H. B., M. R. Hermann, J. Polleux, T. Vignaud, S. Zanivan, C. C. Friedel, Z. Sun et al. 2013. beta1- and alphav-class integrins cooperate to regulate myosin II during rigidity sensing of fibronectin-based microenvironments. *Nat Cell Biol* 15 (6): 625–636. doi:10.1038/ncb2747.

Schlaepfer, D. D., S. K. Hanks, T. Hunter, and P. van der Geer. 1994. Integrin-mediated signal transduction linked to Ras pathway by GRB2 binding to focal adhesion kinase. *Nature* 372 (6508): 786–791.

Schlaepfer, D. D., and T. Hunter. 1997. Focal adhesion kinase overexpression enhances ras-dependent integrin signaling to ERK2/mitogen-activated protein kinase through interactions with and activation of c-Src. *J Biol Chem* 272 (20): 13189–13195.

Schlie-Wolter, S., A. Ngezahayo, and B. N. Chichkov. 2013. The selective role of ECM components on cell adhesion, morphology, proliferation and communication in vitro. *Exp Cell Res* 319 (10): 1553–1561. doi:10.1016/j.yexcr.2013.03.016.

Schneider, P. J., and J. D. Deck. 1981. Tissue and cell renewal in the natural aortic valve of rats: An autoradiographic study. *Cardiovasc Res* 15 (4): 181–189.

Schober, M., S. Raghavan, M. Nikolova, L. Polak, H. A. Pasolli, H. E. Beggs, L. F. Reichardt, and E. Fuchs. 2007. Focal adhesion kinase modulates tension signaling to control actin and focal adhesion dynamics. *J Cell Biol* 176 (5): 667–680. doi:10.1083/jcb.200608010.

Schwartz, M. 2004. Rho signalling at a glance. *J Cell Sci* 117 (Pt 23): 5457–5458. doi:10.1242/jcs.01582.

Schwarzbauer, J. E., and D. W. DeSimone. 2011. Fibronectins, their fibrillogenesis, and in vivo functions. *Cold Spring Harb Perspect Biol* 3 (7). doi:10.1101/cshperspect.a005041.

Scott, M. J., and I. Vesely. 1996. Morphology of porcine aortic valve cusp elastin. *J Heart Valve Dis* 5 (5): 464–471.

Sharma, A., and B. J. Mayer. 2008. Phosphorylation of p130Cas initiates Rac activation and membrane ruffling. *BMC Cell Biol* 9: 50. doi:10.1186/1471-2121-9-50.

Sherratt, M. J. 2009. Tissue elasticity and the ageing elastic fibre. *Age (Dordr)* 31 (4): 305–325. doi:10.1007/s11357-009-9103-6.

Sider, K. L., C. Zhu, A. V. Kwong, Z. Mirzaei, C. F. de Lange, and C. A. Simmons. 2014. Evaluation of a porcine model of early aortic valve sclerosis. *Cardiovasc Pathol* 23 (5): 289–297. doi:10.1016/j.carpath.2014.05.004.

Simionescu, A., D. T. Simionescu, and N. R. Vyavahare. 2007. Osteogenic responses in fibroblasts activated by elastin degradation products and transforming growth factor-beta1: Role of myofibroblasts in vascular calcification. *Am J Pathol* 171 (1): 116–123.

Simmons, C. A., G. R. Grant, E. Manduchi, and P. F. Davies. 2005. Spatial heterogeneity of endothelial phenotypes correlates with side-specific vulnerability to calcification in normal porcine aortic valves. *Circ Res* 96 (7): 792–799. doi:10.1161/01.RES.0000161998.92009.64.

Simon, T., and J. S. Bromberg. 2017. Regulation of the immune system by laminins. *Trends Immunol* 38: 858–871.

Singh, P., C. Carraher, and J. E. Schwarzbauer. 2010. Assembly of fibronectin extracellular matrix. *Annu Rev Cell Dev Biol* 26: 397–419. doi:10.1146/annurev-cellbio-100109-104020.

Soini, Y., J. Satta, M. Maatta, and H. Autio-Harmainen. 2001. Expression of MMP2, MMP9, MT1-MMP, TIMP1, and TIMP2 mRNA in valvular lesions of the heart. *J Pathol* 194 (2): 225–31. doi:10.1002/path.850.

Song, R., D. A. Fullerton, L. Ao, D. Zheng, K. S. Zhao, and X. Meng. 2015. BMP-2 and TGF-beta1 mediate biglycan-induced pro-osteogenic reprogramming in aortic valve interstitial cells. *J Mol Med (Berl)* 93 (4): 403–412. doi:10.1007/s00109-014-1229-z.

Song, R., Q. Zeng, L. Ao, J. A. Yu, J. C. Cleveland, K. S. Zhao, D. A. Fullerton, and X. Meng. 2012. Biglycan induces the expression of osteogenic factors in human aortic valve interstitial cells via Toll-like receptor-2. *Arterioscler Thromb Vasc Biol* 32 (11): 2711–2720. doi:10.1161/ATVBAHA.112.300116.

Sottile, J., and D. C. Hocking. 2002. Fibronectin polymerization regulates the composition and stability of extracellular matrix fibrils and cell-matrix adhesions. *Mol Biol Cell* 13 (10): 3546–3559. doi:10.1091/mbc. E02-01-0048.

Stegemann, J. P., H. Hong, and R. M. Nerem. 2005. Mechanical, biochemical, and extracellular matrix effects on vascular smooth muscle cell phenotype. *J Appl Physiol* (1985) 98 (6): 2321–2327. doi:10.1152/japplphysiol.01114.2004.

Stella, J. A., and M. S. Sacks. 2007. On the biaxial mechanical properties of the layers of the aortic valve leaflet. *J Biomech Eng* 129 (5): 757–766. doi:10.1115/1.2768111.

Stenzel, D., C. A. Franco, S. Estrach, A. Mettouchi, D. Sauvaget, I. Rosewell, A. Schertel et al. 2011. Endothelial basement membrane limits tip cell formation by inducing Dll4/Notch signalling in vivo. *EMBO Rep* 12 (11): 1135–1143. doi:10.1038/embor.2011.194.

Stephens, E. H., C. K. Chu, and K. J. Grande-Allen. 2008. Valve proteoglycan content and glycosaminoglycan fine structure are unique to microstructure, mechanical load and age: Relevance to an age-specific tissue-engineered heart valve. *Acta Biomater* 4 (5): 1148–1160. doi:10.1016/j.actbio.2008.03.014.

Stephens, E. H., J. G. Saltarrelli, L. S. Baggett, I. Nandi, J. J. Kuo, A. R. Davis, E. A. Olmsted-Davis, M. J. Reardon, J. D. Morrisett, and K. J. Grande-Allen. 2011. Differential proteoglycan and hyaluronan distribution in calcified aortic valves. *Cardiovasc Pathol* 20 (6): 334–342. doi:10.1016/j.carpath.2010.10.002.

Stetler-Stevenson, W. G. 2008. Tissue inhibitors of metalloproteinases in cell signaling: Metalloproteinase-independent biological activities. *Sci Signal* 1 (27): re6. doi:10.1126/scisignal.127re6.

Stewart, B. F., D. Siscovick, B. K. Lind, J. M. Gardin, J. S. Gottdiener, V. E. Smith, D. W. Kitzman, and C. M. Otto. 1997. Clinical factors associated with calcific aortic valve disease. Cardiovascular Health Study. *J Am Coll Cardiol* 29 (3): 630–634.

Sundberg, L. J., L. M. Galante, H. M. Bill, C. P. Mack, and J. M. Taylor. 2003. An endogenous inhibitor of focal adhesion kinase blocks Rac1/JNK but not Ras/ERK-dependent signaling in vascular smooth muscle cells. *J Biol Chem* 278 (32): 29783–29791. doi:10.1074/jbc.M303771200.

Sung, D. C., C. J. Bowen, K. A. Vaidya, J. Zhou, N. Chapurin, A. Recknagel, B. Zhou, J. Chen, M. Kotlikoff, and J. T. Butcher. 2016. Cadherin-11 overexpression induces extracellular matrix remodeling and calcification in mature aortic valves. *Arterioscler Thromb Vasc Biol* 36 (8): 1627–1637. doi:10.1161/ATVBAHA.116.307812.

Tadokoro, S., S. J. Shattil, K. Eto, V. Tai, R. C. Liddington, J. M. de Pereda, M. H. Ginsberg, and D. A. Calderwood. 2003. Talin binding to integrin beta tails: A final common step in integrin activation. *Science* 302 (5642): 103–106. doi:10.1126/science.1086652.

Tamkun, J. W., D. W. DeSimone, D. Fonda, R. S. Patel, C. Buck, A. F. Horwitz, and R. O. Hynes. 1986. Structure of integrin, a glycoprotein involved in the transmembrane linkage between fibronectin and actin. *Cell* 46 (2): 271–282.

Tang, Y., R. G. Rowe, E. L. Botvinick, A. Kurup, A. J. Putnam, M. Seiki, V. M. Weaver et al. 2013. MT1-MMP-dependent control of skeletal stem cell commitment via a beta1-integrin/YAP/TAZ signaling axis. *Dev Cell* 25 (4): 402–416. doi:10.1016/j.devcel.2013.04.011.

Thayer, P., K. Balachandran, S. Rathan, C. H. Yap, S. Arjunon, H. Jo, and A. P. Yoganathan. 2011. The effects of combined cyclic stretch and pressure on the aortic valve interstitial cell phenotype. *Ann Biomed Eng* 39 (6): 1654–1667. doi:10.1007/s10439-011-0273-x.

Thubrikar, M. J., J. Aouad, and S. P. Nolan. 1986. Patterns of calcific deposits in operatively excised stenotic or purely regurgitant aortic valves and their relation to mechanical stress. *Am J Cardiol* 58 (3): 304–308.

Thubrikar, M. J., S. P. Nolan, J. Aouad, and J. D. Deck. 1986. Stress sharing between the sinus and leaflets of canine aortic valve. *Ann Thorac Surg* 42 (4): 434–440.

Thubrikar, M. 1990. *The Aortic Valve*. Boca Raton, FL: CRC Press.

Tomakidi, P., S. Schulz, S. Proksch, W. Weber, and T. Steinberg. 2014. Focal adhesion kinase (FAK) perspectives in mechanobiology: Implications for cell behaviour. *Cell Tissue Res* 357 (3): 515–526. doi:10.1007/s00441-014-1945-2.

Tompkins, R. G., J. J. Schnitzer, and M. L. Yarmush. 1989. Macromolecular transport within heart valves. *Circ Res* 64 (6): 1213–1223.

Torr, E. E., C. R. Ngam, K. Bernau, B. Tomasini-Johansson, B. Acton, and N. Sandbo. 2015. Myofibroblasts exhibit enhanced fibronectin assembly that is intrinsic to their contractile phenotype. *J Biol Chem* 290 (11): 6951–6961. doi:10.1074/jbc.M114.606186.

Towler, D. A. 2013. Molecular and cellular aspects of calcific aortic valve disease. *Circ Res* 113 (2): 198–208. doi:10.1161/CIRCRESAHA.113.300155.

van Geemen, D., A. L. Soares, P. J. Oomen, A. Driessen-Mol, M. W. Janssen-van den Broek, A. J. van den Bogaerdt, A. J. Bogers, M. J. Goumans, F. P. Baaijens, and C. V. Bouten. 2016. Age-dependent changes in geometry, tissue composition and mechanical properties of fetal to adult cryopreserved human heart valves. *PLoS One* 11 (2): e0149020. doi:10.1371/journal.pone.0149020.

Vesely, I. 1998. The role of elastin in aortic valve mechanics. *J Biomech* 31 (2): 115–123.

Vesely, I., and R. Noseworthy. 1992. Micromechanics of the fibrosa and the ventricularis in aortic valve leaflets. *J Biomech* 25 (1): 101–113.

Visse, R., and H. Nagase. 2003. Matrix metalloproteinases and tissue inhibitors of metalloproteinases: Structure, function, and biochemistry. *Circ Res* 92 (8): 827–839. doi:10.1161/01.RES.0000070112.80711.3D.

Walker, G. A., K. S. Masters, D. N. Shah, K. S. Anseth, and L. A. Leinwand. 2004. Valvular myofibroblast activation by transforming growth factor-beta: Implications for pathological extracellular matrix remodeling in heart valve disease. *Circ Res* 95 (3): 253–260. doi:10.1161/01.RES.0000136520.07995.aa.

Wang, H., S. M. Haeger, A. M. Kloxin, L. A. Leinwand, and K. S. Anseth. 2012. Redirecting valvular myofibroblasts into dormant fibroblasts through light-mediated reduction in substrate modulus. *PLoS One* 7 (7): e39969. doi:10.1371/journal.pone.0039969.

Wang, H., M. W. Tibbitt, S. J. Langer, L. A. Leinwand, and K. S. Anseth. 2013. Hydrogels preserve native phenotypes of valvular fibroblasts through an elasticity-regulated PI3K/AKT pathway. *Proc Natl Acad Sci U S A* 110 (48): 19336–19341. doi:10.1073/pnas.1306369110.

Wang, H. B., M. Dembo, and Y. L. Wang. 2000. Substrate flexibility regulates growth and apoptosis of normal but not transformed cells. *Am J Physiol Cell Physiol* 279 (5): C1345–C1350.

Wang, J. G., M. Miyazu, E. Matsushita, M. Sokabe, and K. Naruse. 2001. Uniaxial cyclic stretch induces focal adhesion kinase (FAK) tyrosine phosphorylation followed by mitogen-activated protein kinase (MAPK) activation. *Biochem Biophys Res Commun* 288 (2): 356–361. doi:10.1006/bbrc.2001.5775.

Warnock, J. N., C. A. Gamez, S. A. Metzler, J. Chen, S. H. Elder, and J. Liao. 2010. Vasoactive agents alter the biomechanical properties of aortic heart valve leaflets in a time-dependent manner. *J Heart Valve Dis* 19 (1): 86–95; discussion 96.

Watanabe, T., M. Tsuda, S. Tanaka, Y. Ohba, H. Kawaguchi, T. Majima, H. Sawa, and A. Minami. 2009. Adaptor protein Crk induces Src-dependent activation of p38 MAPK in regulation of synovial sarcoma cell proliferation. *Mol Cancer Res* 7 (9): 1582–1592. doi:10.1158/1541-7786.MCR-09-0064.

Weber, K. T., Y. Sun, L. C. Katwa, J. P. Cleutjens, and G. Zhou. 1995. Connective tissue and repair in the heart. Potential regulatory mechanisms. *Ann N Y Acad Sci* 752: 286–299.

Webster, K. D., W. P. Ng, and D. A. Fletcher. 2014. Tensional homeostasis in single fibroblasts. *Biophys J* 107 (1): 146–155. doi:10.1016/j.bpj.2014.04.051.

Wipff, P. J., D. B. Rifkin, J. J. Meister, and B. Hinz. 2007. Myofibroblast contraction activates latent TGF-beta1 from the extracellular matrix. *J Cell Biol* 179 (6): 1311–1323. doi:10.1083/jcb.200704042.

Xing, Y., J. N. Warnock, Z. He, S. L. Hilbert, and A. P. Yoganathan. 2004. Cyclic pressure affects the biological properties of porcine aortic valve leaflets in a magnitude and frequency dependent manner. *Ann Biomed Eng* 32 (11): 1461–1470.

Xu, J., and G. P. Shi. 2014. Vascular wall extracellular matrix proteins and vascular diseases. *Biochim Biophys Acta* 1842 (11): 2106–2119. doi:10.1016/j.bbadis.2014.07.008.

Yap, C. H., H. S. Kim, K. Balachandran, M. Weiler, R. Haj-Ali, and A. P. Yoganathan. 2010. Dynamic deformation characteristics of porcine aortic valve leaflet under normal and hypertensive conditions. *Am J Physiol Heart Circ Physiol* 298 (2): H395–H405. doi:10.1152/ajpheart.00040.2009.

Yap, C. H., N. Saikrishnan, G. Tamilselvan, and A. P. Yoganathan. 2012. Experimental measurement of dynamic fluid shear stress on the aortic surface of the aortic valve leaflet. *Biomech Model Mechanobiol* 11 (1–2): 171–182. doi:10.1007/s10237-011-0301-7.

Yap, C. H., N. Saikrishnan, and A. P. Yoganathan. 2012. Experimental measurement of dynamic fluid shear stress on the ventricular surface of the aortic valve leaflet. *Biomech Model Mechanobiol* 11 (1–2): 231–244. doi:10.1007/s10237-011-0306-2.

Yip, C. Y., J. H. Chen, R. Zhao, and C. A. Simmons. 2009. Calcification by valve interstitial cells is regulated by the stiffness of the extracellular matrix. *Arterioscler Thromb Vasc Biol* 29 (6): 936–942. doi:10.1161/ATVBAHA.108.182394.

Yoshigi, M., L. M. Hoffman, C. C. Jensen, H. J. Yost, and M. C. Beckerle. 2005. Mechanical force mobilizes zyxin from focal adhesions to actin filaments and regulates cytoskeletal reinforcement. *J Cell Biol* 171 (2): 209–215. doi:10.1083/jcb.200505018.

Yutzey, K. E., L. L. Demer, S. C. Body, G. S. Huggins, D. A. Towler, C. M. Giachelli, M. A. Hofmann-Bowman et al. 2014. Calcific aortic valve disease: A consensus summary from the Alliance of Investigators on Calcific Aortic Valve Disease. *Arterioscler Thromb Vasc Biol* 34 (11): 2387–2393. doi:10.1161/ATVBAHA.114.302523.

Zamir, E., and B. Geiger. 2001. Molecular complexity and dynamics of cell-matrix adhesions. *J Cell Sci* 114 (Pt 20): 3583–3590.

Zeke, A., M. Misheva, A. Remenyi, and M. A. Bogoyevitch. 2016. JNK signaling: Regulation and functions based on complex protein-protein partnerships. *Microbiol Mol Biol Rev* 80 (3): 793–835. doi:10.1128/MMBR.00043-14.

Zhao, R., K. L. Sider, and C. A. Simmons. 2011. Measurement of layer-specific mechanical properties in multilayered biomaterials by micropipette aspiration. *Acta Biomater* 7 (3): 1220–1227. doi:10.1016/j.actbio.2010.11.004.

Zhou, J., C. Aponte-Santamaria, S. Sturm, J. T. Bullerjahn, A. Bronowska, and F. Grater. 2015. Mechanism of focal adhesion kinase mechanosensing. *PLoS Comput Biol* 11 (11): e1004593. doi:10.1371/journal.pcbi.1004593.

3

Blood Flow Mechanics

M. Fenech and L. Haya

Contents

3.1 Introduction

Human blood is mostly composed of cells. Typically, red blood cells (RBCs, or erythrocytes) occupy 40%–45% of the blood volume, whereas the white blood cells (WBCs, or leukocytes) and platelets (or thrombocytes) occupy less than 1% of the volume. In flow, RBCs tumble, roll, and deform. Normal RBCs can deform substantially, enabling them to pass through small blood vessels. It was recently shown that RBCs can also adopt highly deformed and polylobed shapes (Lanotte et al. 2016). Under flow conditions inducing low shear, they also tend to stack in two or three dimensions, forming aggregates or rouleaux. In blood circulation, RBCs tend to migrate away from the vessel wall toward the centerline, leaving a cell-depleted region near the wall, known as the cell-free layer (CFL). Blood cells are suspended in plasma, the liquid component of blood. Plasma is mostly composed of water, with salt and proteins in suspension. The composition of plasma is extremely important from a physiological point of view, but regarding fluid mechanics, it is considered a Newtonian fluid with fluid properties comparable to water (Fung 1993). The plasma density is about 1.02 g/L, and its normal viscosity at 37°C is about 1.1–1.3 mPa.s (Késmárky et al. 2008). However, its composition, particularly its concentration of protein and salts, greatly influences the mechanical properties of the suspended cells within plasma and their interactions. The viscosity of whole blood is not constant, as it depends on several factors, such as shear rate (non-Newtonian behavior), plasma composition, the hematocrit[1], as well as the geometry and diameter of the vessels. However, it is commonly accepted that in vessels with diameters larger than 300 μm, which typically present shear rates greater than 50 s^{-1}, the apparent viscosity of blood is nearly constant at approximately $\mu_{app} = 3$ mPa.s (or cP). Therefore, at this scale, blood can be considered a homogeneous mixture with Newtonian fluid properties. The typical density of healthy blood is about 1060 kg/m^3. The representation of blood as a homogenous fluid (either Newtonian or non-Newtonian) is not a new development in fluid mechanics but is an opportunity to introduce useful principles of fluid mechanics and applications specifically related to hemodynamics. More complex approaches, which account for flexible blood vessel walls and blood cell interactions, will be presented in Chapters 6 and 12.

3.2 Conservation Relations

3.2.1 Conservation of Mass

The conservation of mass guarantees that the mass entering a volume over a specific time period is equal to the increase in mass inside the volume plus the mass leaving the volume over the same period of time.

As an application, considering a vascular tree branching into a network of several generations of vessels, if the vessel diameters and characteristic velocities of each generation are known, we can estimate the number of vessels required for each generation to accommodate the total flow passing through them. The conservation of mass, assuming constant mass density, gives the following relationship: the flow in the aorta equals the sum of flows in the daughter branches:

$$Q_{\text{Aorta}} = V_{\text{Aorta}} \frac{\pi D_{\text{Aorta}}^2}{4} = N_b V_b \frac{\pi D_b^2}{4},$$

---

[1] Hematocrit is defined as the percentage by volume of RBCs (denoted by H).

$$N_b = \frac{V_{\text{Aorta}}}{V_b} \left(\frac{D_{\text{Aorta}}}{D_b} \right)^2, \qquad (3.1)$$

where V_b, D_b, and N_b are the characteristic average velocity, the diameter, and the number of vessels of generation b, respectively, and V_{Aorta} and D_{Aorta} are the characteristic average velocity and the diameter of the aorta, respectively. Table 3.1 presents the obtained values typical for the systemic circulation.

Assuming that the scales of interest are much larger than those of local inhomogeneity, that is, ignoring the local cell density or interactions, blood is considered a homogenous, incompressible fluid characterized by constant density ρ. All variables are assumed to be continuous in time t and space x. The flow will be defined by its velocity $u(x,t)$ and the pressure field $p(x,t)$.

The conservation of mass can be written locally, relating ρ and u as:

$$\frac{D\rho}{Dt} = \rho \nabla \cdot u. \qquad (3.2)$$

Here, $D\rho/Dt$ is the material derivative of ρ that computes the time rate of change of ρ for the fluid moving with velocity u. $\nabla \cdot u$ is the divergence of the field of velocity u that computes the rate of expansion of the fluid volume per unit volume. This equation is known as the continuity equation. In the cardiovascular system, blood is considered an incompressible fluid, that is, the blood density is constant in space and time. Then, Equation 3.2 reduces to

$$\nabla \cdot u = 0. \qquad (3.3)$$

This equation means that a volume of fluid does not expand while the blood density is fixed. The divergence of the velocity field ∇u is defined as:

$$\text{in Cartesian coordinates:} \ \nabla \cdot u = \frac{\partial u_x}{\partial x} + \frac{\partial u_y}{\partial y} + \frac{\partial u_z}{\partial z}, \qquad (3.4)$$

TABLE 3.1 Estimation of Numbers of Vessel Based on Vessel Diameters and Average Velocity for the Systemic Circulation. Diameters and Velocity from (Dawson 2008)

	Characteristic Diameter of Single Vessel (mm)	Average Velocity (cm/s)	Estimated Number $N_b = \frac{V_{\text{Aorta}}}{V_b} \left(\frac{D_{\text{Aorta}}}{D_b} \right)^2$
Aorta	22	25	1
Large arteries	6	8.3	40
Small arteries	2	1.2	2500
Arterioles	0.02	0.3	1.0×10^8
Capillaries	0.01	0.03	4.0×10^9

where u_x, u_y, and u_z are the velocity components in directions x, y, and z, respectively;

$$\text{in cylindrical coordinates: } \nabla \cdot \boldsymbol{u} = \frac{1}{r}\frac{\partial(ru_r)}{\partial r} + \frac{1}{r}\frac{\partial u_\theta}{\partial \theta} + \frac{\partial u_z}{\partial z}, \tag{3.5}$$

where u_r, u_θ, and u_z are the velocity components in directions r, θ, and z, respectively.

3.2.2 Conservation of Momentum

Newton's second law of motion can be applied to fluids: the sum of forces (body and surface forces) acting on a fluid is equal to the product of its mass by acceleration. This principle is called the conservation of momentum.

In case of blood flow, the only applied body force is normally due to gravity, equaling $\rho \boldsymbol{g}$; however, for particular cases, other body forces may need to be considered. For example, if the referential frame is accelerating, the force that results from the acceleration of the reference frame must also be considered. Examples of these so-called fictitious forces include the centrifugal force that acts on blood cells during a centrifugation process and the "g-force" that results from the sudden acceleration of a fighter jet, pushing blood away from the pilot's head. The surface forces account for normal and tangential forces and include pressure and viscous forces.

Stresses can act both normal and tangential to the surface of the fluid element. Viscous stresses oppose relative movements between neighboring fluid particles and can be described by tangential shear and normal components. Tangential shear stress can be visualized by considering two neighboring fluid elements flowing at different velocities. Normal viscous stress can be viewed as the "stickiness" of the fluid or the force linking the fluid elements together. By definition, τ_{ij} is the stress per unit surface, that is, the stress acting on the face of the fluid element divided by the area of the face. In this notation, index j indicates the direction of the force and index i indicates the direction normal to the face to which the force is applied, as illustrated in Figure 3.1. The unit of stress is the pascal (Pa), similar to pressure.

As was done for the conservation of mass, the equation of motion resulting from the force balance can be written locally in differential form. This is called Cauchy's equation of motion (Equation 3.6).

$$\rho \frac{D\boldsymbol{u}}{Dt} = -\nabla p + \nabla \cdot \tau + p\boldsymbol{g} + \boldsymbol{f}_b, \tag{3.6}$$

where $\rho\, D\boldsymbol{u}/Dt$ is the product of fluid mass by its acceleration per unit of volume, $-\nabla p$ is the total net pressure force per unit of volume, $\nabla \cdot \tau$ is the net viscous force per unit volume, $p\boldsymbol{g}$ is the net weight force per unit volume, and $\boldsymbol{f}_b$ is the other body forces per unit volume. Acceleration term $D\boldsymbol{u}/Dt$ represents the "global" variation of velocity; it is important to keep in mind that it comprises both the timewise variation of velocity $\partial u/\partial t$ and the spatial variation of velocity $\boldsymbol{u} \cdot \nabla \boldsymbol{u}$.

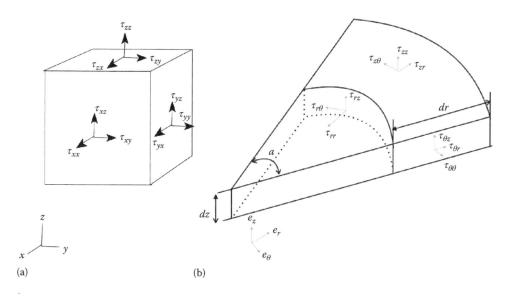

(a)   (b)

Figure 3.1   Unit volume of fluid showing shear stresses in the three coordinate directions in (a) Cartesian and (b) cylindrical reference frames.

In a steady flow, the fluid velocities at each point in the system do not change over time. Therefore, $\partial \boldsymbol{u}/\partial t = 0$; however, a steady flow does not imply that $D\boldsymbol{u}/Dt = 0$, because in most steady flows, velocities change directions. On the other hand, $\boldsymbol{u} \cdot \nabla \boldsymbol{u} = 0$ is typically true for a unidirectional flow, such as in a straight pipe. Although this is an unusual case in nature, it is most often presented in fluid mechanics textbooks because its equations have a simple solution. The mathematical solutions presented in this chapter will be no exceptions, as the examples in Section 3.5 will be for straight vessels. Nevertheless, it is sometimes appropriate to use the equations developed in straight geometries for tortuous geometries, as long as inertial forces are negligible as compared with the other forces present, such as the friction forces (due to viscosity). On the contrary, as will be shown in Section 3.4.3, the formation of the Dean vortices in curved vessels can be described only if inertial forces are not neglected.

Each term in Equation 3.6 can be derived in different coordinate systems. The terms for acceleration forces, pressure forces, and viscous forces are expressed in Cartesian and cylindrical coordinates in Table 3.2.

Cauchy's Equation 3.6 is the general form of the momentum conservation. It is valid for any continuous medium: for compressible or incompressible flow, as well as for Newtonian or non-Newtonian fluids. However, even when the moment equation is coupled with the mass conservation equation, the system is described by only four equations for 11 unknown variables (three components of velocity, six components of shear, the pressure, and the density). Therefore, additional relations and assumptions are required to reduce the number of unknowns. In the following section, particular forms of the equations of fluid motion that are often used for describing blood flow are presented.

TABLE 3.2   Acceleration, Pressure, and Viscous Forces Developed in Cartesian and Cylindrical Coordinates

	Cartesian Coordinates	Cylindrical Coordinates
Acceleration times mass per unit volume $\rho \dfrac{Du}{Dt}$	$\rho\left(\dfrac{\partial u_x}{\partial t}+u_x\dfrac{\partial u_x}{\partial x}+u_y\dfrac{\partial u_x}{\partial y}+u_z\dfrac{\partial u_x}{\partial z}\right)$	$\rho\left(\dfrac{\partial u_r}{\partial t}+u_r\dfrac{\partial u_r}{\partial r}+\dfrac{u_\theta}{r}\dfrac{\partial u_r}{\partial \theta}+u_z\dfrac{\partial u_r}{\partial z}-\dfrac{u_\theta{}^2}{r}\right)$
	$\rho\left(\dfrac{\partial u_y}{\partial t}+u_x\dfrac{\partial u_y}{\partial x}+u_y\dfrac{\partial u_y}{\partial y}+u_z\dfrac{\partial u_y}{\partial z}\right)$	$\rho\left(\dfrac{\partial u_\theta}{\partial t}+u_r\dfrac{\partial u_\theta}{\partial r}+\dfrac{u_\theta}{r}\dfrac{\partial u_\theta}{\partial \theta}+u_z\dfrac{\partial u_\theta}{\partial z}+\dfrac{u_\theta u_r}{r}\right)$
	$\rho\left(\dfrac{\partial u_z}{\partial t}+u_x\dfrac{\partial u_z}{\partial x}+u_y\dfrac{\partial u_z}{\partial y}+u_z\dfrac{\partial u_z}{\partial z}\right)$	$\rho\left(\dfrac{\partial u_z}{\partial t}+u_r\dfrac{\partial u_z}{\partial r}+\dfrac{u_\theta}{r}\dfrac{\partial u_z}{\partial \theta}+u_z\dfrac{\partial u_z}{\partial z}\right)$
Gradient of pressure $-\nabla p$	$-\dfrac{\partial p}{\partial x}$	$-\dfrac{\partial p}{\partial r}$
	$-\dfrac{\partial p}{\partial y}$	$-\dfrac{1}{r}\dfrac{\partial p}{\partial \theta}$
	$-\dfrac{\partial p}{\partial z}$	$-\dfrac{\partial p}{\partial z}$
Viscous forces $\nabla\cdot\tau_{ij}$	$\dfrac{\partial \tau_{xx}}{\partial x}+\dfrac{\partial \tau_{yx}}{\partial y}+\dfrac{\partial \tau_{zx}}{\partial z}$	$\dfrac{1}{r}\dfrac{\partial(r\tau_{rr})}{\partial r}+\dfrac{1}{r}\dfrac{\partial \tau_{r\theta}}{\partial \theta}-\dfrac{\partial \tau_{\theta\theta}}{\partial r}+\dfrac{\partial \tau_{rz}}{\partial z}$
	$\dfrac{\partial \tau_{xy}}{\partial x}+\dfrac{\partial \tau_{yy}}{\partial y}+\dfrac{\partial \tau_{zy}}{\partial z}$	$\dfrac{1}{r^2}\dfrac{\partial(r^2\tau_{\theta r})}{\partial r}+\dfrac{1}{r}\dfrac{\partial \tau_{\theta\theta}}{\partial \theta}+\dfrac{\partial \tau_{\theta z}}{\partial z}$
	$\dfrac{\partial \tau_{xz}}{\partial x}+\dfrac{\partial \tau_{yz}}{\partial y}+\dfrac{\partial \tau_{zz}}{\partial z}$	$\dfrac{1}{r}\dfrac{\partial(r\tau_{zr})}{\partial r}+\dfrac{1}{r}\dfrac{\partial \tau_{z\theta}}{\partial \theta}+\dfrac{\partial \tau_{zz}}{\partial z}$

3.3 Particular Forms of Fluid Motion Equations

3.3.1 Case of Inviscid Flow

An inviscid flow is a flow in which the friction forces can be neglected when compared with the inertial forces. The relation between pressure and velocity in an inviscid incompressible flow can be expressed in the form of Bernoulli's equation. Bernoulli's equation applies to an inviscid flow with no applied body forces. It relates the change in velocity along a streamline to the change in pressure along the same streamline. A streamline in a flow describes a path that is parallel to the velocity vector at all points in the field. The Bernoulli Equation 3.7 is often used to estimate the velocity of a fluid traveling through a narrow orifice of known size.

$$p+\frac{1}{2}\rho v^2+\rho g z = \text{constant}, \tag{3.7}$$

where p is the pressure at a chosen point, ρ is the density of the fluid, v is the fluid flow speed at the chosen point on a given streamline, g is the acceleration due to gravity, and z is the elevation of the point above the reference.

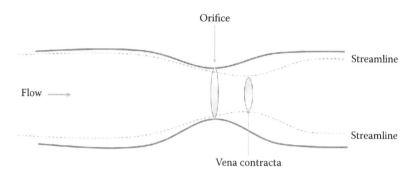

Figure 3.2 Flow through a constriction. Location of the vena contracta compared with the actual larger orifice.

Viscous friction and acceleration can often be ignored under many physiological conditions. Consequently, Bernoulli's equation is widely used in hemodynamics, in particular in echo-Doppler diagnosis to estimate the peak velocity or the transvalvular pressure drop. In hemodynamics, Bernoulli's equation is normally written between two locations (denoted by 1 and 2) and is reduced to

$$\Delta p = 4\left(v_2^{\ 2} - v_1^{\ 2} \right). \tag{3.8}$$

In this expression, Δp is expressed in mmHg, the velocity is expressed in m/s, and the density of blood is taken to be 1.05 g/cm^3. Note that the height difference between the two locations is ignored in this expression.

The degree of an aortic stenosis is often estimated based on Bernoulli's equation, coupled with the equation of mass conservation. In order to assess the severity of cardiac valve stenosis, modified forms of Bernoulli's equation were developed. These specific equations are amended to correct for the assumption of inviscid fluid and the incongruity between the vena contracta and the actual valve orifice, that is, the difference in location and diameter of the vena contracta compared with the larger valve orifice, as shown in Figure 3.2. The aortic valve aperture can be estimated by cardiac catheterization, Doppler echocardiography, or imaging planimetry; the measures of valve aperture provided from these diagnostic techniques are called the Gorlin area, the effective orifice area (EOA), and the geometric orifice area (GOA), respectively (Garcia and Kadem 2006).

3.3.2 Case of Newtonian Fluid

Blood viscosity is a measure of blood's resistance to deformation by shear stress. In layman's terms, it describes the "stickiness" of blood. Blood viscosity is a determining factor in cardiovascular dynamics. For example, the work required for the heart to pump blood increases with higher blood viscosity. In arterial blood flow, in which the shear rate is normally higher than 100 s^{-1}, it is generally assumed that blood is Newtonian, that is, it has a constant viscosity. The Newtonian assumption is widely used in cardiovascular mechanics and generally provides a good estimation of the physiological parameters sought, such as vascular resistance and blood perfusion. The Newtonian approximation assumes that the fluid stress is linearly dependent on the applied rate of strain, where the viscosity is the proportionality coefficient. The relationship between the viscous stress and the deformation rate of the fluid element for an incompressible Newtonian fluid is given by:

$$\tau_{ij} = \mu \left(\frac{\partial u_i}{\partial x_j} + \frac{\partial u_j}{\partial x_i} \right), \tag{3.9}$$

where indices i and j represent directions x, y, and z in Cartesian coordinates and μ is the fluid viscosity. Then, for an incompressible Newtonian fluid, the viscous force per unit volume in the x direction is:

$$f_{x,\text{viscous}} = \frac{\partial \tau_{xx}}{\partial x} + \frac{\partial \tau_{yx}}{\partial y} + \frac{\partial \tau_{zx}}{\partial z} = \mu \left(\frac{\partial^2 u_x}{\partial x^2} + \frac{\partial^2 u_x}{\partial y^2} + \frac{\partial^2 u_x}{\partial z^2} \right). \tag{3.10}$$

The set of equations describing the motion of an incompressible Newtonian fluid is called the Navier–Stokes equations. These equations invoke the conservation equations for mass and momentum as:

$$\nabla \cdot \boldsymbol{u} = 0,$$

$$\rho \frac{D\boldsymbol{u}}{Dt} = -\nabla p + \mu \nabla^2 \boldsymbol{u} + p\boldsymbol{g}. \tag{3.11}$$

The simplification of the Cauchy's equation with the assumption of an incompressible and Newtonian fluid reduces the number of unknowns to four, namely, the velocity components u_x, u_y, and u_z and density ρ. With the four equations (one for continuity and three for momentum), the system can now be solved, given initial and boundary conditions. Table 3.3 presents the Navier–Stokes equations in developed form for both Cartesian and cylindrical coordinates. Solutions for classical problems are given in Section 3.5.

3.3.3 Case of Non-Newtonian Fluid

It has been well established that, under low shear stress, blood does not have a constant viscosity (Bureau et al. 1980). Recent studies have shown the importance of accounting for non-Newtonian fluid behavior, even in large vessels under certain conditions. De Vita et al. (2015) showed that the shear rate in the aorta can be low enough to cause aggregation, which could change the blood viscosity. This was attributed to the pulsatile and transitional properties of the blood flow.

TABLE 3.3 Navier–Stokes Equations in Developed Form

Navier–Stokes Equations in Cartesian Coordinates

$$\frac{\partial u_x}{\partial x} + \frac{\partial u_y}{\partial y} + \frac{\partial u_z}{\partial z} = 0$$

$$\rho \frac{Du_x}{Dt} = -\frac{\partial p}{\partial x} + \rho g_x + \mu \left(\frac{\partial^2 u_x}{\partial x^2} + \frac{\partial^2 u_x}{\partial y^2} + \frac{\partial^2 u_x}{\partial z^2} \right)$$

$$\rho \frac{Du_y}{Dt} = -\frac{\partial p}{\partial y} + \rho g_y + \mu \left(\frac{\partial^2 u_y}{\partial x^2} + \frac{\partial^2 u_y}{\partial y^2} + \frac{\partial^2 u_y}{\partial z^2} \right)$$

$$\rho \frac{Du_z}{Dt} = -\frac{\partial p}{\partial z} + \rho g_z + \mu \left(\frac{\partial^2 u_z}{\partial x^2} + \frac{\partial^2 u_z}{\partial y^2} + \frac{\partial^2 u_z}{\partial z^2} \right)$$

Navier–Stokes equations in cylindrical coordinates

$$\frac{1}{r} \frac{\partial (r u_r)}{\partial r} + \frac{1}{r} \frac{\partial u_\theta}{\partial \theta} + \frac{\partial u_z}{\partial z} = 0$$

$$\rho \left(\frac{\partial u_r}{\partial t} + u_r \frac{\partial u_r}{\partial r} + \frac{u_\theta}{r} \frac{\partial u_r}{\partial \theta} + u_z \frac{\partial u_r}{\partial z} - \frac{u_\theta^2}{r} \right)$$

$$= -\frac{\partial p}{\partial r} + \rho g_r + \mu \left(\frac{\partial}{\partial r} \left(\frac{1}{r} \frac{\partial (r u_r)}{\partial r} \right) + \frac{1}{r^2} \frac{\partial^2 u_r}{\partial \theta^2} - \frac{2}{r^2} \frac{\partial u_\theta}{\partial \theta} + \frac{\partial^2 u_r}{\partial z^2} \right)$$

$$\rho \left(\frac{\partial u_\theta}{\partial t} + u_r \frac{\partial u_\theta}{\partial r} + \frac{u_\theta}{r} \frac{\partial u_\theta}{\partial \theta} + u_z \frac{\partial u_\theta}{\partial z} + \frac{u_r u_\theta}{r} \right)$$

$$= -\frac{1}{r} \frac{\partial p}{\partial \theta} + \rho g_\theta + \mu \left(\frac{\partial}{\partial r} \left(\frac{1}{r} \frac{\partial (r u_\theta)}{\partial r} \right) + \frac{1}{r^2} \frac{\partial^2 u_\theta}{\partial \theta^2} + \frac{\partial^2 u_\theta}{\partial z^2} + \frac{2}{r^2} \frac{\partial u_r}{\partial \theta} \right)$$

$$\rho \left(\frac{\partial u_z}{\partial t} + u_r \frac{\partial u_z}{\partial r} + \frac{u_\theta}{r} \frac{\partial u_z}{\partial \theta} + u_z \frac{\partial u_z}{\partial z} \right)$$

$$= -\frac{\partial p}{\partial z} + \rho g_z + \mu \left(\frac{1}{r} \frac{\partial}{\partial r} \left(r \frac{\partial u_z}{\partial r} \right) + \frac{1}{r^2} \frac{\partial^2 u_z}{\partial \theta^2} + \frac{\partial^2 u_z}{\partial z^2} \right)$$

When blood begins to flow, the RBC aggregates break into smaller aggregates, which reach an equilibrium size for a fixed shear rate. Increases in shear rate lead to a reduction in equilibrium size and lower effective viscosity. At higher shear rates, the viscosity is influenced by the tendency of RBCs to align with the flow direction and deform. Chien (1970) first demonstrated the role of aggregation and disaggregation on blood viscosity. He compared the viscosities of RBCs suspended in plasma and albumin solutions (the latter of which inhibits aggregation). The viscosity of the suspensions in plasma was higher at low shear rates (less than approximately $5s^{-1}$), when RBC aggregation occurred. To analyze the effect of RBC deformation, Chien used a suspension of hardened RBCs in albumin solution for comparison. The ability of

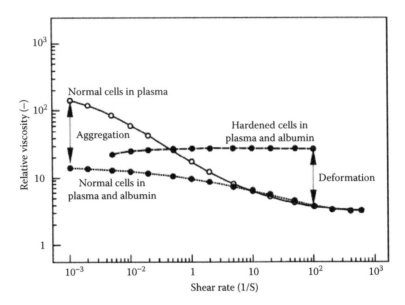

Figure 3.3 Log–log plot of the relative viscosity of RBC suspension (hematocrit, $H = 45\%$) as a function of the shear rate for normal RBC in plasma, normal RBC in albumin solution, and hardened RBCs in albumin solution. (Data from Chien, S., *Science*, 168, 977–979, 1970; Adapted by Vennemann, P. et al., *Exp. Fluids*, 42, 495–511, 2007.)

normal RBCs to deform resulted in a significant decrease in viscosity for all shear rates tested, as shown in Figure 3.3.

3.3.3.1 Power Law
One of the most used non-Newtonian models for blood is the power law. According to this model, the shear stress can be modeled as:

$$\tau_{rz} = K\left(\frac{du_z}{dr}\right)^n, \tag{3.12}$$

where K represents the fluid consistency index in Pa.s^n, n is the non-Newtonian behavior index (dimensionless, <1), u_z is the streamwise velocity of the fluid, and r is the coordinate normal to the vessel wall. When K increases, the viscosity of the fluid increases. K can be influenced by the hematocrit. This model clearly describes a fluid in which the viscosity decreases with increasing shear rate. This fluid is called shear-thinning fluid or pseudoplastic. The advantage of this constitutive model is its simplicity and the possibility of obtaining analytical solutions to the governing equations. However, this model is not capable of predicting the behavior and viscosity of fluids at very high or very low shear rates, because the law is not a bounded function, that is, at zero shear rate, the viscosity is unbounded, and at infinite shear rate, the viscosity tends to be zero (Robertson et al. 2009). Note that $n = 1$ corresponds to Newtonian behavior, in which case K is the viscosity of the fluid. Typically, for blood,

n lies between 0.6 and 0.8 and K is between 0.09 and 0.042 Pa.s^n. Both variables n and K are dependent on the hematocrit and temperature.

3.3.3.2 Carreau Model

The Carreau model was first introduced by Pierre Carreau and was further developed by Kenji Yasuda (1979). Contrary to the power law, the Carreau model predicts finite viscosities at both low and high shear rates. At low shear rates, the model characterizes a fluid with a finite viscosity μ_0, whereas at high shear rates, the model characterizes a fluid that behaves as a Newtonian fluid, with a viscosity μ_∞. The Carreau–Yasuda model expresses shear stress as:

$$\mu_{app} = \mu_\infty + \left(\mu_0 - \mu_\infty\right)\left(1 + \left(\lambda\gamma\right)^a\right)^{\frac{n-1}{a}}, \tag{3.13}$$

where γ represents the shear rate, λ is the relaxation time, n is the power law index, and a is the shape parameter. The Carreau model represents a special case of the Carreau–Yasuda model, where $a = 2$. Figure 3.4 shows the apparent viscosity of blood predicted by the Carreau law when μ_∞ equals the value for the Newtonian model (i.e., 0.0035 Pa.s) at shear 400 s^{-1}, while the value at zero shear is $\mu_0 = 0.056$ Pa.s.

3.3.3.3 Constitutive Law with Hematocrit Dependency

Some models developed for concentrated suspensions have been applied to blood. Among those, some models were developed to predict blood viscosity based on only the hematocrit, while other models also included the effect of viscosity in shear. For instance, the Walburn and Schneck (1976) model is an extension of the power law model, where

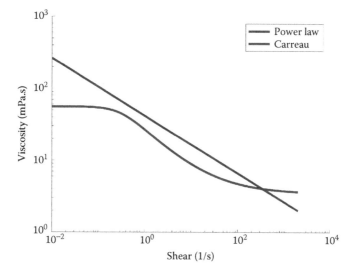

Figure 3.4 Log–log plot of predicted viscosity of blood by Carreau ($\mu_\infty = 0.0035$ Pa.s, $\mu_0 = 0.056$ Pa.s, $\lambda = 3.313$ s, and $n = 0.3568$ [Bauersachs et al. 1989]) and power law model ($K = 0.042$ Pa.s^n and $n = 0.6$) as a function of the shear rate.

K and n are functions of the hematocrit. Quemada's model (Quemada 1978a, 1978b) was formulated from empirical fits of experimental data. To describe the shear-thinning behavior and the dependence of the hematocrit, the apparent viscosity μ_a was defined as:

$$\mu_a = \mu_a\left(k, H\right) = \frac{\mu_q}{\left(1 - \dfrac{1}{2kH}\right)^2}, \tag{3.14}$$

where $\mu_q = 3.5$ mPa, and $k = \dfrac{k_0 + k_\infty \sqrt{\dot{\gamma}/\gamma_c}}{\left(1 + \sqrt{\dot{\gamma}/\gamma_c}\right)}$ is an intrinsic viscosity expressed in terms of Quemada, with parameters $\gamma_c = 1.88$ s^{-1}, $k_0 = 4.33$, and $k_\infty = 2.07$ (Robertson et al. 2009). Figure 3.5 shows the apparent viscosity of blood predicted by Quemada's model. Popel proposed an analytical solution to study the flow of a Quemada's fluid in a circular tube (Popel and Enden 1993).

In the presented models, the dependence of the material properties on the time over which shear is applied (thixotropic behavior) is not taken into account. The thixotropic behavior of blood is largely due to the finite time required for the RBC aggregates to form and break down, as well as, probably at higher shear, due to the transition and relaxation times needed for RBCs to change shapes and orientations. It should be noted that experimental measurements of viscosity are usually discontinuous, such as the one presented in Figure 3.3: for each shear rate, the viscosity is recorded after 2 minutes of applying a constant shear to allow for reaching equilibrium in the structural arrangement. When the shear rate is constantly changing, to the effect that there is no possibility for the aggregates to approach an equilibrium arrangement, the response of the material to variable shear is more complex than

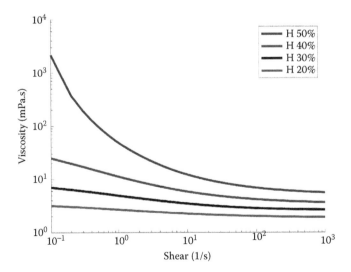

Figure 3.5 Log–log plot of predicted viscosity of blood by Quemada's model as a function of the shear rate for various hematocrits. Computed with parameters $\mu_q = 0.0035$ Pa.s, $\gamma_c = 1.88$ s^{-1}, $k_0 = 4.33$, and $k_\infty = 2.07$.

that under step loading. The thixotropic response was first investigated by Bureau et al. (1980). Later, Owens (2006) developed a new constitutive equation that described blood behavior, including the dynamics of aggregation and disaggregation.

3.4 Dimensional Analysis

Dimensional analysis is a powerful tool to investigate fluid problems. It allows one to analyze the relative contribution of different forces (or factors) and then simplify the equations or choose a set of equations accordingly. In addition, writing dimensionless equations makes it possible to manipulate quantities independently of the units used to measure them, as any consistent set of units will work. As long as the characteristic features are preserved, an experiment can then be conducted in a larger or smaller structure than the original one or by using a different fluid. In computational fluid dynamics, the use of dimensionless equations will prevent round-off errors caused by the manipulation of very large or small numbers. After presenting a selection of useful dimensionless numbers for cardiovascular dynamics, we will present how to write dimensionless equations.

3.4.1 Reynolds Number in Pipe Flows

The Reynolds number may be described as the ratio of inertial forces $\rho V_0^2/2$ to viscous forces $\mu V_0/L_0$, and, consequently, it quantifies the relative importance of these forces for given flow conditions. For a pipe, Re is defined as follows:

$$Re = \frac{\rho L_0 V_0}{\mu},$$
(3.15)

where ρ is the fluid density, μ is the dynamic viscosity of the fluid, V_0 is the characteristic velocity of the flow (usually the maximum or the average velocity), and L_0 is the characteristic length (usually taken as D, the diameter for pipe flow).

3.4.2 Womersley Number in Pipe Flows

The Womersley number α is a dimensionless parameter used to characterize a cyclical flow.

$$\alpha = R\sqrt{\frac{\omega \rho}{\mu}},$$
(3.16)

where R is the vessel radius and ω is the cyclical frequency or the heart rate in radians/sec. Analogous to the Reynolds number in a steady flow, the Womersley number is the ratio of unsteady inertial forces to viscous forces. Further details are presented in Section 3.5.3.

3.4.3 Dean Number in Curved Pipe Flows

The Dean number aims to study the relative importance of centrifugal force in flows in curved pipes and channels. The Dean number may be described as the ratio of inertial forces times the centrifugal force to viscous forces, as follows:

$$De = \frac{\sqrt{\dfrac{\rho V_0^2}{2} \cdot \dfrac{\rho L_0 V_0^2}{R_c}}}{\dfrac{\mu V_0}{L_0}} = \frac{\rho L_0 V_0}{\mu} \sqrt{\frac{L_0}{2 R_c}} = Re \sqrt{\frac{L_0}{2 R_c}}, \tag{3.17}$$

where L_0 is the characteristic length, typically the diameter, and R_c is the radius of curvature of the path of the channel. Typically, for low Dean numbers ($De < 36$), the flow is unidirectional. It has been shown that as the Dean number increases beyond a critical value of about 36, recirculations called Dean cells appear, an example of which is shown in Figure 3.6. These manifest as secondary vortical flow structures, with their axes of rotation in the axial flow direction. Finally, for large Reynolds numbers, these Dean structures become unstable.

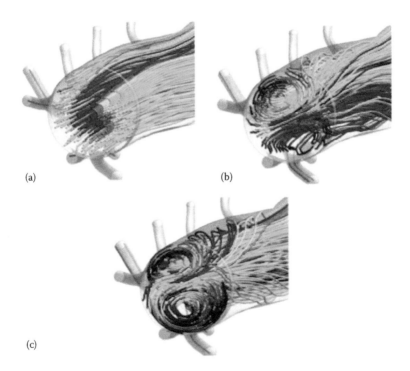

(a)   (b)

(c)

Figure 3.6 Streamlines of blood flow in the descending thoracic rabbit aorta in a posterior–anterior view when (a) $Re = 50$ and $De = 25$, (b) $Re = 300$ and $De = 150$, and (c) $Re = 1300$ and $De = 650$. (Reproduced from Vincent, P. E. et al., *R. Soc. Interface*, 8, 1708–1719, 2011.)

3.4.4 Dimensionless Equations

Based on the principles of dimensional analysis, variables u, p, x, y, z, and t can be written as functions of dimensionless variables denoted by $*$. For example, in Cartesian coordinates: $u_x = u_x^* \cdot V_0$, $u_y = u_y^* \cdot V_0$, $u_z = u_z^* \cdot V_0$, $x = x^* \cdot L_0$, $y = y^* \cdot L_0$, $y = y^* \cdot L_0$, and $t = t^* \cdot V_0/L_0$, where L_0 and V_0 are the characteristic length and velocity, respectively. Note that depending on the flow characteristic that one wishes to emphasize, the dimensionless value of p will be different. For a creeping flow where viscous effects dominate, one could choose $p = p^* \mu V_0/L_0$, whereas for an inertial flow, one will go with $p = p^* \rho V_0^2$.

By changing these variables, the conservation of momentum for a Newtonian incompressible flow, neglecting the effect of gravity, could be rewritten by using the dimensionless numbers defined previously.

$$Re \frac{Du^*}{Dt^*} = -\nabla p^* + \Delta^2 u^* \text{ with } p^* = \frac{pL_0}{\mu V_0}, \tag{3.18}$$

$$\frac{Du^*}{Dt^*} = -\nabla p^* + \frac{1}{Re} \Delta^2 u^* \text{ with } p^* = \frac{p}{\rho V_0^2}. \tag{3.19}$$

For very low Reynolds numbers (<1), a typical situation in flows where the fluid velocities are very low, the viscosities are very large, or the length scales of the flow are very small, the first term of Equation 3.18 could be neglected, giving the so-called Stokes equation that describes creeping flow:

$$\nabla p^* = \Delta^2 u^*. \tag{3.20}$$

When the inertial forces are negligible, time disappears from the equation, leading to an interesting property of Stokes flow, called the reversibility of the flow. This phenomenon is often illustrated by the Taylor–Couette experiment. Another consequence is the difficulty in mixing flows. It should be noted that these properties are true for only incompressible Newtonian fluids, and they do not apply to microcirculation, even if the Reynolds number can be as low as 10^{-2}. Indeed, in microcirculation, blood flow cannot generally be modeled as Newtonian because of nonlinear and time-dependent effects.

For very large Reynolds numbers, a typical situation in flows where the fluid velocities are very high, the viscosities are very low, or the length scales of the flow are very large, the viscous term in Equation 3.19 can be neglected with respect to inertial effects, giving the so-called Euler equation that describes inviscid flow:

$$\nabla p^* + \frac{Du^*}{Dt^*} = 0. \tag{3.21}$$

3.5 Applications

In this section, the solutions to the above equations will be presented for different cases relevant in hemodynamics. For the sake of conciseness, the complete derivations are not presented, but they can be found in classical fluid mechanics textbooks. Therefore, only relevant results will be introduced and discussed from the perspective of their physiological significance.

3.5.1 Flow of a Newtonian Fluid in Simple Geometries

The assumption of blood flow circulating in rigid pipes is commonly used for the analysis of the cardiovascular system. In particular, to estimate the shear rate at the wall and the maximum and average blood velocities, the pressure–flow relationship, commonly called the Poiseuille equation, is used. The Poiseuille equation can be used to estimate the resistance to flow in blood vessels.

For a Newtonian incompressible flow, the velocity profile must satisfy the Navier-Stokes equations. Invoking the no-slip condition, that is, assuming that the velocity is null at the wall of the pipe $(u_z(R)=0)$, axisymmetric flow develops, implying that the shear is null at the center of the pipe $(du_z/dr(0)=0)$; the velocity profile in the pipe is then given by Equation 3.22 in cylindrical coordinates:

$$u_z(r) = -\frac{R^2}{4\mu}\left(\frac{dp}{dz}\right)\left(1 - \frac{r^2}{R^2}\right), \tag{3.22}$$

where R is the radius of the vessel.

By integrating the velocity profile over the pipe cross-section, the so-called Poiseuille equation is then obtained:

$$Q = -\frac{\pi R^4}{8\mu}\left(\frac{dp}{dz}\right). \tag{3.23}$$

Note that the pressure gradient dp/dz is negative because of the pressure drop along the pipe, and this results in a positive flow rate Q. The equation is commonly expressed in the form

$$Q = \frac{\Delta p \pi R^4}{8\mu L},$$

where $\Delta p/L = -dp/dz$. Additional results from the Poiseuille solution for pipes of different-shaped cross-sections are given in Table 3.4. These include the average velocity, maximum velocity at the center of the pipe, and shear stress in the direction of the flow. Similar equations can be written for vessels having other cross-sections. For example, an ellipsoidal-shaped tube will better reflect the geometry of veins, while a parallel-plate geometry is useful to model in vitro endothelial flow chambers. The relations for these shapes are compared in Table 3.4.

TABLE 3.4 Newtonian, Incompressible Flow in Pipes of Different Shapes

	Circular Cross-Section (Cylinder)	Elliptical Cross-Section	Parallel Plates (length L and width w)
Velocity profile	$u_z(r) = \dfrac{\Delta p}{L}\dfrac{R^2}{4\mu}\left(1-\dfrac{r^2}{R^2}\right)$	$u_z(x,y) = \dfrac{\Delta p}{2\mu L}\dfrac{a^2 b^2}{a^2+b^2}\left(1-\dfrac{x^2}{a^2}-\dfrac{y^2}{b^2}\right)$	$u_z(x) = \dfrac{h^2}{2\mu}\dfrac{\Delta p}{L}\left(1-\dfrac{x^2}{h^2}\right)$
Average velocity	$\bar V = \dfrac{\Delta p R^2}{8\mu L}$	$\bar V = \dfrac{\Delta p}{4\mu L}\dfrac{a^2 b^2}{a^2+b^2}$	$\bar V = \dfrac{\Delta p h^2}{3\mu L}$
Maximum velocity	$2\bar V$	$2\bar V$	$\dfrac{3}{2}\bar V$
Pressure–flow relationship	$Q = \dfrac{\pi \Delta p R^4}{8\mu L}$	$Q = \dfrac{\pi \Delta p}{4\mu L}\dfrac{a^3 b^3}{a^2+b^2}$	$Q = \dfrac{2\Delta p w h^3}{3\mu L}$
Shear stress	$\tau_{rx} = -\dfrac{\Delta p}{2L}r$ $\tau_{rx} = -Q\dfrac{4\mu}{\pi R^4}r$	$\tau_{xz} = -\dfrac{\Delta p}{L}\dfrac{b^2}{a^2+b^2}x = -Q\dfrac{4\mu}{\pi a^3 b}x$ $\tau_{yz} = -\dfrac{\Delta p}{L}\dfrac{a^2}{a^2+b^2}y = -Q\dfrac{4\mu}{\pi b^3 a}y$	$\tau_{xz} = -\dfrac{\Delta p}{L}x$ $= -Q\dfrac{3\mu}{wh^3}x$
Axial wall shear stress (WSS)	$|WSS| = \dfrac{\Delta p}{2L}R$ $= Q\dfrac{4\mu}{\pi R^3}$	$\|\tau_{nz}\|_{wall} = \dfrac{\Delta p}{L}\dfrac{ab}{a^2+b^2}\sqrt{(b\cos\Phi)^2+(a\sin\Phi)^2}$ $= \dfrac{4\mu Q}{\pi a^2 b^2}\sqrt{(b\cos\Phi)^2+(a\sin\Phi)^2}$	$|WSS| = \dfrac{\Delta p}{L}h$ $= Q\dfrac{3\mu}{wh^2}$

Fluid shear stress is implicated in biological phenomena such as hemolysis, arteriosclerosis formation, and changes in the shape of endothelial cells. For instance, the shape of human endothelial cells changes with the magnitude of fluid shear stress present at the blood vessel wall. One common theory purports that this wall shear stress is a key player in the formation of atherosclerosis, which will be discussed in detail in Chapter 7. It has been observed that low magnitude and oscillating wall shear stress may be related to atherosclerosis (David et al. 1985). To study these physiological phenomena, experiments are performed using culture plates. Typically, a fluid medium (considered Newtonian) is pumped through a rectangular flow chamber, where cells are attached at the bottom. The channel is usually much wider than deep, thereby approximating a flow between parallel plates, where side walls do not have a significant role. The effect of fluid shear stress on endothelial cells can be observed under the microscope. The estimation of shear stress is obtained from the resolution of the Navier–Stokes equations, from which the stress at the wall can be evaluated using the channel dimension and, depending on the experimental setup, either the pressure drop or the flow rate that is imposed on the channel (Table 3.4).

3.5.2 Flow of a Power-Law Fluid in a Circular Pipe

The simplification of the general form of the momentum Equation 3.6 in the z direction, assuming that the Reynolds number is small enough so that inertial effects may be neglected and there is no gravity and other forces, leads to:

$$0 = -\frac{\partial p}{\partial z} + \frac{1}{r}\frac{\partial\left(r\tau_{zr}\right)}{\partial r}. \tag{3.24}$$

After integration, assuming zero shear at the center of the capillary, one obtains $\frac{r}{2}\frac{\partial p}{\partial z} = \tau_{zr}$. Combining this momentum equation with the power law (Equation 3.12) leads to

$$\frac{r}{2}\frac{\partial p}{\partial z} = K\left(\frac{du_z}{dr}\right)^n. \tag{3.25}$$

The velocity profile is then obtained by integration, invoking the no-slip boundary condition at the wall, according to which $u_z = 0$ at $r = R$:

$$u_z = \left(\frac{\Delta p}{2KL}\right)^{1/n}\frac{n}{n+1}\left[R^{(n+1)/n} - r^{(n+1)/n}\right]. \tag{3.26}$$

One can then integrate the velocity to obtain the flow rate:

$$Q = \frac{n\pi R^3}{3n+1}\left(\frac{R\Delta p}{2KL}\right)^{1/n}. \tag{3.27}$$

Resulting from these relations, expressions for the average velocity, maximum velocity, and shear stress are obtained as functions of n and K:

$$\bar{V} = \frac{nR}{3n+1}\left(\frac{R\Delta p}{2KL}\right)^{1/n},$$

$$V_{max} = \frac{3n+1}{n+1}\bar{V},$$

$$\tau_{zr} = -\frac{r}{2}\frac{\Delta p}{L} = -r\left(\frac{Q(3n+1)}{n\pi}\right)^{n}\frac{K}{R^{(3n+1)}}$$

3.5.3 Pulsatile Newtonian Flow in a Pipe

The solutions presented earlier in this chapter were for steady flows in rigid tubes, in which the driving pressure gradient was constant in time. While these approximations are useful to study blood flow in veins or through an extracorporeal circuit during hemodialysis or surgery, it is well known that blood flow in the circulatory system is unsteady, that is, not constant in time. More specifically, blood flow is pulsatile, meaning that the pressure and flow velocities vary periodically. Womersley described the dimensionless parameter α, the Womersley number (Equation 3.16), which characterizes the nature of an unsteady flow. He also developed a method to solve the Navier–Stokes equations for any given pressure wave in a rigid pipe (Womersley 1955).

Typical Womersley numbers are presented in Table 3.5 for various locations within the circulation and for various animal species. As α increases (e.g., as vessel size and heart rate increase), the unsteady inertial forces become more dominant. The inertial forces initiate at the center of the tube and result in blunter velocity profiles across the vessel diameter, while the viscous effects are confined near the walls of the vessel. A delay in the bulk fluid velocity exists relative to the driving pressure gradient.

TABLE 3.5 Typical Womersley Numbers for Different Vessels in the Human Circulation and in the Aortas of Different Animals

Species/Vessel	r (mm)	HR (bpm)	μ (cP)	α
Human adult aorta at rest	12.5	72	3.5	19
Arteriole	0.4	72	3.5	0.3
Capillary	0.008	72	<3.5	<0.01
Mouse aorta	0.7	550	4.9[a]	2.5
Dog aorta (Labrador retriever)	7.5	90	5.6[a]	10
Horse aorta	18.5	36	5.2[a]	16

Source: Windberger, U. et al., *Exp. Physiol.*, 88, 431–440, 2003.

r is the vessel radius in mm, and HR is the heart rate in beats per minute (bpm).

[a] Blood viscosities at shear rate $\gamma = 94\ \text{s}^{-1}$.

In capillaries, α is very small ($\ll 1$) and the flow is quasi-steady (i.e., the effects of pulsatility can be neglected). Indeed, the pulsatile fluctuations that are strong in the aorta, at the outlet of the left ventricle, are dampened by the vascular compliance as the flow progresses through the arteries and the arterioles and diminish as the vessels become smaller, until blood flow is nearly steady by the time blood reaches the capillaries and returns to the lungs through the veins.

Note that the normal resting heart rates increase with decreasing animal size. The heart of a mouse beats more than seven times faster than that of a human. Heart rates in babies are also normally higher than those in adults. This helps offset the effects of smaller blood vessel sizes in small animals, which causes a significant decrease in the Womersley number and change in the balance between inertial and viscous forces. Even so, Womersley numbers tend to be higher in larger animals, meaning that the inertial fluid forces are relatively more significant than in the circulation of smaller mammals.

3.5.3.1 Womersley Solution to Estimate the Unsteady Blood Velocity in a Straight, Rigid Tube
Herein, blood vessels are assumed to be rigid and axisymmetric (cylindrical). The time-varying velocity profile in a straight, rigid tube can be solved for a pulsatile flow by starting from the continuity and Navier–Stokes equations in cylindrical coordinates for the unsteady flow of an incompressible Newtonian fluid, in the z direction, with no body forces.

Assuming that the radial and azimuthal velocities are zero and that the flow is fully developed in the z direction, from applying the continuity equation, the Navier–Stokes equations reduce to:

$$\frac{\partial u_z}{\partial t} = -\frac{1}{\rho}\frac{\partial p}{\partial z} + \frac{\mu}{\rho}\left(\frac{\partial^2 u_z}{\partial r^2} + \frac{1}{r}\frac{\partial u_z}{\partial r}\right).$$

It is reasoned that the pressure in the tube is a function of only t and z. The axial pressure gradient $\partial p/\partial z$ can then be written as a Fourier series, as:

$$\frac{\partial p}{\partial z} = \mathbb{R}\left(\sum_{n=0}^{\infty} a_n e^{i\omega nt}\right),$$

where a_n is a constant representing the amplitude of the harmonic n of the pressure gradient, ω is the fundamental frequency, i is the unit complex number, and $\mathbb{R}$ denotes the real component. Each component of the axial pressure gradient can then be written as:

$$\left.\frac{\partial p}{\partial z}\right|_n = a_n e^{i\omega nt}.$$

Recalling that the axial pressure gradient is the driving force dictating the flow velocity, velocity u_z will then take a similar form:

$$u_z = \mathbb{R}\left(\sum_{n=0}^{\infty} u_{z,n} \right),$$

with

$$u_{z,n} = f_n(r)e^{i\omega nt}.$$

Taking the partial derivatives of velocity u_z gives

$$\left. \frac{\partial u_z}{\partial t} \right|_n = \frac{\partial}{\partial t}\left(f_n(r)e^{i\omega nt} \right) = i\omega n f_n(r)e^{i\omega nt},$$

$$\left. \frac{\partial u_z}{\partial r} \right|_n = \frac{\partial}{\partial r}\left(f_n(r)e^{i\omega nt} \right) = e^{i\omega nt}\frac{\partial f_n}{\partial r},$$

and

$$\left. \frac{\partial^2 u_z}{\partial r^2} \right|_n = e^{i\omega nt}\frac{\partial^2 f_n}{\partial r^2}.$$

These expressions can then be substituted into the reduced Navier–Stokes equation, and after some simple mathematical manipulation, they provide a set of n equations:

$$\frac{d^2 f_n(r)}{dr^2} + \frac{1}{r}\frac{df_n(r)}{dr} + \lambda^2 f_n(r) = B, \tag{3.28}$$

where $\lambda^2 = -in\omega\rho/\mu$ and $B = a_n/\mu$. These equations can further be solved for $f_n(r)$ by using a zero-order Bessel function. The velocity profile as a function of radius r and time t, for a given driving pressure, is obtained by adding together the n harmonics $f_n(r)e^{i\omega nt}$. When Equation 3.28 is made dimensionless, the Womersley number appears and characterizes the term that brings the nonlinear effect:

$$\frac{d^2 f_n(r)}{dr^{*2}} + \frac{1}{r^*}\frac{df_n(r)}{dr^*} - in\alpha^2 f_n(r) = BR^2.$$

Indeed, when α is small, one can neglect the third term, and the solutions for each harmonic are parabolic, resulting in a succession of parabolic profiles independent of time.

3.6 Flows in Networks: Electrical Analogies

3.6.1 Flow Resistance

The term "electrical current" is derived from hydraulic equivalents, because electricity was originally understood to be a type of fluid. Hydraulic resistance is related to the fluid pressure and the flow rate of the fluid in a way that is similar to how resistance in electrical circuits is related to voltage and current, as illustrated in Figure 3.7. The equivalent hydraulic resistance of a complex flow network depends on the viscosity of the fluid flowing through the channels and on the geometry of the channels. The equivalent hydraulic resistance is computed by summing up the individual resistances in series or in parallel, as with electrical circuits, by using the following equations:

$$R_{eq_{series}} = R_1 + R_2 + \ldots + R_n,$$

$$R_{eq_{parallel}}^{-1} = R_1^{-1} + R_2^{-1} + \ldots + R_n^{-1}.$$

These simple additive laws are valid only in the limit of low Reynolds numbers ($Re \to 0$) and for long narrow channels.

In the overall circuit, the pressure drop (Δp) of a fluidic feature is equal to the flow rate (Q) multiplied by the hydraulic resistance (R_{hyd}). The hydraulic resistance is then defined as $R_{hyd} = \Delta p / Q$. Recalling the Poiseuille flow developed earlier for a straight circular rigid pipe, with Newtonian incompressible flow, the hydraulic resistance is then:

$$R_{hyd} = \frac{8\mu L}{\pi R^4}.$$

Note that the unit of R_{hyd} is Pa.s/m^3. Since R_{hyd} is based on the viscosity of the fluid, it can be represented by the viscosity multiplied by a resistance factor X_{hyd}, such that $R_{hyd} = \mu_{app} X_{hyd}$. X_{hyd} is then a constant based on only geometrical parameters and is expressed in m^{-3}. The equations for the hydraulic resistance factors

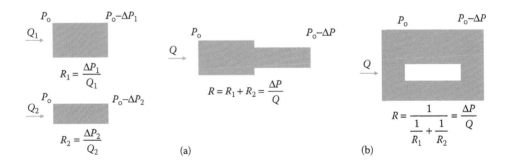

Figure 3.7 Series (a) and parallel (b) coupling of two channels with hydraulic resistances R_1 and R_2.

TABLE 3.6   List of Hydraulic Resistance Factors X_{hyd} for Straight Channels with Different Cross-Sectional Shapes

Shape	X_{hyd}
Circle	

$$\frac{8}{\pi} L \frac{1}{R^4}$$

| Ellipse | |

$$\frac{4}{\pi} L \frac{a^2 + b^2}{a^3 b^3}$$

Parallel plates (length L and width w)

$$\frac{3L}{2wh^3}$$

Rectangle

$$\frac{12L}{1 - 0.63(h/w)} \frac{1}{wh^3}$$

Square

$$\frac{12L}{1 - 0.917(0.63)} \frac{1}{h^4}$$

of individual vessel segments or flow channels having different cross-sectional geometries are tabulated in Table 3.6.

In Chapter 1, we described the anatomy and physiology of blood vessels, as well as the mechanisms that enable them to adjust the system resistance in order to restrict or enable blood flow and regulate blood pressure. This resistance, primarily regulated by the arterioles, is analogous to electrical resistance R. The total resistance of a circulatory system, often called the peripheral resistance R_p, can be calculated as $R_p = P_a - P_v/CO \approx P_a/CO$, where P_a and P_v are the average aortic and venous pressures, respectively, and CO is the cardiac output (Westerhof et al. 2009).

3.6.2 System Compliance

In Chapter 1, we also discussed the elasticity of blood vessels, which is an important characteristic of larger arteries. The ability of arteries to stretch under pressure and hold additional fluid volume in reserve is described as compliance, denoted as C.

A measure of an artery's compliance or distensibility is defined as $C = dV/dP$, where dV is the unit change in volume for unit change in pressure dP. The compliance of a circulation system is analogous to the capacitance of an electrical circuit, that is, the ability to store an electric charge. Because of their thinner walls, veins have a much higher compliance than arteries. Among other methods, arterial compliance can be evaluated by measuring the arterial diameter by ultrasound imaging, while simultaneously monitoring blood pressure. As discussed in Chapter 15, compliance diminishes with age. A change in arterial compliance may indicate an alteration of the elastic and collagen fibers in the arterial wall, an accumulation of deposits in the vessel, or alterations in muscular tone.

3.6.3 Analogy to Electric RLC Circuits

It is often useful to model the circulatory system as a network by using analogies to electric RLC circuits (circuits consisting of resistance (R), inductance (L), and capacitance (C) elements) to predict an output response to specific system inputs, conditions, or changes to these conditions. In such representations, blood flow rate Q is analogous to electrical current I (consider electrical current as the flow rate of electrons). The pressure gradient P driving the flow is analogous to the voltage potential V across a circuit. The first lumped parameter model of the arterial system was formulated by Otto Frank (1899). Consisting of one resistance and one compliance element (Figure 3.8), it has since then been called the two-element Windkessel model. The name came from an earlier analogy made by Westerhof (2009), in which the volume elasticity of the large arteries was compared to the German Windkessels (literally meaning air chambers) that were used to dampen pressure fluctuations of water in eighteenth-century fire engines.

These simplified models of the circulation are referred to as "lumped parameter" models, as only the net properties of the system are considered (e.g., compliance and resistance) instead of the continuous distribution of these parameters throughout

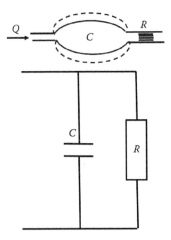

Figure 3.8   The two-element Windkessel model.

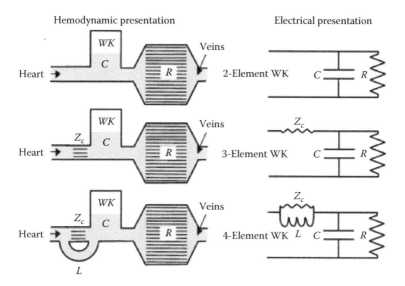

Figure 3.9 The two-element Windkessel, the three-element Windkessel, and the four-element Windkessel models presented in hydraulic and electrical forms. Z_c is the aortic characteristic impedance and equals $\rho PWV/A$. It connects Frank's Windkessel model with wave transmission models. PWV is the pulse wave velocity in the proximal aorta, ρ is blood density, and A is the area of the proximal aorta. (Reproduced from Westerhof, N. et al., *Med. Biol. Eng. Comput.*, 47, 131–141, 2009.)

the system, and these properties are represented as single lumped elements. As such, they are useful for lower-resolution analyses but are not capable of modeling the local behavior of the circulatory system, which requires high spatial resolution.

The two-element Windkessel model was improved by considering resistance and/or inertance terms and by considering the effects of reflected waves (three- and four-elements models). These models are briefly presented in Figure 3.9 and are discussed in more detail by Westerhof et al. (2009).

3.7 Conclusion

The cardiovascular system encompasses a wide range of flow types, from near-turbulent and pulsatile flows in the large arteries (or turbulent for some pathological cases) to the highly laminar, quasi-steady flows in the microcirculation. The complete understanding of the relationship between pressure, flow, and cardiovascular symptoms remains a critical problem. Models of blood flow should be often coupled with structural dynamics (e.g., of vessel walls and cells), involving intricate problem resolution of fluid–structure interactions. The complexity of the fluid flow in the cardiovascular system requires the power of advanced simulation tools, which will be presented in Chapter 6. The accuracy of the predictions from blood flow mechanics are fundamentally dependent on the assumptions made in the transport equations. Whether for mathematical resolution or when using numerical tools, correct modeling of a problem is the starting point to success. The objective in this chapter was to introduce some tools to define blood flow problems. Current research is taking a new look at this vital issue by accounting for the complexity of blood as a suspension and investigating phenomena at the micro scale, as will be discussed in Chapter 12. Important discoveries regarding the importance of the deformability of RBCs in blood flow continue to be made (Abkarian and Viallat 2016).

References

Abkarian, M., and A. Viallat. 2016. Chap 10: On the importance of the deformability of red blood cells in blood flow. In C. Duprat and H. A. Stone (Eds.), *Fluid–Structure Interactions in Low-Reynolds-Number Flows*. Cambridge, UK: The Royal Society of Chemistry, pp. 347–462.

Bauersachs, R. M., R. B. Wenby, and H. J. Meiselman. 1989. Determination of specific red blood cell aggregation indices via an automated system. *Clin Hemorheol* 9(1):1–25.

Bruus, H. 2006. *Theoretical Microfluidics*. Lecture notes third edition. Copenhagen, Denmark: MIC – Department of Micro and Nanotechnology, Technical University of Denmark.

Bureau, M., J. C. Healy, D. Bourgoin, and M. Joly. 1980. Rheological hysteresis of blood at low shear rate. *Biorheology* 17(1–2):191–203.

Chien, S. 1970. Shear dependence of effective cell volume as a determinant of blood viscosity. *Science* 168:977–979.

David, N. K., D. P. Giddens, C. K. Zarins, and S. Glagov. 1985. Pulsatile flow and atherosclerosis in the human carotid bifurcation. Positive correlation between plaque location and low and oscillating shear stress. *Arterosclerosis* 5(3):293–302.

Dawson, T. H. 2008. Modeling the vascular system and its capillary networks. In P. J. Yim (Ed.), *Vascular Hemodynamics: Bioengineering and Clinical Perspectives*. New Brunswick, NJ: John Wiley, pp. 1–35.

De Vita, F., M. de Tullio, and R. Verzicco. 2015. Numerical simulation of the non-Newtonian blood flow through a mechanical aortic valve. *Theor Comput Fluid Dyn* 30:129–138.

Frank, O. 1899. Die Grundform des arteriellen Pulses. *Z Biol* 37:483–526.

Fung, Y. C. 1993. *Biomechanics Mechanical Properties of Living Tissues*. Berlin, Germany: Springer-Verlag.

Garcia, D., and L. Kadem. 2006. What do you mean by aortic valve area: Geometric orifice area, effective orifice area, or gorlin area? *J Heart Valve Dis* 15(5):601–608.

Késmárky, G., P. Kenyeres, M. Rábai, and K. Tóth. 2008. Plasma viscosity: A forgotten variable. *Clin Hemorheol Microcirc* 39(1–4):243–246.

Lanotte, L., M. Mauer, S. Mendez, D. A. Fedosov, J. M. Fromental, V. Claveria, F. Nicoud, G. Gompper, and M. Abkariana. 2016. Red cells' dynamic morphologies govern blood shear thinning under microcirculatory flow conditions. *Proc Natl Acad Sci U S A* 113(47):13289–13294.

Owens, R. G. 2006. A new microstructure-based constitutive model for human blood. *J Non-Newton Fluid Mech* 140(1–3):57–70.

Popel, A. S., and G. Enden. 1993. An analytical solution for steady flow of a Quemada fluid in a circular tube. *Rheol Acta* 32(4):422–426.

Quemada, D. 1978a. Rheology of concentrated dispersed systems: II. A model for non-Newtonian shear viscosity in shear flows. *Rheol Acta* 17:632–642.

Quemada, D. 1978b. Rheology of concentrated dispersed systems: III. General features of proposed non-Newtonian model: Comparison with experimental data. *Rheol Acta* 17:643–653.

Robertson, A. M., A. Sequeira, and R. G. Owens. 2009. Chap 6: Rheological models for blood. In L. Formaggia, A. Quarteroni, and A. Veneziani (Eds.), *Cardiovascular Mathematics: Modeling and Simulation of the Circulatory System*. Milano, Italy: Springer-Verlag Italia.

Vennemann, P., R. Lindken, and J. Westerweel. 2007. In vivo whole-field blood velocity measurement techniques. *Exp Fluids* 42:495–511.

Vincent, P. E., A. M. Plata, A. A. E. Hunt, P. D. Weinberg, and S. J. Sherwin. 2011. Blood flow in the rabbit aortic arch and descending thoracic aorta. *R Soc Interface* 8:1708–1719.

Walburn, F. J., and D. J. Schneck. 1976. A constitutive equation for whole human blood. *Biorheology* 13(3):201–210.

Westerhof, N., J. W. LankhaarBerend, and E. Westerhof. 2009. The arterial Windkessel. *Med Biol Eng Comput* 47(2):131–141.

Windberger, U., A. Bartholovitsch, R. Plasenzotti, K. J. Korak, and G. Heinze. 2003. Whole blood viscosity, plasma viscosity and erythrocyte aggregation in nine mammalian species: reference values and comparison of data. *Exp Physiol* 88(3):431–440.

Womersley, J. R. 1955. Method for the calculation of velocity, rate of flow and viscous drag in arteries when the pressure gradient is known. *J Physiol* 127(3):553–563.

Yasuda, K. 1979. Investigation of the analogies between viscometric and linear viscoelastic properties of polystyrene fluids. PhD thesis, Massachusetts Institute of Technology, Department of Chemical Engineering.

4

Experimental Methods in Cardiovascular Mechanics

M. R. Labrosse and L. Kadem

Contents

4.1 Introduction

This chapter focuses on those investigative methods that belong in the laboratory rather than in the clinic. This means that tissues and organs may be excised and tested at will and that the invasiveness of the method to obtain samples is usually not an issue. However, the availability and dimensions of the samples are typically limited. The fundamental goals of experimental testing in the context of cardiovascular mechanics may be multifold. For instance, while the main driver may be to understand how normal tissues or organs work (basic science), a secondary driver may be to differentiate between the workings of normal tissues or organs and the diseased ones, to be able to tell them apart (diagnosis), or to mitigate the effects of the disease (treatment). Normal tissues or organs may also be studied to establish target values in reparative processes or in the design of prostheses for organ replacement. In addition, experimental measurements on in vitro models are of primary importance for the validation of clinical parameters used in the diagnosis of cardiovascular diseases and in the development of cardiovascular medical devices.

As pointed out by epistemologists, experimentation, as opposed to mere observation, presupposes the existence, at least in a tentative fashion, of a game plan, theory, or model to be tested and quantified, or otherwise disproved (this is the "why?" of the experiments). As such, experimentation is a concerted act of probing the unknown. Obviously, great attention to detail and meticulousness are required, along with the choice of proper experimental techniques (this is the "how?" of the experiments).

Whether at the tissue level or organ level, challenges arise from cardiovascular tissues featuring highly nonlinear stress–strain relationships (i.e., Hooke's law does not apply), large deformations with respect to the unpressurized configuration (the definitions of linear strains, as often used in engineering, do not apply), heterogeneity (material differences at different locations in the sample), marked anisotropy (differences in mechanical behavior in different orientations of the sample), frequent presence of residual loads (internal loads, understood as stresses or strains, that exist in the absence of external loading), and complex boundary conditions (tissues may be prestretched in vivo, in a way that may or may not be easy to reproduce in the laboratory). In experiments involving blood flow, additional challenges arise, for example, from the need for appropriate equipment design and blood analogs to enable the use of the optical methods required to investigate the details of the flow. In any event, variability has to be expected, not only between samples from the same source but also depending on the source of the sample, owing to, for instance, gender, age, and medical history. Importantly, for statistical analyses, the sample size should refer to the number of subjects from which the samples have been analyzed, such that multiple samples from the same subjects do not skew the results.

At the tissue level, quantification of the biomechanical behavior falls under the umbrella of material characterization and needs to adhere to strict requirements from continuum mechanics. For instance, one is not interested in developing or using constitutive equations that violate the laws of thermodynamics! At the organ level, quantification of the biomechanical behavior is usually synonymous with the assessment of organ function, which may need to be carried out in ways compatible with clinical practice. For example, a new prosthetic heart valve will be tested for its opening and closing characteristics under a range of cardiac outputs that are physiologically meaningful. Indeed, experiments in cardiovascular mechanics must generally explore behaviors that, at minimum, include those found under physiological conditions.

Regarding the recording and analysis of measurements, accuracy refers to the closeness of a measured value to a standard or known (true) value (ISO 2008). Accuracy is achieved when statistical bias, the amount of inaccuracy with respect to the true value, is small. Practically, accuracy is quantified by a measurement tolerance and requires the calibration of the measurement system at regular intervals. The resolution of a measurement is the smallest change in the underlying physical quantity that produces a response in the measurement. Precision, on the other hand, refers to the closeness of two or more measurements to each other (ISO 2008). Precision is achieved when statistical variability is small. Therefore, it includes repeatability and reproducibility. A measurement system can be accurate but not precise, precise but not accurate, neither accurate nor precise, or both accurate and precise, as desired. It is also worth pointing out that, in numerical analysis, accuracy is the closeness of a calculation to the true value (Macneal and Harder 1985), as expected, while precision is the resolution of the representation, typically defined by the number of decimal or binary digits.

Although cardiovascular tissues are, at the microscopic level, multiphasic materials in that they contain fluids and solids in various proportions, their biomechanical testing is usually carried out at the macroscopic level, where the solid and fluid phases can be considered separately. The outline of the present chapter will reflect this, by separately presenting experimental methods for solids and fluids that exist in the context of cardiovascular mechanics, before discussing animal models.

4.2 Solids Aspects

4.2.1 General Considerations

4.2.1.1 Storage
Proper storage of cardiovascular soft tissues is of practical concern if the tissues are harvested relatively far away from the location of testing and/or if availability of the testing equipment is limited. Tissues are typically considered fresh for testing purposes, as long as they are stored for less than 24 hours, in saline or phosphate-buffered

saline (PBS) solution, at a temperature of 4°C. By using pressurization testing, it was determined that storage in physiological saline at 4°C up to 28 days did not significantly alter the passive mechanical properties of common carotid arteries of mice (Amin et al. 2011). However, the authors noticed that significant effects on stretch ratio and stress were due to decreases in the unloaded dimensions with storage time, when measured from cut arterial rings; alternatively, they reported that there were no significant changes with storage time when the unloaded dimensions were measured from histology sections instead. Similar findings were obtained by others (Adham et al. 1996). Nevertheless, for storage longer than 24 hours, many investigators recommend freezing at −80°C, as it has been reported to not significantly affect the mechanical properties of tissues for up to a year (Stemper et al. 2007; Chow et al. 2011), even though cold storage may be expected to result in bulk redistribution of water, damage to the collagen network from ice crystals, and breaking of crosslinks in the extracellular matrix (ECM) (Narine et al. 2006; Schenke-Layland et al. 2007). Alternatively, more advanced cryopreservation techniques are available to mitigate these aspects and preserve tissue properties (Lisy et al. 2017).

4.2.1.2 Temperature During Testing

Soft tissues are best kept moist or immersed at all times during testing, so as not to affect their high water content and artificially alter their properties. Conditions close to the in vivo environment can be replicated at a temperature of 37°C, along with the use of a physiological solution such as saline, PBS, and Krebs-Ringer solution. Several studies reported complex changes in the mechanical properties of human aorta and carotid artery with changes in temperature during testing (namely, 17°C, 27°C, 37°C, and 42°C) (Guinea et al. 2005; Atienza et al. 2007). The authors also pointed out the need for further study, as some surgical procedures involving major arteries are performed using systemic hypothermia, sometimes down to 18°C–20°C. When dealing with these important issues, it is most important to keep in mind that the theory of hyperelasticity for soft tissues, as it is most commonly known, was developed with the assumption of isothermal transformations (Humphrey 2002).

When the tissues being tested need to be kept alive for an extended period, say for days or weeks, for example, to study the effect of the mechanical environment on remodeling, organ culture systems or bioreactors that can accommodate the ongoing testing are required (Macrae et al. 2016).

4.2.1.3 Viscoelasticity and Preconditioning

Soft tissues are generally viscoelastic, and they are expected to exhibit different loading and unloading paths, corresponding to the dissipation of energy (hysteresis) during one cyclic loading. Determining the viscoelastic response of cardiovascular tissues, from dynamic shear testing (Courtial et al. 2016) or dynamic pressure–diameter tests (Abé et al. 1986), may be important to design better blood vessel phantoms or prostheses. However, for many other modeling purposes, viscoelastic properties of cardiovascular tissues may be simplified according to the concept of pseudoelasticity, whereby two different elastic behaviors are assumed: one during loading and another during unloading (Fung et al. 1979; Holzapfel et al. 2002). In addition, viscoelasticity may also be ruled out if variations in the strain rate by several orders of magnitude do not affect the stress–strain behavior of interest.

Preconditioning—the repeated cyclic loading and unloading of a specimen—is used to overcome the effects of soft tissue handling and to establish a repeatable reference state from which a pseudoelastic behavior can be hypothesized (Fung et al. 1979). Although the mechanisms underlying the preconditioning effects remain unknown (Zhang et al. 2015), the following observations have been made:

1. Varying the preconditioning protocols can affect the mechanical response of many biological materials, such as porcine aortic valve (Carew et al. 2000) and bovine pericardium (Sacks 2000).
2. The effect of preconditioning is largely dependent on the maximum strain imposed, with larger strains during preconditioning resulting in a decrease in soft tissue stiffness (Cheng et al. 2009; Weisbecker et al. 2012).
3. The effect of preconditioning is similar to a permanent set but different in that a long relaxation time between tests at different strain levels (~24 hours) may result in a "reset" of the material behavior (Sacks 2000).

Based on these observations, it was recently recommended that for arterial tissues, "the preconditioning protocol should be as similar to the testing protocol as possible in terms of maximum strain level and rate, so as not to influence the test data with inconsistent loading patterns. Similarly, during biaxial preconditioning, the ratio between axial stretches should be kept consistent with intended test ratios. If multiple tests are to be carried out on a single specimen, then the preconditioning strain level should be the maximum strain level intended for testing" (Macrae et al. 2016). These investigators also noted that a wide range of preconditioning cycles have been reported in the literature, but to ensure repeatability, 10 cycles should be conducted on the sample before testing, as 10 cycles are more than sufficient to generate repeatable data.

Testing of other cardiovascular tissues (namely porcine aortic valve leaflets, as well as different grades of porcine and bovine pericardia, in their fresh or chemically fixed states), according to these guidelines, produced consistent results under a strain rate of approximately 0.04 s^{-1} (Labrosse et al. 2016). No significant effect on the stress–strain behavior is expected by changing this strain rate value by at least one order of magnitude (Sauren et al. 1983; Naimark 1996).

4.2.2 Histology

Although a direct connection between soft tissue microstructure and mechanical properties has proven largely elusive (Humphrey 2002, pp. 97–99) or require a large amount of data (Hollander et al. 2011), gathering information about the constituents present in a tissue is extremely valuable, not only to pathologists but also to biomedical engineers, to distinguish between healthy and diseased tissues or to qualitatively discuss the mechanical behavior of samples, whether of natural origin or tissue-engineered.

4.2.2.1 Extracellular Matrix (Collagen/Elastin/Glycosaminoglycans)
        and Cell Content

Histology, the study of the microscopic anatomy of cells and tissues (Hillman 2000), has spawned many useful techniques since the second half of the nineteenth century (Table 4.1). These techniques have progressively combined with methods from physics and materials science such as electron microscopy, polarized light microscopy, Fourier-transform infrared spectroscopy, optical coherence tomography, confocal laser scanning microscopy, second harmonic generation, and two-photon excited fluorescence (Bergholt et al. 2016). However, these methods remain qualitative or semiquantitative in nature, and although they might, under the right circumstances, provide insight into the relative spatial distributions of the major constituents of the ECM, they are usually limited by the spatial resolution that they can achieve (Bergholt et al. 2016).

4.2.2.2 Fiber Orientation

Over the years, there has been a shift in interest from phenomenological to structural constitutive modeling (Auricchio 2014), putting a premium on the determination of the microstructural organization of soft tissues, rather than merely curve fitting the mechanical response of the same. As a result, several methods have been proposed to

TABLE 4.1   Stains Used in Cardiovascular Histology and Illustrative References

Stain Name and Cardiovascular Examples	What Does It Stain? In What Color?
Hematoxylin and eosin (H&E) (Iliopoulos et al. 2013; Sassani 2015)	Cell nuclei—blue ECM—pink
Verhoeff–Van Gieson's stain (Holzapfel 2006; Martin et al. 2011)	Cell nuclei and elastic fibers—black Collagen—pink Smooth muscle cells (SMCs)—brown
Sirius red (Iliopoulos et al. 2013; Sassani 2015)	Collagen—red
Masson's trichrome (Pichamuthu et al. 2013)	Cell nuclei and elastic fibers—black Collagen—blue
Russell–Movat's pentachrome (Rego and Sacks 2017)	Cell nuclei and elastic fibers—black Collagen—yellow Glycosaminoglycans (GAGs)—blue Fibrin—bright red Muscle—red
Alcian blue (Narine et al. 2006)	GAGs—blue
Von Kossa (Pham and Sun 2014)	Calcific deposits—black or brown
4,6-diamidino-2-phenylindole (DAPI) (Della Corte et al. 2008)	Cellular DNA—blue under fluorescence
CNA35/OG488 labeling (Megens et al. 2007)	Collagen—green under fluorescence

determine the distributions of collagen fiber orientations in cardiovascular tissues—some destructive and some nondestructive.

In Holzapfel (2006), specimens cut from the human aorta were embedded while maintaining their planar geometry and sectioned serially at 3 mm across the thickness to reveal the fiber orientations in the local circumferential–axial plane. Sixty representative collagen fibers in the intima and adventitia and oblate nuclei of smooth muscle cells in the media were selected per specimen from the histological images. Mean fiber angles and standard deviations were determined numerically from the data by assuming normal distribution and symmetrical arrangement with respect to the circumferential direction.

Optical, nondestructive methods have also been proposed. In small-angle light scattering (SALS), a beam of laser light is passed through tissue, which scatters due to the underlying fiber structure. By using a laser of wavelength close to that of the diameter of collagen/elastin fibers and by using the distribution of intensity of the scattered beam, quantitative measurements of fiber orientation were made in planar tissues such as porcine heart valves (Kunzelman and Cochran 1992; Sacks et al. 1997) and bovine pericardium (Hiester and Sacks 1998). Small-angle light scattering requires specimens to have a thickness less than 500 μm and to be relatively translucent, such that optical clearing (e.g., using a hyperosmotic sugar solution) may be required; SALS measurements are also limited to static states of deformation (Waldman et al. 2002).

Polarized light microscopy is a contrast-enhancing technique that can be useful for analyzing birefringent (or optically anisotropic) materials. Collagen has a molecular structure that is anisotropic, making it linearly birefringent. It can be stained with Picrosirius red dye to enhance its birefringence and visibility under polarized light. The appearance of type I collagen goes from red to yellow as the fiber diameter decreases, and this effect is associated with a decreased level of birefringence (Whittaker et al. 1994). This optical technique has been used for decades to assess the structure of collagenous tissues and has been combined with uniaxial mechanical testing of tissues such porcine heart valves (Hilbert et al. 1996). However, it is limited in that it provides only qualitative information of the spatial distribution and anisotropy of collagen.

Quantitative polarized light microscopy uses the contrast-enhancing technique of polarized light microscopy and adapts it for quantitative analysis by examining multiple polarization states of birefringent materials (Massoumian et al. 2003; Dixon 2015). Another optical technique derived from optical coherence tomography, called optical polarization tractography, was used to reveal the high-resolution fiber orientation and alignment throughout the whole bovine common carotid artery (Azinfar et al. 2017). Two-photon microscopy was used to determine the through-the-thickness orientation of collagen fibers in vascular tissues (Keyes et al. 2011, 2013). Raman spectroscopy, which also primarily reveals information about the relative composition of samples, was tweaked to extract information on the orientation of collagen fibers across the depth of tissues in articular cartilage (Bergholt et al. 2016). This technique may also open new horizons for cardiovascular tissues.

4.2.3 Thickness Measurements

With stress being loosely defined as a force divided by a unit area, it is clear that thickness measurements are crucial to the accurate estimation of stresses in soft tissue samples. Using the incompressibility assumption, the measurement of the variation in thickness during testing is usually not needed, as long as the thickness in the undeformed reference state can be established. In a landmark comparative study of thickness measurement methods, including Vernier calipers, micrometer, thickness gauge, glass slide technique coupled with Vernier calipers and micrometers, and a noncontact laser displacement sensor, O'Leary et al. (2013) investigated the accuracy of the methods against ground-truth measurements. These reference measurements were obtained from a photogrammetric approach, whereby the tissue was sliced with a surgical scalpel at three evenly spaced locations, and the thickness was measured at six equidistant locations on each length by using calibrated photographs and edge detection software. The measurements were performed on two tissue types: porcine aorta and human intraluminal thrombus from an abdominal aortic aneurysm (AAA). The interrater and retest reliabilities of Vernier calipers, micrometer, and thickness gauge were also investigated. This study showed that errors in tensile stress estimations of more than 10% could easily be caused by inaccuracies in thickness measurement. In addition, from the multipronged findings of the study, it was recommended that a thickness gauge be used to measure structured tissue such as the aorta and a micrometer be used for unstructured tissue such as AAA intraluminal thrombus.

4.2.4 Elastic Behavior

In the following discussion, full material characterization means that all the modes of deformation, that is, all three direct strains and all three shear strains, of the material are resolved in terms of the corresponding stress components. Full material characterization allows for the computation of stress distribution in tissues under any type of loading. Using the continuum mechanics theory, Holzapfel and Ogden showed that full material characterization is possible for an isotropic hyperelastic material from planar biaxial testing and that, conversely, it is impossible for an anisotropic material from such testing alone (Holzapfel and Ogden 2009). Specifically, "the minimum (ideal) test portfolio that allows full characterization of the properties of transversely isotropic materials consists of either

- Planar biaxial tests with an in-plane shear and separate through-thickness shear tests
- Extension and inflation tests on a tubular specimen combined with torsion and separate through-thickness shear tests (axial shear, azimuthal shear, or simple shear of a patch cut from the tube)" (Holzapfel and Ogden 2009)

If—and this is a common occurrence—one commits to a specific constitutive model, without thoroughly considering the guidelines mentioned from the beginning of

Section 4.2.4 and others, for example (Humphrey 2002), one is intrinsically, and perhaps unwittingly, limited by the underlying assumptions associated with that model. Specifically, equations based on fundamentally two-dimensional (2D) approaches often followed to process results from biaxial testing should be distinguished from the thin sheet or "membrane" approximation, which is a 2D specialization within the framework of a three-dimensional (3D) theory. In a fundamentally 2D theory, a significant part of the 3D constitutive law is missing, and no distinction can be made between compressible and incompressible materials (Holzapfel and Ogden 2009).

These observations are not meant to diminish the value of planar biaxial testing. Indeed, full material characterization is needed only in computer simulations where all the modes of deformation are present. When the focus of a study is rather the differentiation between various levels of tissue properties (e.g., health vs. disease and the effect of age), full material characterization is most likely not required, especially because the associated material constants may neither have any physical meaning nor allow for direct comparisons between samples. This happens mainly if the associated constitutive models are phenomenological. In this respect, stress–strain curves obtained in a well-documented fashion, and over a range that includes but is not limited to physiological values, may be all that is needed. As always, it is especially important to clearly state the nature of the membrane tensions or stresses (e.g., engineering, Cauchy, first Piola-Kirchhoff, and second Piola-Kirchhoff) and stretch ratios or strains reported (e.g., engineering, Green-Lagrange, and Almansi). For cardiovascular tissues, only quantities suited for the description of large deformations should be used, thereby excluding linear elasticity (engineering) descriptors.

In many relevant situations, such as in the study of blood vessels, several modes of deformation can be neglected for the study of function under physiological conditions, relieving some constraints on the experimentalist or analyst regarding full material characterization (Humphrey 2002; Holzapfel and Ogden 2009). However, it is important to keep in mind that cardiovascular surgical procedures such as balloon angioplasty, stenting, and bypass create mechanical loads that are significantly different from physiological loads; in such cases, full material characterization of the relevant blood vessels may be required for modeling.

In general, the state of stress in a deformable solid depends on its geometry (shape), boundary conditions (how it is held in place), material properties, and the loads applied to the sample (here, loads are understood as displacements/rotations or forces/moments). The point in experimental mechanical testing is to achieve a homogeneous state of stress (at least in some portion of the sample) that is independent of the material properties, such that stress and strain can be independently evaluated and then correlated by a constitutive equation. Testing standards have been designed to achieve this goal to high accuracy and repeatability for engineering materials, where all the specimen dimensions and testing conditions are prescribed. However, as far as soft tissues are concerned, this goal has largely remained out of reach.

Figure 4.1 presents a graphical summary of the most common experimental testing methods for cardiovascular tissues.

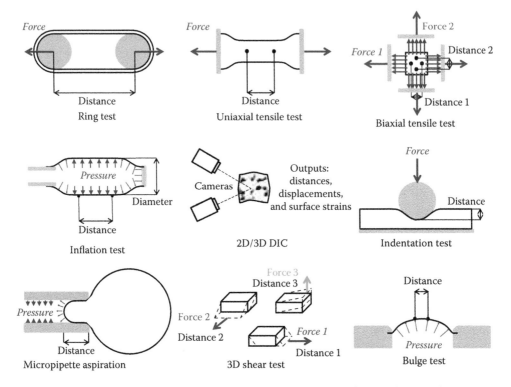

Figure 4.1 Most common experimental testing methods for cardiovascular tissues. Indicated in the figure are the quantities that will be varied during the experiments and that need monitoring, such that stresses and strains in the sample may be derived.

4.2.4.1 Ring Test

The ring tensile test may be used when ring sections can be cut from cylindrical tissue specimens, especially from small arterial tissues (Macrae et al. 2016). The ring is mounted on two parallel pins, which are then separated in a controlled fashion, while the associated reaction force is also recorded. Humphrey pointed out that exact finite strain solutions for this test do not exist in the literature (Humphrey 2002). Not surprisingly, therefore, investigators have combined its use with that of finite element (FE) analyses to solve for the complex loading conditions, including severe bending and crushing of the sample near the fixtures, not to mention the possible residual stresses in the unloaded ring (Askari et al. 2017). In Bustos et al. (2016), the ring tensile test was employed to validate a constitutive model developed for a Dacron graft otherwise based on uniaxial tests. The FE simulation was able to accurately reproduce the experimental findings in terms of force versus displacement of the pins during the ring test. Finally, let us note that given the exclusive uniaxial nature of the test, the ring test cannot be used for full material characterization of cardiovascular tissues.

4.2.4.2 Uniaxial Testing

The ring test described in the previous subsection can be seen as one variant of uniaxial testing, whereby a rectangular strip of tissue (or a dog-bone-shaped sample) is tested along its longitudinal dimension. Since the other two dimensions are uncontrolled, the use of the incompressibility assumption is insufficient to identify the stretch ratios or strains in all three directions of anisotropic samples. However, if the assumption of isotropy can be made, then all the deformations in the axes of the machine may be quantified. Even then, from the theory of continuum mechanics, the stress in the longitudinal direction (the only nonzero stress component) can be expressed in terms of two unknown scalar functions (e.g., derivatives of the strain energy function with respect to the first and second invariants of the right Cauchy-Green tensor) (Humphrey 2002). Obviously, one equation with two unknowns cannot be solved uniquely, which renders uniaxial testing improper for full material characterization of isotropic hyperelastic materials (Humphrey 2002); this statement holds a fortiori for anisotropic hyperelastic materials. However, Holzapfel showed that uniaxial information could be exploited for full material characterization if certain restrictive assumptions can be made about the material's microstructure and behavior and if the orientation of the constitutive fibers could be measured (Holzapfel 2006).

4.2.4.3 Planar Biaxial Testing

As a tool for material characterization of rubber-like and biological membranes, planar biaxial testing has been used for decades, resulting from the understanding, grounded in continuum mechanics, that uniaxial testing is generally insufficient when one's goal is a more advanced, if not full, material characterization of anisotropic hyperelastic materials (Lanir and Fung 1974; Sacks 2000). Planar biaxial testing makes it possible to explore a wide range of loads, understood as forces or displacements, applied at once in two orthogonal directions. The loads applied in both directions may be the same (equibiaxial loading), may be kept in constant proportion between both directions (proportional loading), or may be independent from each other (general biaxial loading). The work from the pioneers of planar biaxial testing strongly supports that series of protocols, including equibiaxial and proportional loadings, should be used for more robust material characterization (Lanir and Fung 1974; Humphrey et al. 1992; Brossollet and Vito 1996; Sacks 2000).

Most experimental setups used to date have been custom-designed, to the effect that a wide disparity in experimental conditions has been the norm (e.g., displacement- vs. force-controlled protocols, grip displacements vs. optical tracking for determination of strains, and rigid grips vs. suture lines). However, integrated biaxial testing equipment specially designed for biological soft tissues has now become commercially available, such as the BioTester (CellScale, Waterloo, Canada).

Regardless of whether one piece of testing equipment is intrinsically better suited to carry out displacement- or force-controlled protocols, it is interesting to note the following: with equibiaxial displacement testing (green dashed line in Figure 4.2), it is possible to miss the upward turn in the curve for the softer direction of the material (and possibly that in the curve for the stiffer direction as well) if the range of displacements is not large enough, or if the capacity of the force gauge is too low in the axis of the stiffer direction of the material. With equibiaxial force testing (black dashed line in Figure 4.2), one could miss both upward turns if the applied force is not high

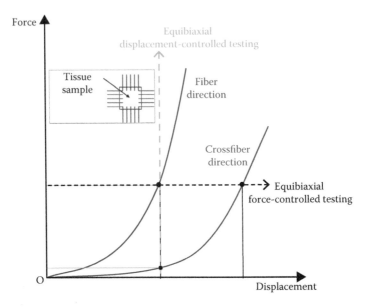

Figure 4.2 Illustrative example of force–displacement curves expected from anisotropic soft tissues under equibiaxial planar biaxial testing. As detailed in the main text, force-controlled biaxial testing is more likely to capture the main features of the curves than displacement-controlled testing.

enough, but if it is high enough, assuming that displacements are not restricted, the upward turns of the curves for both the softer and stiffer directions of the material will be properly captured. Based on these observations, efficient testing protocols can be devised to simulate equibiaxial and general force-controlled testing by using displacement-controlled equipment (Labrosse et al. 2016).

In Waldman and Lee (2002), the authors demonstrated that the method of sample gripping affects not only how the load is transferred to the sample but also how the load is transmitted throughout the rest of the material, thereby influencing the resulting mechanical behavior of the tissue. They compared the biaxial mechanical response of pericardial tissue samples under two different gripping methods: (1) sutures around the sample edges, and (2) a biaxial clamping method. The tissue samples appeared to be stiffer and less extensible when mechanically tested with clamped sample edges, as opposed to when tested with sutured sample edges. They also concluded that it is doubtful that any in vitro mechanical testing method could be used to determine the "real" properties of the tissue, since the boundary conditions of the tissue in situ are unknown. This is an important reminder that, after characterizing specific materials, it is highly desirable, albeit often quite difficult, to verify whether or not the whole organ made up of these materials behaves as expected when simulated. For instance, no stress–strain curves for aortic leaflets should be considered definitive until a trustworthy FE model implementing material properties consistent with these curves reproduces the experimentally observed dynamic opening and closing of the valve (which are also influenced by the properties of the supporting aortic root).

Although rigid clamps can indeed be expected to overconstrain soft tissue samples, the experience shows that sutures and rigid rakes are associated with mechanical behaviors that are reasonably close to those expected to happen physiologically. What seems to matter the most is which configuration is taken as the reference configuration for the calculation of strains. Indeed, in Martin et al. (2012) and Labrosse et al. (2016), the authors achieved close agreements between both sutures and rigid rakes, as long as the reference configuration taken to analyze the data was obtained at the end of the preconditioning cycles.

Let the original domain (within the grips of the apparatus) be defined as: $-L_1/2 \leq X_1 \leq L_1/2$, $-L_2/2 \leq X_2 \leq L_2/2$, and $-H/2 \leq X_3 \leq H/2$, where H is the undeformed thickness. After deformation, the material originally at location X_1, X_2, X_3 in the unloaded, stress-free configuration can be mapped to x_1, x_2, x_3 as follows: $x_1 = \lambda_1 X_1 + F_{12} X_2$, $x_2 = F_{21} X_1 + \lambda_2 X_2$, $x_3 = (h/H) X_3$. The biaxial testing equipment allows one to monitor stretch ratios λ_1, λ_2, as well as the forces applied in each direction, say f_1 and f_2. Assuming the material to be incompressible (due to its large water content), the determinant of the second-order transformation gradient tensor $\overline{F} = \partial x / \partial X$ associated with general planar biaxial testing must be equal to 1. Therefore, unknown current thickness h can be expressed in terms of measurable quantities, as $h = H/J_{2D}$, where $J_{2D} = \lambda_1 \lambda_2 - F_{12} F_{21}$ and the Cartesian components of $\overline{F}$ are given as:

$$\left[\overline{F} \right] = \begin{bmatrix} \lambda_1 & F_{12} & 0 \\ F_{21} & \lambda_2 & 0 \\ 0 & 0 & 1/J_{2D} \end{bmatrix}.$$

From experience, it is known that the displacements of the attachments are not representative of those within the central region of the sample. This has led to the widespread use of an overhead video camera to track fiducial markers or surface texture. Once the displacements of these landmarks are known, local strains can be computed using interpolation methods borrowed from FE analysis (Humphrey 1992; Labrosse et al. 2016). As a result, stretch ratios λ_1, λ_2 as well as components F_{12} and F_{21} over a region of interest of the sample can be obtained. The Green (or St. Venant or Lagrangian) strain tensor can then be derived from F by $E = 1/2(\overline{F}^T . F - I)$, where "." denotes the dot or scalar product and "T" means transpose. Note that by definition, $\overline{E}$ is symmetric.

Curves of second Piola-Kirchhoff (P-K) membrane tensions versus Green strains are often reported, as such curves are unaffected by thickness measurements. The components of second P-K stress resultant (or membrane tension, in N/m) tensor are $T_{11}^S = \lambda_2 f_1 / (J_{2D} L_2)$, $T_{22}^S = \lambda_1 f_2 / (J_{2D} L_1)$ and, owing to the symmetry of S, $T_{12}^S = -F_{21} f_1 / (J_{2D} L_2) = T_{21}^S = -F_{12} f_2 / (J_{2D} L_1)$, where external forces f_1 and f_2 are applied in directions 1 and 2 (Labrosse et al. 2016).

Interestingly, an elegant solution was recently proposed to calculate the resulting stresses in planar biaxial experiments by using sutures when specimens undergo shear and exhibit substantial inelastic effects (Zhang et al. 2015). However, for simplicity of processing and accuracy of the results, it has long been recommended that shear should be minimized by aligning the sample's preferred directions with those of the biaxial testing machine (Humphrey 1990; Holzapfel and Ogden 2009). The use of rigid rakes, as available with the CellScale BioTester, to mount the tissue samples greatly simplifies the testing and removes at least one source of inconsistency during experiments. Still, care must be taken to keep the tines of the rakes evenly spaced to promote homogeneous stress and strain distributions in the central portion of the sample, as desirable for material characterization (Eilaghi et al. 2009).

Finally, let us note that planar biaxial testing is ill-suited for samples obtained from originally cylindrical organs, such as arteries, in which case inflation testing, discussed in Section 4.2.4.4, is more natural.

4.2.4.4 Inflation Testing of a Tube

In inflation or pressurization testing, a tube-like sample can be stretched longitudinally and simultaneously inflated in a controlled manner. Since the original shape of the sample can be preserved and in vivo longitudinal stretching can be implemented, inflation testing is better than biaxial testing in terms of reproducing physiological geometries and boundary conditions.

To promote robust material characterization, different testing protocols have been devised, whereby different values of longitudinal stretches are applied statically, and then, pressurization is applied over physiological or supraphysiological range. Humphrey et al. and Deng et al. showed the possibility and value of adding longitudinal torsion to the experiment, in order to analyze shear properties of blood vessels (Humphrey et al. 1993; Deng et al. 1994; Humphrey 2002; Lu et al. 2003). Other authors (Labrosse et al. 2009; Badel et al. 2012) proposed a simplification of inflation test, wherein one end of the blocked sample is let to expand freely in the longitudinal direction as inflation occurs. This automatically applies varying levels of longitudinal stretch while pressure is applied. It was verified that this method yields identical results regarding material characterization as inflation testing, with arbitrarily defined sets of stretches applied statically (Labrosse et al. 2009). However, the method excludes the application of longitudinal torsion.

Whether with or without longitudinal torsion, or with or without retesting of the sample after inversion, exact finite strain solutions for all these variants in testing configuration exist in the literature (Humphrey 2002), which has made the pressurization approach to material characterization so valuable. The mathematical derivation to describe the pressurization of an assumed axisymmetric, thick-walled, closed-end cylinder with homogeneous hyperelastic anisotropic and incompressible material properties is briefly repeated here for the case of fresh aortic segments pressurized under closed-end and free extension conditions (Labrosse et al. 2009, 2013).

In cylindrical coordinates, let a material particle located at (r, θ, z) in the deformed vessel be mapped to (R, Θ, Z) in the undeformed body, such that $r = r(R)$, $\theta = \Theta$, and $z = z(Z)$ in the radial, circumferential, and longitudinal directions, respectively. In these notations, $r_i \leq r \leq r_o$, where r_i and r_o are the inner and outer radii, respectively, of the deformed vessel. Similarly, $R_i \leq R \leq R_o$, where R_i and R_o are the inner and outer radii, respectively, in the undeformed vessel (Figure 4.3). The deformations are induced by loads consisting of gauge pressure p and applied axial force F_z, which represents the force necessary to keep the pressurized sample at constant length. As the

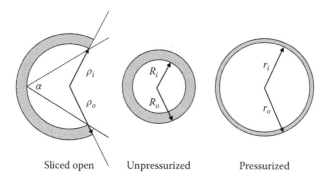

Sliced open   Unpressurized   Pressurized

Figure 4.3 Schematic of a blood vessel cross-section in the three configurations considered for modeling purposes: sliced open, unpressurized, and pressurized. The geometric parameters used in the equations in the main text are represented.

closed end of the sample is assumed to be free to move longitudinally, $F_z \equiv 0$ herein, even though internal axial forces compensate for the pressure acting on the cap.

Assuming transverse isotropic or orthotropic behavior of the aortic tissue, with the principal material and deformation directions being radial, circumferential, and longitudinal, the strain energy function used to describe the hyperelastic material behavior depends a priori on the strains in all three directions (e.g., Green strains E_r, E_θ, and E_z). However, material incompressibility is assumed and imposes $(2E_r +1)(2E_\theta +1)(2E_z +1) \equiv 1$. Therefore, strain energy function W can be made to depend on only two strains instead of three strains. For instance, we take $W = W(E_\theta, E_z)$, with $E_i = 1/2(\lambda_i^2 -1)$ for $i = \theta, z$, where the circumferential and longitudinal stretch ratios are defined as $\lambda_\theta = r / R$ and $\lambda_z = l / L$, respectively. Then, one can demonstrate that $p = \int_{r_i}^{r_o} 1/r\lambda_\theta^2 (\partial W/\partial E_\theta) dr$ and $F_z = \pi \int_{r_i}^{r_o} \left(2\lambda_z^2 (\partial W/\partial E_z) - \lambda_\theta^2 (\partial W/\partial E_\theta) \right) r dr$.

Modeling can also be simplified by considering that the tubular sample is thin, instead of thick, in which case the circumferential stress reduces to that predicted by the Laplace law and is assumed uniform across the vessel wall thickness.

When the stress distribution across the vessel wall is the focus of the study, the finite strain solution for pressurization can be modified to include the three constitutive layers of blood vessels. Although each layer can be made to carry individual levels of residual stresses, in both the circumferential and longitudinal directions (Holzapfel et al. 2007), when, for simplicity, the circumferential residual stress is taken into account through a unique opening angle α (Figure 4.2), the circumferential stretch ratio becomes $\lambda_\theta = \pi/(\pi -\alpha)r/\rho$, where $\rho = \sqrt{\pi / (\pi -\alpha)\lambda_z(r^2 -r_i^2) + \rho_i^2}$ and ρ_i is the inner radius of the unpressurized open aorta (Figure 4.3). For the midline length l_m of the ring to be the same before the cut ($l_m = 2\pi \times 1/2(R_o + R_i)$, Figure 4.3) and afterward ($l_m = 2(\pi -\alpha) \times 1/2(\rho_o + \rho_i)$, Figure 4.3), one must have $\alpha = (1-(R_o + R_i/\rho_o + \rho_i))\pi$, where ρ_o is the outer radius of the unpressurized open aorta. Note that if the ring opens up into a straight line, $\alpha = \pi$ (i.e., 180 degrees) and both ρ_i and ρ_o theoretically become infinite; for α greater than 180 degrees, both ρ_i and ρ_o become negative, reflecting the change in sign of the curvature of the aortic wall.

In an insightful study, Keyes et al. (2013) examined variations in FE simulations driven from planar or tubular testing of the same porcine coronary arteries to determine what differences may exist between these testing techniques. Arteries were first tested in tube form and then in planar form, with each mechanical response fitted to a 2D Fung-type strain energy density function. When performing FE simulations of tube inflation from a planar-derived constitutive model, the systolic diameter was underpredicted by 12.3% and the circumferential stresses were higher by 50.4% compared with the results directly obtained from inflation testing data. However, this difference reduced to 3.9% when the sample with planar-derived properties was first rolled into a tube and then inflated with tube-derived properties. The authors noticed collagen uncrimping in the microstructure of the flattened planar samples. It remains to be seen whether or not similar discrepancies would be observed in arteries of larger caliber, where flattening would incur a lesser change in curvature than in arteries about 2.5 mm in diameter; in addition, it would seem important to use a 3D material model rather than a 2D model.

Another form of pressurization testing, known as bulge inflation, consists of inflating a flat membrane. As the membrane is assumed to be thin compared to its other dimensions, the tension in it can be determined without the use of a constitutive model to describe the elastic properties of the membrane. Instead, detailed knowledge of the deformed geometry (as allowed by full-field or point-based analyses, using digital image correlation (DIC), as discussed in Section 4.2.4.6) and pressure information can be used in combination with interpolations methods borrowed from FE analysis to identify the three components of the Cauchy stress in the local basis attached to the nodes of an arbitrary mesh made of the membrane's surface (Romo et al. 2014). The bulge inflation method has been especially favored toward the determination of rupture properties of cardiovascular tissues, as will be discussed in Section 4.2.6 (Mohan and Melville 1983; Duprey et al. 2016).

4.2.4.5 Flexural Testing

The mechanical tests discussed so far do not make it possible to assess the flexural properties of tissues; however, such properties may be extremely relevant, especially in the context of heart valve leaflets in their open–close movement. Importantly, in-plane properties cannot be directly used to derive out-of-plane (i.e., flexural) properties, unless certain material symmetry or isotropy conditions are assumed, and this is one reason why models based on 2D constitutive equations should not be trusted for the simulation of the bending behavior of heart valve leaflets (Kim et al. 2006; Kim et al. 2008). Merryman et al. (2006) used three-point bending to determine the effects of cellular contraction on the flexural stiffness of porcine aortic valve leaflet. The data were reduced to bending moment-curvature curves according to the procedure worked out in (Engelmayr et al. 2003). Mirnajafi et al. (2006) used cantilever beam-bending experiments to measure the flexural rigidity of porcine aortic valve leaflets in the commissural region. Nicosia (2007) identified the lack of a theoretical framework for fitting bending data to constitutive models and proposed one for isotropic hyperelastic materials with finite deformations. Ragaert et al. (2012) used what they referred to as a flexural indentation test, wherein the sample was placed over a round hole and indented by a descending ball probe. However, the properties that they measured were not related to bending. Fan and Sacks (2014) used the experimental moment-curvature curve from the three-point bending experiments carried out by Mirnajafi et al. (2005), in combination with tensile biaxial and inflation testing data, to validate their modeling and FE implementation in the context of heart valve tissue engineering. Similarly, Murdock et al. (2018) recently used cantilever beam-bending experiments on samples of pericardium to quantify their flexural behavior and, in combination with biaxial testing data from another study, to identify material constants that could capture both the flexural and biaxial responses. As can be seen, despite sporadic, albeit valuable, efforts, a comprehensive experimental, theoretical, and computational framework for the treatment of bending for the material characterization of anisotropic hyperelastic tissues has yet to be achieved. It would potentially provide ways to standardize testing procedures and processing methods while increasing the accuracy of computational simulations.

4.2.4.6 Three-Dimensional Digital Image Correlation and Motion Capture Systems

As already mentioned previously, DIC permits the tracking of a naturally occurring (e.g., surface texture) or applied (e.g., fiducial markers) surface pattern during an experiment. This is done by analyzing the displacement of the pattern within subsets of the whole image. Once limited to 2D analyses, DIC has now been generalized to three dimensions, requiring two cameras trained on the same scene from two different viewpoints. Three-dimensional DIC allows for the noncontact acquisition of strain maps at the surface of planar or nonplanar samples (Sutton et al. 2008; Kim and Baek 2011; Badel et al. 2012). Such measurements can be combined with previous testing techniques to remove assumptions about the homogeneity of the strain field and carry out detailed inverse methods for local material characterization.

The same stereoscopic principles used in 3D DIC have also been used to monitor the 3D displacements of fiducial markers placed on the leaflets of porcine aortic valves tested in a pulse duplicator with a clear fluid (Weiler et al. 2011). From the displacements of these markers, timewise strain maps were constructed for the basal, belly, and coaptation regions of the leaflets, across a cardiac cycle.

4.2.4.7 Indentation Testing

Indentation testing measures the force needed to drive an indenter of known dimensions into a material over a certain depth. At its simplest, it can be used to extract the isotropic, small-strain elastic or viscoelastic properties of biological tissues. Thankfully, several investigators have developed a theoretical framework for indentation testing that is relevant to anisotropic and hyperelastic materials such as cardiovascular tissues (Bischoff 2004). For porcine aortic valve leaflets, Cox et al. used an inverse FE method to resolve the force-displacement information obtained from indentation, along with the fiber orientation information obtained separately, and to identify the material parameters of an anisotropic hyperelastic constitutive relation (Cox et al. 2006). Alternatively, in the absence of independent fiber orientation information, they showed the feasibility of using first and second principal strain information at the center of indentation, obtained from confocal microscopy by tracking the deformation of the collagen fibers in the bottom plane of the samples. The method was used again by Oomen et al. (2016) to investigate the age-dependent changes of stress and strain in the human heart valve and their relationship with collagen remodeling. To reduce the significant computational overhead incurred by the inverse FE method, Zhang et al. (2014) leveraged dimensional analysis and the Pi theorem to reduce the number of forward computations required in the full nonlinear optimization. Although promising, their analysis was limited to isotropic hyperelastic constitutive models.

4.2.4.8 Micropipette Aspiration

In micropipette aspiration, the projection of the aspirated tongue inside a micropipette of known inner radius is measured as a function of the suction pressure to correlate it to the local elastic properties of the cells or soft tissues of interest (Sato et al. 1987; Hochmut 2000). In a study of bovine endothelial cells under different levels of shear stress, Theret et al. (1988) developed a small-strain model of an infinite homogeneous half-space drawn into a micropipette from which an equivalent elastic modulus of cells can be readily extracted. Many other investigators have used this model in different contexts (Haga et al. 1998; Hochmuth 2000; Merryman et al. 2006; Shojaei-Baghini et al. 2013). Baaijens et al. and Zhou et al. independently expanded the model to accommodate neo-Hookean solid material properties, of relevance primarily for chondrocytes and epithelial cells (Baaijens et al. 2005; Zhou et al. 2005). For donut-shaped red blood cells, consistent with observations that their membranes do not noticeably stretch under micropipette aspiration ("preservation of cell membrane areal strain" assumption), the finite elasticity frameworks developed in Evans et al. (1973) and Skalak et al. (1973) were brought to bear for processing the results from micropipette aspiration (Chien et al. 1978; Haga et al. 1998). McGrath et al. (2011) developed another finite elasticity model for inactive murine and human platelets of oblate spheroidal (i.e., discoidal) shape, based on their observation that the volume bounded by the platelet membrane was constant during micropipette experiments ("preservation of cell volume" assumption).

4.2.4.9 Three-Dimensional Shear Testing

Dokos et al. (2000) reported on the design of a triaxial shear test device. The device makes it possible to apply simple shear separately in two orthogonal directions while the resulting forces along the three axes are measured. Simple shear can be applied independently on the six faces of a cubic sample; therefore, repeated rotations by 90 degrees of the sample in the device allow for the coverage of all six modes of simple shear deformation. The device was used to determine the shear properties of passive porcine ventricular myocardium (Dokos et al. 2002).

4.2.5 Tear Propagation

The study of tear propagation is especially relevant to aortic dissection, wherein blood infiltrates an initial injury of the inner layer of the aorta, causing the inner and middle layers of the aorta to separate (dissect). If the blood-filled channel ruptures through the outer layer of the aorta, aortic dissection can be fatal. Usual tensile or inflation tests induce unstable dynamic failures, in which controlled tear propagation cannot be achieved. Therefore, these methods are poorly suited to quantify the fracture properties of soft biological tissue. Several other approaches have been developed instead.

Purslow investigated the fracture toughness (resistance to tear propagation) in both the circumferential and longitudinal directions of porcine thoracic aortas (Purslow 1983). The tear tests were carried out on a standard uniaxial testing machine. During the tests, an initial tear of known dimensions was propagated along almost the entire length of the sample before unloading, and the energy under the load–extension curve was noted. Interestingly, the author remarked that when attempting to propagate cracks in the longitudinal direction of the aorta, the toughness in this direction was much greater than that in the circumferential direction, causing the longitudinal propagation of cracks to invariably deviate into the weaker circumferential direction and tear out through the side of the specimen.

In a technique later referred to as media splitting test (Sommer et al. 2008), Carson and Roach carried out pressure–volume measurements, as a dilute suspension of India ink was infused into the tunica media of porcine thoracic aortas by using a constant flow pump attached to a 20 G needle (Carson and Roach 1990). They recorded the maximum pressure required to tear the media and the average distensibility of the media, along with the work per unit area of tissue required to propagate a tear in the aorta. These values were found to be independent of the tear depth.

MacLean et al. and Sommer et al. measured the radial extensibility and the dissection strength across the lamellae of the aortic media in the radial direction of porcine thoracic aortas (MacLean et al. 1999) and human abdominal aortas (Sommer et al. 2008) by tailoring a classical tensile test to relatively very thin samples. Sommer et al. made incisions to promote the initiation of failure at locations "away" from the fixtures.

Sommer et al. (2008) also performed peeling tests on the aortic media of human abdominal aortas to investigate the fracture energy required to propagate a dissection. The specimens were split at one end to get two layers of about equal thickness and 8–10 mm in length. Each of the layers was mounted into the grips of a uniaxial tensile testing machine. Separation of the grips induced controlled peeling of the media. The peeling force divided by the width of the layers was recorded as a function of length of the peeling path. Tests were carried out on aortic specimens cut either longitudinally or circumferentially.

Chu et al. (2013) designed and implemented a lubricated cutting test (guillotine) to assess the fracture toughness (resistance to crack growth and propagation) of porcine aortas. Compared with other testing methods, this method was particularly well suited for the relative small dimensions of the accessible aortic samples. A two-pass approach was used: in the first pass, a razor blade cut the sample, while in the second pass, the razor blade was reinserted into the cut, without extending it, to measure the frictional force between the walls of the cut and the blade. The force required to drive the razor blade during the passes and the resulting displacement were monitored. Shahmansouri et al. (2015) used the same setup and determined the energy required for steady-state Mode-I crack progression (i.e., tensile opening), also in porcine aortic tissue.

4.2.6 Rupture Properties

Usual biaxial tensile tests of soft biological tissue rely on the use of suture lines or rakes to attach the samples. These sharp implements typically tear through the sample at the higher loads needed to test the samples until failure. Therefore, rupture properties of cardiovascular tissues are typically measured by uniaxial testing (Mohan and Melvin 1982; see Table 1 in Duprey et al. 2016) or, better yet, bulge inflation testing (Mohan and Melvin 1983). The method is especially interesting, as it creates a biaxial load, similar to what the bulging tissues of aneurysms experience in vivo. Duprey et al. combined bulge inflation with full-field optical measurements to determine the values at failure for the stress and stretch ratios in both the circumferential and longitudinal directions of human ascending thoracic aortic aneurysm samples (Duprey et al. 2016).

Note that the measurement of the rupture properties of blood vessels in the radial direction was already discussed in Section 4.2.5 (Sommer et al. 2008).

4.3 Fluids Aspects

4.3.1 In Vitro Experimental Models

Experimental measurements on in vitro models are of primary importance for the validation of clinical parameters used in the diagnosis of cardiovascular diseases and in the development of cardiovascular medical devices. In vitro testing offers a cost-affordable environment free of patient-to-patient variability and where a large portfolio of clinically relevant scenarios can be tested. Several heart duplicators have already been developed (Balducci et al. 2004; Scotten and Walker 2004; Tanné et al. 2010; Keshavarz-Motamed et al. 2012; Keshavarz-Motamed et al. 2014; Yoganathan et al. 2015; Okafor et al. 2017). Most of the duplicators reproduce only the left heart function. Designs vary significantly between duplicators, but an ideal duplicator should have at least the following characteristics: (1) It should include anatomically correct elastic models of left heart cavities; (2) it should include a double-activation mechanism, that is, ventricular activation and atrial activation; (3) it should allow for invasive data recording, including pressure and flow waveforms; (4) it should allow for noninvasive recordings, for example, using Doppler echocardiographic measurements; and (5) it should allow for optical-based velocity recordings by using particle image velocimetry (PIV). An important aspect to consider when developing a heart duplicator is to perform a validation step at least in terms of pressure and flow waveforms in the time domain. Ideally, a frequency domain validation should also be performed by computing the aortic input and characteristic impedances (Segers et al. 1998; Mouret et al. 2000). An additional validation step requires the computation of the most important parameters characterizing the flow behavior (Table 4.2).

TABLE 4.2   Some Characteristic Dimensionless Parameters for the Evaluation of Cardiovascular Flows

Reynolds number (Re)	$Re = \dfrac{\rho v d}{\mu}$	Ratio between the inertial and viscous forces.
Womersley number (Wo)	$Wo = d\left(\dfrac{\omega \rho}{\mu}\right)^{1/2}$	Ratio between the transient and viscous forces.
Shapiro number (Sh)	$Sh = \dfrac{v}{C}$, with $c = 1/\sqrt{\rho \delta}$	Ratio between the velocities of the fluid flow and the wave speed velocity.
Dean number (De)	$De = \sqrt{\dfrac{d}{2R}}\, Re$	Ratio between the viscous forces acting on the fluid in a curved pipe and the centrifugal force.

v is the velocity of the fluid; d is the characteristic length (tube diameter); ω is the frequency of the pulsatile flow; μ is the dynamic viscosity of the fluid flow; ρ is the density; δ is the distensibility of the aorta $\delta = A^{-1}(\delta A / \delta p)$, where A and p are the pressure and cross-sectional area, respectively; and R is radius of curvature of the tube.

4.3.2 Blood Analogs

Blood consists of a complex mixture of cells, proteins, lipoproteins, and ions (Ku 1997). As discussed in Chapter 3, blood typically exhibits a non-Newtonian behavior; however, the assumption of Newtonian behavior is reasonable in large arteries (blood vessel >1 mm) and in heart cavities, where the shear rate is generality greater than $100 \ s^{-1}$ (Pedley and Luo 1995; Fung 1997; Berger and Jou 2000). Finding the most appropriate blood analog, mostly for optical-based velocity measurement techniques, is a challenging task. This is because there is a need for matching both the dynamic viscosity and density of the blood analog with those of blood while also matching the refractive index of the blood analog with that of the transparent experimental model. Several blood-analog models have been suggested in the literature, including water and glycerol (Keshavarz-Motamed et al. 2012; Keshavarz-Motamed et al. 2014); diethyl phthalate and ethanol (Nguyen et al. 2004); and water, glycerol, and sodium iodide (Grigioni et al. 2001; Yousif et al. 2011).

4.3.3 Cardiovascular Flow Velocity Measurements

The experimental determination of the velocity field in vivo or in vitro is of paramount importance for the hemodynamic evaluation of heart function and for testing the ability of medical devices to adequately reproduce healthy blood flow conditions. Currently, several techniques can be used to accurately measure whole plane velocity fields in cardiovascular cavities. The focus here will be on the three most widely used techniques: phase-contrast magnetic resonance imaging (MRI), PIV, and echocardiographic particle image velocimetry (echo-PIV).

4.3.3.1 Phase-Contrast Magnetic Resonance Imaging

Phase-contrast MRI is a noninvasive technique that allows for flow characterization and velocity field mapping in patients (Lotz et al. 2002). It is mentioned for its high clinical relevance but is typically not an in vitro method. Briefly, it relies on the application of gradient pulses that induce phase shifts in the moving protons existing in the flow. Pulse sequences are capable of velocity recordings in directions perpendicular or parallel to the direction of the flow (Srichai et al. 2009). Most recent sequences are capable of time-resolved 3D determination of the velocity field in heart cavities (Markl et al. 2007; Garcia et al. 2015). Phase-contrast MRI has already been applied to the evaluation of several pathological conditions, including aortic coarctation (Keshavarz-Motamed et al. 2013), aortic stenosis (Garcia et al. 2012; Garcia et al. 2014; Larose 2014), and tetralogy of Fallot (Geiger et al. 2011; Hirtler et al. 2016).

4.3.3.2 Particle Image Velocimetry

Particle image velocimetry is an optical velocity measurement technique that uses a laser, digital cameras, and seeding particles. Two consecutive images of the illuminated particles are taken by the high-speed camera. The images are divided into small interrogation regions, typically between 8×8 pixels and 64×64 pixels in size. A cross-correlation is then applied on the interrogation regions to identify the direction and displacement of the seeding particles. The timing between the two images, or laser pulses, and the estimated displacement lead to the determination of the velocity vector in each interrogation region (Adrian 1991; Keane and Adrian 1992; Raffel et al. 2013). Particle image velocimetry allows for the determination of time-resolved 2D and 3D velocity fields. More recent techniques, such as tomographic PIV (tomo-PIV), allow for direct time-resolved volumetric measurements (Elsinga et al. 2005; Hasler and Obrist 2016). Because PIV is an optical-based technique requiring a transparent fluid, its application is limited to experimental, in vitro, velocity measurements. Its application to cardiovascular flows includes the investigation of flow characteristics in models of the left and right ventricles, the aorta, the pulmonary artery, the left atrium, the carotid artery, and aneurysms of the abdominal aorta. Particle image velocimetry has also been used to investigate the performance of medical devices and surgical procedures, including various heart valves, left ventricular assist devices, and the total cavopulmonary connection.

4.3.3.3 Ultrasound-Based Particle Image Velocimetry

Velocity field determination by using ultrasound is based on speckle tracking. In echo-PIV, microbubbles are added to the flow to increase the signal-to-noise ratio (Kim et al. 2004; Jensen et al. 2016). However, in velocity flow mapping (VFM), color Doppler and speckle tracking data are directly used, without a need for microbubble injection (Garcia et al. 2010). Both techniques have been used extensively, mostly to evaluate blood flow structures in the left ventricle during the diastolic phase. Important results regarding the characteristics of the vortices in the left ventricle have been correlated with the development of pathological conditions such as cardiomyopathy and aortic regurgitation (Hong et al. 2008; Kheradvar et al. 2010; Pedrizzetti et al. 2014; Stugaard et al. 2015).

TABLE 4.3   Examples of Flow Characteristics That Can Be Extracted from Two-Dimensional Velocity Field Measurements

Viscous shear stress (VSS)	$VSS = \mu\left(\dfrac{\partial u}{\partial y} + \dfrac{\partial v}{\partial x}\right)$
Viscous energy dissipation (P)	$P = \dfrac{\mu}{2}\displaystyle\int_A \left[\sum_{\forall i,j}\left(\dfrac{\partial u}{\partial y} + \dfrac{\partial v}{\partial x}\right)^2\right] dA$
Turbulent kinetic energy (TKE)	$TKE = \dfrac{1}{2}\rho\left(\overline{u'^2} + \overline{v'^2}\right)$, with
	$u' = \sqrt{\dfrac{1}{N}\sum\left(u - \overline{u}\right)^2}\;;\; \overline{u} = \dfrac{1}{N}\sum u$
	$v' = \sqrt{\dfrac{1}{N}\sum\left(v - \overline{v}\right)^2}\;;\; \overline{v} = \dfrac{1}{N}\sum v$
Reynolds shear stress (RSS)	$RSS = \rho\sqrt{\left(\dfrac{\overline{u'u'} - \overline{v'v'}}{2}\right)^2 + \left(\overline{u'v'}\right)^2}$

4.3.3.4 *Cardiovascular Flow Velocity Characterization*

The velocity fields obtained from phase-contrast MRI, PIV, or ultrasound-based PIV can be used to determine important characteristics of the flow field. Of main interest are the characteristics that provide useful information regarding shear stress, turbulence characteristics, and viscous energy dissipation. Table 4.3 lists some of the important flow characteristics that can be extracted from 2D velocity field recordings. The underlying assumption is that these parameters are optimal under healthy conditions and change significantly and monotonically with the severity of pathological conditions. Note that it is recommended for the evaluation of velocity gradients to use the fourth-order noise-minimizing Richardson extrapolation scheme (Etebari and Vlachos 2005; Garcia et al. 2013). Also note that it is important to consider the limitations of each measurement technique used in terms of spatial and temporal resolutions before extracting higher-order flow characteristics from the velocity fields.

4.4 Application of Singular-Value Decomposition to Cardiovascular Flows

The complex nature of cardiovascular flows under healthy and pathological conditions requires the use of advanced postprocessing techniques to provide deeper fundamental insight and more accurate characterization of coherent flow structures. Of interest are the characteristic coherent structures that contribute the most to the dynamics and the spectral signature of the flow (Lusseyran et al. 2011). Identifying the key flow structures can ultimately lead to better diagnosis of cardiovascular disease and may also contribute to the design of more efficient medical devices. This section will specifically deal with singular-value decomposition of cardiovascular velocity fields. More specifically, proper orthogonal decomposition (POD) and dynamic mode decomposition (DMD) are briefly introduced.

4.4.1 Proper Orthogonal Decomposition

Proper orthogonal decomposition has been used for the analysis of cardiovascular flows in the works of Grinberg et al. (2009), using in vivo phase-contrast MRI data on occluded arteries; Kefayati and Poepping (2013), who investigated the flow dynamics in normal and stenosed arteries; Abulkhair (2016), who processed experimental data in models of AAAs; and Di Labbio et al. (2017), who investigated coherent structures in pulsatile flows subjected to sudden body forces. The main concept behind POD is to create a mathematical model capable of decoupling the spatial from the temporal evolutions of an unsteady flow (Andrianne et al. 2009). It was initially introduced to identify the dominant energetic coherent structures, in terms of kinetic energy, in a turbulent velocity field. Significant variations in energy associated with the eigenvalues of the modes or the number of modes required to correctly reconstruct the original velocity data set might be an early indication of pathological cardiovascular conditions. Table 4.4 shows the algorithm for POD applied to a 2D velocity field. Figure 4.4 shows the first three most energetic modes in the case of experimental measurements in an AAA (Abulkhair 2016).

4.4.1.1 Dynamic Mode Decomposition

Dynamic mode decomposition is a data reduction method introduced to investigate the dynamical behavior of a system. The main concept behind DMD is to identify a linear mapping that better represents the nonlinear flow process (Tu et al. 2013). It leads to the decomposition of the flow field into a set of modes that represent the main characteristic frequencies of the flow (Schmid 2010). Dynamic mode decomposition

TABLE 4.4   Proper Orthogonal Decomposition Algorithm

1. Arrange the velocity vectors.	$A = \begin{bmatrix} u^1 u^2 \ldots \ldots u^N \end{bmatrix} = \begin{bmatrix} u_1^1 & u_1^2 & \cdots & u_1^N \\ \vdots & \vdots & \vdots & \vdots \\ u_m^1 & u_m^2 & \cdots & u_m^N \\ v_1^1 & v_1^2 & \cdots & v_1^N \\ \vdots & \vdots & \vdots & \vdots \\ v_m^1 & v_m^2 & \cdots & v_m^N \end{bmatrix}$
2. Calculate the covariance matrix.	$C = A^T A$
3. Evaluate the eigenvalues and eigenvectors.	$SVD(C) = U \Sigma V^T$
4. Find the POD modes.	$\phi_i = \dfrac{A U^i}{\|A U^i\|}, \quad i = 1, \ldots, N$
5. Find the temporal modes.	$a_i^n = \phi_i A$

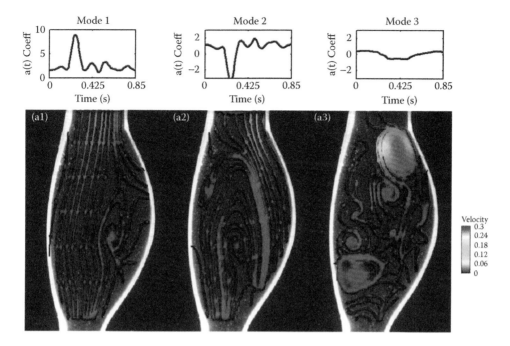

Figure 4.4 First three most energetic modes from experimental measurements of a pulsatile flow in an elastic model of an AAA. The top row represents temporal modes, while the bottom row represents spatial modes. The fractional kinetic energy associated with each mode is 86.81% for Mode 1 (the average mode), 12.86% for Mode 2, and 2.43% for Mode 3. (From Abulkhair, H., Experimental investigation of the flow dynamics in a model of an abdominal aortic aneurysm, Doctoral dissertation, Concordia University, 2016.)

can identify both the main dynamical coherent structures in the flow field and their temporal evolution (Tirunagari et al. 2012). It has been used for the analysis of cardiovascular flows by Delorme et al. (2014) in the context of an idealized total cavopulmonary connection and by Abulkhair (2016), who performed DMD of the flow in an AAA model. Dynamic mode decomposition has the ability to provide useful information regarding the stability of the main coherent structures in the flow. This can be a powerful tool for the design and optimization of cardiovascular devices. Table 4.5 shows the algorithm for DMD of velocity fields. Figure 4.5 shows the first three most energetic modes in the case of experimental measurements in an AAA.

4.5 Animal Models

The information that can be gleaned from in vitro or computational studies is limited, as, most likely, these studies cannot be used to understand long-term effects in detail. Thankfully, animal models are available to study a large number of specific

TABLE 4.5   Dynamic Mode Decomposition Algorithm

1. Arrange the velocity vectors based on D_1.	$D_1 = \{v_1,\ v_2, \ldots\ldots\ldots, v_{N-1}\}$
2. Arrange the velocity vectors based on D_2.	$D_2 = \{v_2,\ v_{23}, \ldots\ldots\ldots, v_N\}$
3. Find the correlation between D_1 and D_2.	$A_{\Delta t} D_1 = D_2$
4. Assume linear mapping between the snapshots.	$A_{\Delta t} D_1 = D_2 \approx D_1 S$
5. Find the companion matrix.	$S \approx U^H A U = U^H D_2 V \Sigma^{-1}$
6. Calculate the eigenvalues of S.	$[\Lambda_i, \lambda_i] = eiv(S)$
7. Find DMD modes.	$\Phi_i = U\Lambda_i$
8. Find the mode frequency and the growth/decay rate.	$real(\lambda_i) \sim \text{growth / decay}$
	$imag(\lambda_i)/2\pi \sim \text{frequency}$

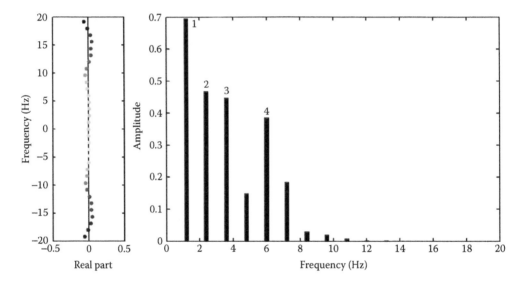

Figure 4.5   Dynamic mode decomposition of experimental measurements of a pulsatile flow in an elastic model of an AAA. The left figure shows mode spectrum, and the right figure shows modal energy distribution. (From Abulkhair, H., Experimental investigation of the flow dynamics in a model of an abdominal aortic aneurysm, Doctoral dissertation, Concordia University, 2016.)

conditions (Table 4.6), not only in acute setting but also over a period spanning up to several months (chronic setting). As such, they constitute an integral part of the experimental armamentarium available to investigate specific aspects of cardiovascular mechanics, such as, among many other examples, the long-term efficacy of new drug-eluting stents (Granada et al. 2009). Moreover, animal testing is one of the many requirements set by regulatory bodies to provide data such as the biocompatibility, toxicity, thrombogenicity, and/or inflammatory responses induced by implanted devices.

TABLE 4.6 Animal Models for Cardiovascular Function and Diseases. Given the Large Number of Publications Involving Animal Models, Mostly Only Recent Review Articles are Referenced, for Illustrative Purposes

Target in Humans	Animal Models	Comments and/or References
Heart (younger)	Pigs	Native absence of anastomoses between adjacent coronary perfusion beds (Hearse and Sutherland 2000)
Heart (older, with ischemic heart disease)	Dogs	Native collateralization (Hearse and Sutherland 2000)
Myocardial infarction	Dogs, fetal sheep, pigs, nonhuman primates	(Dixon and Spinale 2009; Camacho et al. 2016)
Healing infarct scar	Rats, sheep, pigs	(Camacho et al., 2016; Clarke et al. 2016)
Chronic ischemic heart failure/nonischemic heart failure, sudden cardiac death, arrhythmogenic right ventricular cardiomyopathy	Dogs	(Camacho et al. 2016)
Duchenne muscle dystrophy	Gene-mutated Golden Retriever dogs	Spontaneous (Camacho et al. 2016)
Dilated cardiomyopathy	Giant dog breeds	Spontaneous (Camacho et al. 2016)
Tetralogy of Fallot	Pigs	(Camacho et al. 2016)
Tachycardia-induced congestive heart failure	Nonhuman primates	(Camacho et al. 2016)
Aortic valve	Isolated pig valve	Aside from more subtle differences in regional dimensions (Sim et al. 2003), the muscle shelf at the base of the right coronary cusp of the porcine AV, which prevents this cusp from completely opening, is a major difference with the human AV
Calcific aortic valve disease	Mice, rabbits, dogs, pigs	(Sider et al. 2011)

(Continued)

TABLE 4.6 (*Continued*) Animal Models for Cardiovascular Function and Diseases. Given the Large Number of Publications Involving Animal Models, Mostly Only Recent Review Articles are Referenced, for Illustrative Purposes

Target in Humans	Animal Models	Comments and/or References
Aortic valve (AV) replacement, mitral valve repair	Pigs, sheep	Sheep preferred for percutaneous AV devices (Suzuki et al. 2009)
Mitral valve regurgitation	Middle-aged to older small- and medium-sized dogs, sheep	Spontaneous in dogs (Dixon and Spinale 2009; Camacho et al. 2016)
Coronary atherosclerosis and plaque	Pigs, Watanabe heritable hyperlipidemic rabbits, dogs	(Granada et al. 2009; Zaragoza et al. 2011; Tsang et al. 2016)
Coronary interventions	Rabbits, pigs	(Suzuki et al. 2009)
Atherosclerosis	low density lipoprotein receptor (LDLR) -/- and apolipoprotein E (apoE) -/- mice, rats, rabbits, pigs	(Zaragoza et al. 2011; Tsang et al. 2016)
Vascular calcification	Pigs, horses, cows	(Tsang et al. 2016)
Abdominal aortic aneurysm	Broad-breasted white turkeys, blotchy mice, rats, rabbits, pigs	Spontaneous in turkeys (Boucek et al. 1983) and blotchy mice (Zaragoza et al. 2011; Tsang et al. 2016)
Thoracic aortic aneurysm/Marfan syndrome	Mice, cattle	(Zaragoza et al. 2011; Tsang et al. 2016)
Gene therapy	Pigs	(Dixon and Spinale 2009; Tsang et al. 2016)
Stem cell therapy	Pigs, sheep, dogs	(Dixon and Spinale 2009)

Animal studies require that a number of technical and logistical hurdles be overcome, as handling of animals is complex, and necessitate skilled personnel and specialized facilities; they also require ethical approvals by local research ethics boards. In addition, selection of a proper animal model can be challenging. As noted by Hearse and Sutherland (2000), "the further one moves away from the study of human tissues, the greater becomes the quantity, quality and reproducibility of the data and the lower becomes the cost and time-to-result, but unfortunately this is usually offset by the model becoming increasingly less relevant to the human condition [...]. The art of designing a good experiment, therefore, requires not only the ability to identify the most appropriate investigative model and species to answer the question but also the ability to balance, as well as possible, the inevitable conflict between the quality of measured endpoints and their clinical relevance." Milani-Nejad and Janssen recently reviewed the advantages and disadvantages of the most common animal models used in the context of cardiac contraction research (Milani-Nejad and Janssen 2014). As can be surmised from such reviews, no gold standard animal model exists, and financial aspects are bound to influence the decision of which animal model is selected, as daily housing fees for rabbits, pigs, sheep, and canines are respectively about 30, 60, 80, and 90 times higher than those for mice (Milani-Nejad and Janssen 2014). As a result, large animal models usually feature low sample sizes, reducing the statistical power of the analyses. However, it is also known that any result from studies in rodents needs to be confirmed in large animal models for relevance to humans (Camacho et al. 2016).

Despite the invaluable insights and hard data that can be obtained from animal models, there are also limitations to the spectrum of pathologies that can be reproduced. For instance, bicuspid aortic valves, whether isolated or combined with ascending aortic aneurysms, do not have animal models. This creates an opportunity for yet-to-be designed more advanced, high-fidelity, tunable organ simulators to fill the gap between human physiology and pathology and computational models.

4.6 Conclusion

As can be appreciated in this chapter (Chapter 4), the armamentarium available to experimentalists in cardiovascular mechanics is extensive, from the animal, hardware, and data-processing perspectives. By presenting the characteristics, known limitations, and potential pitfalls of the most prevalent tools and models, the motivation in this chapter was to provide the reader with arguments to make informed decisions. With time and increasingly better protocols and equipment, it is hoped that some level of standardization can be introduced in soft tissue and organ testing at large and in cardiovascular mechanics in particular. In turn, this will provide stronger data sets to verify and validate computational simulations, which will improve their predictive capabilities with respect to clinical applications.

References

Abé H, Hayashi K. Data book on mechanical properties of living cells, tissues, and organs. Sato M, editor. Springer, Tokyo, Japan, 1996.

Abulkhair H. Experimental investigation of the flow dynamics in a model of an abdominal aortic aneurysm. Doctoral dissertation, Concordia University, 2016.

Adham M, Gournier JP, Favre JP, De La Roche E, Ducerf C, Baulieux J, Barral X, Pouyet M. Mechanical characteristics of fresh and frozen human descending thoracic aorta. *Journal of Surgical Research* 1996;64(1):32–34.

Adrian RJ. Particle-imaging techniques for experimental fluid mechanics. *Annual Review of Fluid Mechanics* 1991;23(1):261–304.

Amin M, Kunkel AG, Le VP, Wagenseil JE. Effect of storage duration on the mechanical behavior of mouse carotid artery. *Journal of Biomechanical Engineering* 2011;133(7):071007.

Askari F, Shafieian M, Solouk A, Hashemi A. A comparison of the material properties of natural and synthetic vascular walls. *Journal of the Mechanical Behavior of Biomedical Materials* 2017;71:209–215.

Atienza JM, Guinea GV, Rojo FJ, Burgos RJ, García-Montero C, Goicolea FJ, Aragoncillo P, Elicesa M. The influence of pressure and temperature on the behavior of the human aorta and carotid arteries. *Revista Española de Cardiología (English Edition)* 2007;60(3):259–267.

Auricchio F, Conti M, Ferrara A. How constitutive model complexity can affect the capability to fit experimental data: a focus on human carotid arteries and extension/inflation data. *Archives of Computational Methods in Engineering* 2014;21(3):273–292.

Azinfar L, Ravanfar M, Wang Y, Zhang K, Duan D, Yao G. High resolution imaging of the fibrous microstructure in bovine common carotid artery using optical polarization tractography. *Journal of Biophotonics* 2017;10(2):231–241.

Baaijens FP, Trickey WR, Laursen TA, Guilak F. Large deformation finite element analysis of micropipette aspiration to determine the mechanical properties of the chondrocyte. *Annals of Biomedical Engineering* 2005;33(4):494–501.

Badel P, Avril S, Lessner S, Sutton M. Mechanical identification of layer-specific properties of mouse carotid arteries using 3D-DIC and a hyperelastic anisotropic constitutive model. *Computer Methods in Biomechanics and Biomedical Engineering* 2012;15(1):37–48.

Balducci A, Grigioni M, Querzoli G, Romano GP, Daniele C, D'Avenio G, Barbaro V. Investigation of the flow field downstream of an artificial heart valve by means of PIV and PTV. *Experiments in Fluids* 2004;36(1):204–213.

Berger SA, Jou LD. Flows in stenotic vessels. *Annual Review of Fluid Mechanics* 2000;32(1):347–382.

Bergholt MS, St-Pierre JP, Offeddu GS, Parmar PA, Albro MB, Puetzer JL, Oyen ML, Stevens MM. Raman spectroscopy reveals new insights into the zonal organization of native and tissue-engineered articular cartilage. *ACS Central Science* 2016;2(12):885–895.

Bischoff JE. Static indentation of anisotropic biomaterials using axially asymmetric indenters-a computational study. *Journal of Biomechanical Engineering* 2004;126(4):498–505.

Boucek RJ, Gunja-Smith Z, Noble NL, Simpson CF. Modulation by propranolol of the lysyl cross-links in aortic elastin and collagen of the aneurysm-prone turkey. *Biochemical Pharmacology* 1983;32(2):275–280.

Brossollet LJ, Vito RP. A new approach to mechanical testing and modeling of biological tissues, with application to blood vessels. *Journal of Biomechanical Engineering* 1996;118:433.

Bustos CA, García-Herrera CM, Celentano DJ. Mechanical characterisation of Dacron graft: Experiments and numerical simulation. *Journal of Biomechanics* 2016;49(1):13–18.

Camacho P, Fan H, Liu Z, He JQ. Large mammalian animal models of heart disease. *Journal of Cardiovascular Development and Disease* 2016;3(4):30.

Carew EO, Barber JE, Vesely I. Role of preconditioning and recovery time in repeated testing of aortic valve tissues: Validation through quasilinear viscoelastic theory. *Annals of Biomedical Engineering* 2000;28(9):1093–1100.

Carson MW, Roach MR. The strength of the aortic media and its role in the propagation of aortic dissection. *Journal of Biomechanics* 1990;23(6):579–588.

Cheng S, Clarke EC, Bilston LE. The effects of preconditioning strain on measured tissue properties. *Journal of Biomechanics* 2009;42(9):1360–1362.

Chien S, Sung KL, Skalak R, Usami S, Tözeren A. Theoretical and experimental studies on viscoelastic properties of erythrocyte membrane. *Biophysical Journal* 1978;24(2):463–487.

Chow MJ, Zhang Y. Changes in the mechanical and biochemical properties of aortic tissue due to cold storage. *Journal of Surgical Research* 2011;171(2):434–442.

Chu B, Gaillard E, Mongrain R, Reiter S, Tardif JC. Characterization of fracture toughness exhaustion in pig aorta. *Journal of the Mechanical Behavior of Biomedical Materials* 2013;17:126–136.

Clarke SA, Richardson WJ, Holmes JW. Modifying the mechanics of healing infarcts: is better the enemy of good? *Journal of Molecular and Cellular Cardiology* 2016;93:115–124.

Courtial EJ, Fanton L, Orkisz M, Douek PC, Huet L, Fulchiron R. Hyper-viscoelastic behavior of healthy abdominal aorta. *IRBM* 2016;37(3):158–164.

Cox MA, Driessen NJ, Bouten CV, Baaijens FP. Mechanical characterization of anisotropic planar biological soft tissues using large indentation: A computational feasibility study. *Journal of Biomechanical Engineering* 2006;128(3):428–436.

Della Corte A, Quarto C, Bancone C, Castaldo C, Di Meglio F, Nurzynska D, De Santo LS, De Feo M, Scardone M, Montagnani S, Cotrufo M. Spatiotemporal patterns of smooth muscle cell changes in ascending aortic dilatation with bicuspid and tricuspid aortic valve stenosis: Focus on cell–matrix signaling. *The Journal of Thoracic and Cardiovascular Surgery* 2008;135(1):8–18.

Delorme YT, Kerlo AE, Anupindi K, Rodefeld MD, Frankel SH. Dynamic mode decomposition of Fontan hemodynamics in an idealized total cavopulmonary connection. *Fluid Dynamics Research* 2014;46(4):041425.

Deng SX, Tomioka J, Debes JC, Fung YC. New experiments on shear modulus of elasticity of arteries. *American Journal of Physiology-Heart and Circulatory Physiology* 1994;266(1):H1–H10.

Dixon AW. An optomechanical instrument for pericardial tissue selection in bioprosthetic heart valves. Master of Engineering in Biomedical Engineering's thesis, University of Auckland, 2015.

Di Labbio G, Keshavarz-Motamed Z, Kadem L. Numerical simulation of flows in a circular pipe transversely subjected to a localized impulsive body force with applications to blunt traumatic aortic rupture. *Fluid Dynamics Research* 2017;49(3):035510.

Dixon JA, Spinale FG. Large animal models of heart failure. *Circulation: Heart Failure* 2009;2(3):262–271.

Dokos S, LeGrice IJ, Smaill BH, Kar J, Young AA. A triaxial-measurement shear-test device for soft biological tissues. *Journal of Biomechanical Engineering* 2000;122(5):471–478.

Dokos S, Smaill BH, Young AA, LeGrice IJ. Shear properties of passive ventricular myocardium. *American Journal of Physiology-Heart and Circulatory Physiology* 2002;283(6):H2650–H2659.

Duprey A, Trabelsi O, Vola M, Favre JP, Avril S. Biaxial rupture properties of ascending thoracic aortic aneurysms. *Acta Biomaterialia* 2016;42:273–285.

Eilaghi A, Flanagan JG, Brodland GW, Ethier CR. Strain uniformity in biaxial specimens is highly sensitive to attachment details. *Journal of Biomechanical Engineering* 2009;131(9):091003.

Elsinga GE, Wieneke B, Scarano F, Van Oudheusden BW. Assessment of Tomo-PIV for three-dimensional flows. In *Proceedings of 6th International Symposium on Particle Image Velocimetry*, Pasadena, CA, September 21, 2005, pp. 21–23.

Engelmayr GC, Hildebrand DK, Sutherland FW, Mayer JE, Sacks MS. A novel bioreactor for the dynamic flexural stimulation of tissue engineered heart valve biomaterials. *Biomaterials* 2003;24(14):2523–2532.

Etebari A, Vlachos PP. Improvements on the accuracy of derivative estimation from DPIV velocity measurements. *Experiments in Fluids* 2005;39(6):1040–1050.

Evans EA. A new material concept for the red cell membrane. *Biophysical Journal* 1973;13(9):926–940.

Fan R, Sacks MS. Simulation of planar soft tissues using a structural constitutive model: Finite element implementation and validation. *Journal of Biomechanics* 2014;47(9):2043–2054.

Fung YC, Fronek K, Patitucci P. Pseudoelasticity of arteries and the choice of its mathematical expression. *American Journal of Physiology-Heart and Circulatory Physiology* 1979;237(5):H620–H631.

Fung YC. Blood flow in arteries. In *Biomechanics* (pp. 108–205). Springer, New York, 1997.

Garcia D, del Álamo JC, Tanné D, Yotti R, Cortina C, Bertrand É, Antoranz JC et al. Two-dimensional intraventricular flow mapping by digital processing conventional color-Doppler echocardiography images. *IEEE Transactions on Medical Imaging* 2010;29(10):1701–1713.

Garcia J, Jarvis KB, Schnell S, Malaisrie SC, Clennon C, Collins JD, Carr JC, Markl M, Barker AJ. 4D flow MRI of the aorta demonstrates age-and gender-related differences in aortic size and blood flow velocity in healthy subjects. *Journal of Cardiovascular Magnetic Resonance* 2015;17(S1):P39.

Garcia J, Larose E, Pibarot P, Kadem L. On the evaluation of vorticity using cardiovascular magnetic resonance velocity measurements. *Journal of Biomechanical Engineering* 2013;135(12):124501.

Garcia J, Markl M, Schnell S, Allen B, Entezari P, Mahadevia R, Malaisrie SC, Pibarot P, Carr J, Barker AJ. Evaluation of aortic stenosis severity using 4D flow jet shear layer detection for the measurement of valve effective orifice area. *Magnetic Resonance Imaging* 2014;32(7):891–898.

Garcia J, Marrufo OR, Rodriguez AO, Larose E, Pibarot P, Kadem L. Cardiovascular magnetic resonance evaluation of aortic stenosis severity using single plane measurement of effective orifice area. *Journal of Cardiovascular Magnetic Resonance* 2012;14(1):23.

Geiger J, Markl M, Jung B, Grohmann J, Stiller B, Langer M, Arnold R. 4D-MR flow analysis in patients after repair for tetralogy of Fallot. *European Radiology* 2011;21(8):1651–1657.

Granada JF, Kaluza GL, Wilensky RL, Biedermann BC, Schwartz RS, Falk E. Porcine models of coronary atherosclerosis and vulnerable plaque for imaging and interventional research. *EuroIntervention* 2009;5(1):140–148.

Grigioni M, Daniele C, D'Avenio G, Barbaro V. The influence of the leaflets' curvature on the flow field in two bileaflet prosthetic heart valves. *Journal of Biomechanics* 2001;34(5):613–621.

Grinberg L, Yakhot A, Karniadakis GE. Analyzing transient turbulence in a stenosed carotid artery by proper orthogonal decomposition. *Annals of Biomedical Engineering* 2009;37(11):2200–2217.

Guinea GV, Atienza JM, Elices M, Aragoncillo P, Hayashi K. Thermomechanical behavior of human carotid arteries in the passive state. *American Journal of Physiology-Heart and Circulatory Physiology* 2005;288(6):H2940–H2945.

Haga JH, Beaudoin AJ, White JG, Strony J. Quantification of the passive mechanical properties of the resting platelet. *Annals of Biomedical Engineering* 1998;26(2):268–277.

Hasler D, Obrist D. 3D flow topology behind an aortic valve bioprosthesis. In *18th International Symposium on the Application of Laser and Imaging Techniques to Fluid Mechanics*, Lisbon, Portugal, July 4–7, 2016.

Hearse DJ, Sutherland FJ. Experimental models for the study of cardiovascular function and disease. *Pharmacological Research* 2000;41(6):597–603.

Hiester ED, Sacks MS. Optimal bovine pericardial tissue selection sites. I. Fiber architecture and tissue thickness measurements. *Journal of Biomedical Materials Research Part A* 1998;39(2):207–214.

Hilbert SL, Sword LC, Batchelder KF, Barrick MK, Ferrans VJ. Simultaneous assessment of bioprosthetic heart valve biomechanical properties and collagen crimp length. *Journal of Biomedical Materials Research Part A* 1996;31(4):503–509.

Hillman H. Limitations of clinical and biological histology. *Medical Hypotheses* 2000; 54(4):553–564.

Hirtler D, Garcia J, Barker AJ, Geiger J. Assessment of intracardiac flow and vorticity in the right heart of patients after repair of tetralogy of Fallot by flow-sensitive 4D MRI. *European Radiology* 2016;26(10):3598–3607.

Hochmuth RM. Micropipette aspiration of living cells. *Journal of Biomechanics* 2000;33(1):15–22.

Hollander Y, Durban D, Lu X, Kassab GS, Lanir Y. Experimentally validated microstructural 3D constitutive model of coronary arterial media. *Journal of Biomechanical Engineering* 2011;133(3):031007.

Holzapfel GA, Gasser TC, Stadler M. A structural model for the viscoelastic behavior of arterial walls: continuum formulation and finite element analysis. *European Journal of Mechanics-A/Solids* 2002;21(3):441–463.

Holzapfel GA, Ogden RW. On planar biaxial tests for anisotropic nonlinearly elastic solids. A continuum mechanical framework. *Mathematics and Mechanics of Solids* 2009;14(5):474–489.

Holzapfel GA, Sommer G, Auer M, Regitnig P, Ogden RW. Layer-specific 3D residual deformations of human aortas with non-atherosclerotic intimal thickening. *Annals of Biomedical Engineering* 2007;35(4):530–545.

Holzapfel GA. Determination of material models for arterial walls from uniaxial extension tests and histological structure. *Journal of Theoretical Biology* 2006;238(2):290–302.

Hong GR, Pedrizzetti G, Tonti G, Li P, Wei Z, Kim JK, Baweja A, Liu S, Chung N, Houle H, Narula J. Characterization and quantification of vortex flow in the human left ventricle by contrast echocardiography using vector particle image velocimetry. *JACC: Cardiovascular Imaging* 2008;1(6):705–717.

Humphrey JD, Kang T, Sakarda P, Anjanappa M. Computer-aided vascular experimentation: a new electromechanical test system. *Annals of Biomedical Engineering* 1993;21(1):33–43.

Humphrey JD, Strumpf RK, Yin FC. A constitutive theory for biomembranes: Application to epicardial mechanics. *Journal of Biomechanical Engineering* 1992;114(4):461–466.

Humphrey JD, Strumpf RK, Yin FC. Determination of a constitutive relation for passive myocardium: I. A new functional form. *Journal of Biomechanical Engineering* 1990;112(3):333–339.

Humphrey JD. *Cardiovascular Solid Mechanics: Cells, Tissues, and Organs*. Springer Science & Business Media, Berlin, Germany, 2002.

Iliopoulos DC, Kritharis EP, Boussias S, Demis A, Iliopoulos CD, Sokolis DP. Biomechanical properties and histological structure of sinus of Valsalva aneurysms in relation to age and region. *Journal of Biomechanics* 2013;46(5):931–940.

ISO. International vocabulary of basic and general terms in metrology (VIM). *International Organization* 2004;2004:9–14.

Jensen JA, Nikolov SI, Alfred CH, Garcia D. Ultrasound vector flow imaging—Part I: Sequential systems. *IEEE Transactions on Ultrasonics, Ferroelectrics, and Frequency Control* 2016;63(11):1704–1721.

Keane RD, Adrian RJ. Theory of cross-correlation analysis of PIV images. *Applied Scientific Research* 1992;49(3):191–215.

Kefayati S, Poepping TL. Transitional flow analysis in the carotid artery bifurcation by proper orthogonal decomposition and particle image velocimetry. *Medical Engineering and Physics* 2013;35(7):898–909.

Keshavarz-Motamed Z, Garcia J, Gaillard E, Maftoon N, Di Labbio G, Cloutier G, Kadem L. Effect of coarctation of the aorta and bicuspid aortic valve on flow dynamics and turbulence in the aorta using particle image velocimetry. *Experiments in Fluids* 2014;55(3):1696.

Keshavarz-Motamed Z, Garcia J, Kadem L. Fluid dynamics of coarctation of the aorta and effect of bicuspid aortic valve. *PLoS One* 2013;8(8):e72394.

Keshavarz-Motamed Z, Garcia J, Maftoon N, Bedard E, Chetaille P, Kadem L. A new approach for the evaluation of the severity of coarctation of the aorta using Doppler velocity index and effective orifice area: in vitro validation and clinical implications. *Journal of Biomechanics* 2012;45(7):1239–1245.

Keyes JT, Haskett DG, Utzinger U, Azhar M, Geest JP. Adaptation of a planar microbiaxial optomechanical device for the tubular biaxial microstructural and macroscopic characterization of small vascular tissues. *Journal of Biomechanical Engineering* 2011;133(7):075001.

Keyes JT, Lockwood DR, Utzinger U, Montilla LG, Witte RS, Geest JP. Comparisons of planar and tubular biaxial tensile testing protocols of the same porcine coronary arteries. *Annals of Biomedical Engineering* 2013;41(7):1579–1591.

Kheradvar A, Houle H, Pedrizzetti G, Tonti G, Belcik T, Ashraf M, Lindner JR, Gharib M, Sahn D. Echocardiographic particle image velocimetry: A novel technique for quantification of left ventricular blood vorticity pattern. *Journal of the American Society of Echocardiography*, 2010;23(1):86–94.

Kim H, Lu J, Sacks MS, Chandran KB. Dynamic simulation of bioprosthetic heart valves using a stress resultant shell model. *Annals of Biomedical Engineering* 2008;36(2):262–275.

Kim H, Lu J, Sacks MS, Chandran KB. Dynamic simulation pericardial bioprosthetic heart valve function. *Journal of Biomechanical Engineering* 2006;128(5):717–724.

Kim HB, Hertzberg JR, Shandas R. Development and validation of echo PIV. *Experiments in Fluids* 2004;36(3):455–462.

Kim J, Baek S. Circumferential variations of mechanical behavior of the porcine thoracic aorta during the inflation test. *Journal of Biomechanics* 2011;44(10):1941–1947.

Ku DN. Blood flow in arteries. *Annual Review of Fluid Mechanics* 1997;29(1):399–434.

Kunzelman KS, Cochran R. Stress/strain characteristics of porcine mitral valve tissue: Parallel versus perpendicular collagen orientation. *Journal of Cardiac Surgery* 1992;7(1):71–78.

Labrosse MR, Beller CJ, Mesana T, Veinot JP. Mechanical behavior of human aortas: Experiments, material constants and 3-D finite element modeling including residual stress. *Journal of Biomechanics* 2009;42(8):996–1004.

Labrosse MR, Gerson ER, Veinot JP, Beller CJ. Mechanical characterization of human aortas from pressurization testing and a paradigm shift for circumferential residual stress. *Journal of the Mechanical Behavior of Biomedical Materials* 2013;17:44–55.

Labrosse MR, Jafar R, Ngu J, Boodhwani M. Planar biaxial testing of heart valve cusp replacement biomaterials: Experiments, theory and material constants. *Acta Biomaterialia* 2016;45:303–320.

Lanir Y, Fung YC. Two-dimensional mechanical properties of rabbit skin—I. Experimental system. *Journal of Biomechanics* 1974;7(1):29–34.

Larose E. MRI evaluation of aortic stenosis. In *Multimodality Imaging for Transcatheter Aortic Valve Replacement* (pp. 179–187). Springer, London, UK, 2014.

Lisy M, Kalender G, Schenke-Layland K, Brockbank KG, Biermann A, Stock UA. Allograft heart valves: Current aspects and future applications. *Biopreservation and Biobanking* 2017;15(2):148–157.

Lotz J, Meier C, Leppert A, Galanski M. Cardiovascular flow measurement with phase-contrast MR imaging: basic facts and implementation. *Radiographics* 2002;22(3):651–671.

Lu X, Yang J, Zhao JB, Gregersen H, Kassab GS. Shear modulus of porcine coronary artery: Contributions of media and adventitia. *American Journal of Physiology-Heart and Circulatory Physiology* 2003;285(5):H1966–H1975.

Lusseyran F, Guéniat F, Basley J, Douay CL, Pastur LR, Faure TM, Schmid PJ. Flow coherent structures and frequency signature: Application of the dynamic modes decomposition to open cavity flow. In *Journal of Physics: Conference Series* (Vol. 318, No. 4, p. 042036). IOP Publishing, Warsaw, Poland, 2011.

MacLean NF, Dudek NL, Roach MR. The role of radial elastic properties in the development of aortic dissections. *Journal of Vascular Surgery* 1999;29(4):703–710.

Macneal RH, Harder RL. A proposed standard set of problems to test finite element accuracy. *Finite Elements in Analysis and Design* 1985;1(1):3–20.

Macrae RA, Miller K, Doyle BJ. Methods in mechanical testing of arterial tissue: A review. *Strain* 2016;52(5):380–399.

Markl M, Harloff A, Bley TA, Zaitsev M, Jung B, Weigang E, Langer M, Hennig J, Frydrychowicz A. Time-resolved 3D MR velocity mapping at 3T: Improved navigator-gated assessment of vascular anatomy and blood flow. *Journal of Magnetic Resonance Imaging* 2007;25(4):824–831.

Martin C, Pham T, Sun W. Significant differences in the material properties between aged human and porcine aortic tissues. *European Journal of Cardio-Thoracic Surgery* 2011;40(1):28–34.

Martin C, Sun W. Biomechanical characterization of aortic valve tissue in humans and common animal models. *Journal of Biomedical Materials Research Part A* 2012;100(6):1591–1599.

Massoumian F, Juškaitis R, Neil MA, Wilson T. Quantitative polarized light microscopy. *Journal of Microscopy* 2003;209(1):13–22.

McGrath B, Mealing G, Labrosse MR. A mechanobiological investigation of platelets. Biomechanics and modeling in mechanobiology. 2011;10(4):473–484.

Megens RT, Egbrink MG, Cleutjens JP, Kuijpers MJ, Schiffers PH, Merkx M, Slaaf DW, Van Zandvoort MA. Imaging collagen in intact viable healthy and atherosclerotic arteries using fluorescently labeled CNA35 and two-photon laser scanning microscopy. *Molecular Imaging* 2007;6(4):247–260.

Merryman WD, Huang HY, Schoen FJ, Sacks MS. The effects of cellular contraction on aortic valve leaflet flexural stiffness. *Journal of Biomechanics* 2006;39(1):88–96.

Milani-Nejad N, Janssen PM. Small and large animal models in cardiac contraction research: Advantages and disadvantages. *Pharmacology & Therapeutics* 2014;141(3):235–249.

Mirnajafi A, Raymer J, Scott MJ, Sacks MS. The effects of collagen fiber orientation on the flexural properties of pericardial heterograft biomaterials. *Biomaterials* 2005;26(7):795–804.

Mirnajafi A, Raymer JM, McClure LR, Sacks MS. The flexural rigidity of the aortic valve leaflet in the commissural region. *Journal of Biomechanics* 2006;39(16):2966–2973.

Mohan D, Melvin JW. Failure properties of passive human aortic tissue. I—uniaxial tension tests. *Journal of Biomechanics* 1982;15(11):887895–893902.

Mohan D, Melvin JW. Failure properties of passive human aortic tissue. II—Biaxial tension tests. *Journal of Biomechanics* 1983;16(1):3139–3744.

Mouret F, Garitey V, Gandelheid T, Fuseri J, Rieu R. A new dual activation simulator of the left heart that reproduces physiological and pathological conditions. *Medical and Biological Engineering and Computing* 2000;38(5):558–561.

Murdock K, Martin C, Sun W. Characterization of mechanical properties of pericardium tissue using planar biaxial tension and flexural deformation. *Journal of the Mechanical Behavior of Biomedical Materials* 2018;77:148–156.

Naimark WA. Structure/function relations in mammalian pericardial tissue: Implications for comparative and developmental physiology. *Journal of Physiology* 1996;150:153–160.

Narine K, Ing EC, Cornelissen M, Desomer F, Beele H, Vanlangenhove L, De Smet S, Van Nooten G. Readily available porcine aortic valve matrices for use in tissue valve engineering. Is cryopreservation an option? *Cryobiology* 2006;53(2):169–181.

Nguyen TT, Biadillah Y, Mongrain R, Brunette J, Tardif JC, Bertrand OF. A method for matching the refractive index and kinematic viscosity of a blood analog for flow visualization in hydraulic cardiovascular models. *Journal of Biomechanical Engineering* 2004;126(4):529–535.

Nicosia MA. A theoretical framework to analyze bend testing of soft tissue. *Journal of Biomechanical Engineering* 2007;129(1):117–120.

O'Leary SA, Doyle BJ, McGloughlin TM. Comparison of methods used to measure the thickness of soft tissues and their influence on the evaluation of tensile stress. *Journal of Biomechanics* 2013;46(11):1955–1960.

Okafor I, Raghav V, Condado JF, Midha PA, Kumar G, Yoganathan AP. Aortic regurgitation generates a kinematic obstruction which hinders left ventricular filling. *Annals of Biomedical Engineering* 2017;45(5):1305–1314.

Oomen PJ, Loerakker S, Van Geemen D, Neggers J, Goumans MJ, Van Den Bogaerdt AJ, Bogers AJ, Bouten CV, Baaijens FP. Age-dependent changes of stress and strain in the human heart valve and their relation with collagen remodeling. *Acta Biomaterialia* 2016;29:161–169.

Pedley TJ, Luo XY. Fluid mechanics of large blood vessels. Shaanxi People's Press, China, 1995.

Pedrizzetti G, La Canna G, Alfieri O, Tonti G. The vortex an early predictor of cardiovascular outcome? *Nature Reviews Cardiology* 2014;11(9):545–553.

Pham T, Sun W. Material properties of aged human mitral valve leaflets. *Journal of Biomedical Materials Research Part A* 2014;102(8):2692–2703.

Pichamuthu JE, Phillippi JA, Cleary DA, Chew DW, Hempel J, Vorp DA, Gleason TG. Differential tensile strength and collagen composition in ascending aortic aneurysms by aortic valve phenotype. *The Annals of Thoracic Surgery* 2013;96(6):2147–2154.

Purslow PP. Positional variations in fracture toughness, stiffness and strength of descending thoracic pig aorta. *Journal of Biomechanics* 1983;16(11):947–953.

Raffel M, Willert CE, Wereley ST, Kompenhans J. *Particle Image Velocimetry: A Practical Guide*. Springer, Berlin, Germany, 2013.

Ragaert K, De Somer F, Somers P, De Baere I, Cardon L, Degrieck J. Flexural mechanical properties of porcine aortic heart valve leaflets. *Journal of the Mechanical Behavior of Biomedical Materials* 2012;13:78–84.

Rego BV, Sacks MS. A functionally graded material model for the transmural stress distribution of the aortic valve leaflet. *Journal of Biomechanics* 2017;54:88–95.

Romo A, Badel P, Duprey A, Favre JP, Avril S. In vitro analysis of localized aneurysm rupture. *Journal of Biomechanics* 2014;47(3):607–616.

Sacks MS, Smith DB, Hiester ED. A small angle light scattering device for planar connective tissue microstructural analysis. *Annals of Biomedical Engineering* 1997;25(4):678–689.

Sacks MS. Biaxial mechanical evaluation of planar biological materials. *Journal of Elasticity* 2000;61(1):199.

Sassani SG, Tsangaris S, Sokolis DP. Layer-and region-specific material characterization of ascending thoracic aortic aneurysms by microstructure-based models. *Journal of Biomechanics* 2015;48(14):3757–3765.

Sato M, Levesque MJ, Nerem RM. Micropipette aspiration of cultured bovine aortic endothelial cells exposed to shear stress. *Arteriosclerosis, Thrombosis, and Vascular Biology* 1987;7(3):276–286.

Sauren AA, Van Hout MC, Van Steenhoven AA, Veldpaus FE, Janssen JD. The mechanical properties of porcine aortic valve tissues. *Journal of Biomechanics* 1983;16(5):327–337.

Schenke-Layland K, Xie J, Heydarkhan-Hagvall S, Hamm-Alvarez SF, Stock UA, Brockbank KG, MacLellan WR. Optimized preservation of extracellular matrix in cardiac tissues: Implications for long-term graft durability. *The Annals of Thoracic Surgery* 2007;83(5):1641–1650.

Scotten LN, Walker DK. New laboratory technique measures projected dynamic area of prosthetic heart valves. *The Journal of Heart Valve Disease* 2004;13(1):120–132.

Schmid PJ. Dynamic mode decomposition of numerical and experimental data. *Journal of Fluid Mechanics* 2010;656:5–28.

Segers P, Dubois F, De Wachter D, Verdonck P. Role and relevancy of a cardiovascular simulator. *Cardiovascular Engineering* 1998;3:48–56.

Shahmansouri N, Cartier R, Mongrain R. Characterization of the toughness and elastic properties of fresh and cryopreserved arteries. *Journal of Biomechanics* 2015;48(10):2205–2209.

Shojaei-Baghini E, Zheng Y, Sun Y. Automated micropipette aspiration of single cells. *Annals of Biomedical Engineering* 2013;41(6):1208–1216.

Sider KL, Blaser MC, Simmons CA. Animal models of calcific aortic valve disease. *International Journal of Inflammation* 2011;2011:364310.

Sim EK, Muskawad S, Lim CS, Yeo JH, Hiang Lim K, Grignani RT, Durrani A, Lau G, Duran C. Comparison of human and porcine aortic valves. *Clinical Anatomy* 2003;16(3):193–196.

Skalak R, Tozeren A, Zarda RP, Chien S. Strain energy function of red blood cell membranes. *Biophysical Journal* 1973;13(3):245–264.

Sommer G, Gasser TC, Regitnig P, Auer M, Holzapfel GA. Dissection properties of the human aortic media: an experimental study. *Journal of Biomechanical Engineering* 2008;130(2):021007.

Srichai MB, Lim RP, Wong S, Lee VS. Cardiovascular applications of phase-contrast MRI. *American Journal of Roentgenology* 2009;192(3):662–675.

Stemper BD, Yoganandan N, Stineman MR, Gennarelli TA, Baisden JL, Pintar FA. Mechanics of fresh, refrigerated, and frozen arterial tissue. *Journal of Surgical Research* 2007;139(2):236–242.

Stugaard M, Koriyama H, Katsuki K, Masuda K, Asanuma T, Takeda Y, Sakata Y, Itatani K, Nakatani S. Energy loss in the left ventricle obtained by vector flow mapping as a new quantitative measure of severity of aortic regurgitation: A combined experimental and clinical study. *European Heart Journal-Cardiovascular Imaging* 2015;16(7):723–730.

Sutton MA, Ke X, Lessner SM, Goldbach M, Yost M, Zhao F, Schreier HW. Strain field measurements on mouse carotid arteries using microscopic three-dimensional digital image correlation. *Journal of Biomedical Materials Research Part A* 2008;84(1):178–190.

Suzuki Y, Yeung AC, Ikeno F. The pre-clinical animal model in the translational research of interventional cardiology. *JACC: Cardiovascular Interventions* 2009;2(5):373–383.

Tanné D, Bertrand E, Kadem L, Pibarot P, Rieu R. Assessment of left heart and pulmonary circulation flow dynamics by a new pulsed mock circulatory system. *Experiments in Fluids* 2010;48(5):837–850.

Theret DP, Levesque MJ, Sato M, Nerem RM, Wheeler LT. The application of a homogeneous half-space model in the analysis of endothelial cell micropipette measurements. *Journal of Biomechanical Engineering* 1988;110(3):190–199.

Tirunagari S, Vuorinen V, Kaario O, Larmi M. Analysis of proper orthogonal decomposition and dynamic mode decomposition on les of subsonic jets. *CSI Journal of Computing* 2012;1(3):20–26.

Tsang HG, Rashdan NA, Whitelaw CB, Corcoran BM, Summers KM, MacRae VE. Large animal models of cardiovascular disease. *Cell Biochemistry and Function* 2016;34(3):113–132.

Tu JH, Rowley CW, Luchtenburg DM, Brunton SL, Kutz JN. On dynamic mode decomposition: theory and applications. arXiv preprint arXiv:1312.0041. 2013 Nov 29.

Waldman SD, Lee JM. Boundary conditions during biaxial testing of planar connective tissues. Part 1: dynamic behavior. *Journal of Materials Science: Materials in Medicine* 2002;13(10):933–938.

Waldman SD, Sacks MS, Lee JM. Boundary conditions during biaxial testing of planar connective tissues Part II Fiber orientation. *Journal of Materials Science Letters* 2002;21(15):1215–1221.

Weiler M, Yap CH, Balachandran K, Padala M, Yoganathan AP. Regional analysis of dynamic deformation characteristics of native aortic valve leaflets. *Journal of Biomechanics* 2011;44(8):1459–1465.

Weisbecker H, Pierce DM, Regitnig P, Holzapfel GA. Layer-specific damage experiments and modeling of human thoracic and abdominal aortas with non-atherosclerotic intimal thickening. *Journal of the Mechanical Behavior of Biomedical Materials* 2012;12:93–106.

Whittaker P, Kloner RA, Boughner DR, Pickering JG. Quantitative assessment of myocardial collagen with picrosirius red staining and circularly polarized light. *Basic Research in Cardiology* 1994;89(5):397–410.

Yoganathan AP, Barker AJ, Garcia C, Okafor II, Oshinski J. A physiologic flow phantom for the evaluation of 4D flow MRI in the left ventricle. *Journal of Cardiovascular Magnetic Resonance* 2015;17(1):Q106.

Yousif MY, Holdsworth DW, Poepping TL. A blood-mimicking fluid for particle image velocimetry with silicone vascular models. *Experiments in Fluids* 2011;50(3):769–774.

Zaragoza C, Gomez-Guerrero C, Martin-Ventura JL, Blanco-Colio L, Lavin B, Mallavia B, Tarin C, Mas S, Ortiz A, Egido J. Animal models of cardiovascular diseases. *BioMed Research International* 2011;2011:497841.

Zhang MG, Cao YP, Li GY, Feng XQ. Spherical indentation method for determining the constitutive parameters of hyperelastic soft materials. *Biomechanics and Modeling in Mechanobiology* 2014;13(1):1–1.

Zhang W, Feng Y, Lee CH, Billiar KL, Sacks MS. A generalized method for the analysis of planar biaxial mechanical data using tethered testing configurations. *Journal of Biomechanical Engineering* 2015;137(6):064501.

Zhou EH, Lim CT, Quek ST. Finite element simulation of the micropipette aspiration of a living cell undergoing large viscoelastic deformation. *Mechanics of Advanced Materials and Structures* 2005;12(6):501–512.

5

Computational Methods in Cardiovascular Mechanics

F. Auricchio, M. Conti, A. Lefieux, S. Morganti,
A. Reali, G. Rozza, and A. Veneziani

Contents

5.1 Introduction: The Role and Development of Computational Methods

The introduction of computational models in cardiovascular sciences has progressively brought new and unique tools for the investigation of pathophysiology. Together with the dramatic improvement in imaging and measuring devices on the one hand and in computational architecture on the other hand, mathematical and numerical models have provided a new, clearly noninvasive approach for understanding not only basic mechanisms but also patient-specific conditions and for supporting the design and development of new therapeutic options. The in silico terminology is nowadays commonly accepted for referring to this new source of knowledge, added to traditional in vitro and in vivo investigations. The advantages of in silico methodologies include the low cost in terms of infrastructures and facilities, the reduced invasiveness, and, in general, the intrinsic predictive capabilities based on the use of mathematical models. The disadvantages are generally stated as the gaps between the real cases and their virtual counterparts; this gap, which comes in part from the idealization required by conceptual modeling, may be detrimental to the reliability of numerical simulations.

In this respect, the terrific development of new devices and algorithms for image and data retrieval and processing has allowed the migration from (over)simplified, idealized descriptions to high-fidelity patient-specific models, in a critical, still ongoing process of merging measurement and conceptualization. Meanwhile, the progressive improvement of computational resources provides the infrastructure to perform numerical simulations of complex dynamics in reasonable times. Complementary to these advances is the development of novel specific modeling techniques and solvers in the field of computational mechanics, in an exciting process involving mathematics, engineering, computer science, and biomedical knowledge. This process already has an impact not only on research but also on clinical practice. As a matter of fact, as the example of the HeartFlow company (Taylor et al., 2013) demonstrates, mathematical and computational modeling can be more than research tools and can be integrated in products for the clinical market.

The aim of this chapter is to give an introduction to the computational methods used in cardiovascular mechanics and not to be exhaustive. Thus, our goal is to provide basic concepts and examples for a minimal acquaintance with several important references to the recent literature, possibly with a view to a deeper investigation of the subject. Accordingly, the first part of this chapter is devoted to the numerical simulation of tissues and structures in cardiovascular mechanics. In particular, we will deal with cardiovascular diseases (CVDs) and the structural simulations of the corresponding endovascular treatments. We will also discuss the main steps and issues inherent with such simulations. Regarding applications, we will focus on the simulation of shape-memory alloy (SMA) stents for carotid arteries on the one hand, and consider the important problem of the simulation of transcatheter aortic valve implantation (TAVI) on the other hand. Finite element analysis represents by far the most used simulation tool for the prediction of the structural behavior of tissues and devices, and the results presented will be obtained from this classical simulation framework. However, this section will be completed by a digression on a promising extension of the finite element (FE) method known as isogeometric analysis (IGA).

In the second part of the chapter, the reader will be provided with a "survival kit" for entering the fascinating world of the numerical modeling of human hemodynamics. As a matter of fact, the complexity of the systems to be modeled is reflected in the significant complexity of the mathematical and numerical problems to be solved. In the last several decades, computational hemodynamics has provided a practical framework for many theoretical and methodological developments relevant to a much wider range of applications (in fact, this is also true for the celebrated Euler equations, initially introduced by the Swiss mathematician for describing blood flow in compliant arteries, and is eventually used for describing gas dynamics in pipes such as in internal combustion engines). In particular, we will consider basic concepts for the numerical modeling of blood as a fluid in three-dimensional (3D) domains.

We will then complement the first two parts of the chapter with a discussion on specific methods to simulate the complexity that may arise when considering fluid–structure interaction problems occurring in computational hemodynamics, such as the interaction between blood and the vascular walls, and in heart valve dynamics. Moreover, as the computational cost of the numerical approximations of the problems is generally high, their complexity may need to be conveniently reduced, calling for specific model reduction techniques based on the online/ offline paradigm. These techniques take advantage of the available high-fidelity results from previous simulations to perform new and fast simulations of different cases. Therefore, the final part of this chapter will be a primer on reduced-order model methods and especially those that look particularly promising to fulfill clinical timelines.

5.2 Simulating Tissues and Structures in Cardiovascular Mechanics

5.2.1 Cardiovascular Diseases and Endovascular Treatments

Cardiovascular disease is the generic name given to dysfunctions of the cardiovascular system such as atherosclerosis, hypertension, coronary heart disease, heart failure, and stroke. Cardiovascular disease is still the main cause of death in Europe, leading to almost twice as many deaths as cancer across the continent (Townsend et al., 2015). In particular, within the broad family of CVD, we will refer in the following text to focal obstructive lesions or stenosis of the arteries (coronaries, carotid, and limb arteries) and heart valves or the abnormal localized bulging of the aorta called aneurysm. The use of endovascular approaches has revolutionized the treatment of this class of vascular diseases, which used to be treated by combining open surgery with medical management. In fact, in recent decades, endovascular therapy of vascular diseases has broadened its field of applications—from coronary stenting to treat atherosclerotic stenosis to the endovascular replacement of aortic valve. As mentioned earlier, the broadening of indications for endovascular therapy has been supported by improvements in the design and technological content of endovascular devices. Such advancements have been supported by dedicated biomechanical analyses of the artery–device interactions through computational tools, such as structural finite element analysis (FEA) and computational fluid dynamics (CFD), which are nowadays extensively used during the design of devices (Alaimo et al., 2017), for preoperative planning (Morganti et al., 2016, de Jaegere et al., 2016), or in diagnostics (Gasser et al., 2016; Gaur et al., 2017), as discussed in the following text, which deals with different aspects of simulating tissues and structures in cardiovascular mechanics. In particular, we will focus herein on the simulation of endovascular treatments of peripheral arteries (e.g., carotid artery) and the aortic valve, and we will neglect coronary stenting, which deserves a dedicated dissertation, as reported in (Morlacchi et al., 2013).

5.2.2 Simulation Framework: From Medical Images to Virtual Endovascular Implant

In the recent years, numerical methods and scanning technology such as computed tomography (CT) and magnetic resonance imaging (MRI) have advanced rapidly, making it possible to generate high-quality meshes directly from images and enabling the analysis of complex biomedical phenomena. In common approaches to generate vascular meshes, boundary surfaces are extracted using isocontouring (Yushkevich et al., 2006), which usually involves manual interaction, and then, tetrahedral (Antiga et al., 2008) or hexahedral (hex) meshes (De Santis et al., 2011; Bols et al., 2016) are constructed. Dedicated algorithms have been proposed (Zhang et al., 2007) to generate hexahedral solid nonuniform rational B-splines (NURBS) meshes for patient-specific vascular geometric models from imaging data for use in IGA (Hughes et al., 2005) as well.

The direct assessment of arterial wall thickness, which is an important part of the computational modeling of the vessel wall, by using CT and MRI is a nontrivial task in most cases, because of the limitations of imaging resolution and lack of contrast. Many approaches have been proposed in the literature. Johnson and colleagues (2011) deformed a healthy vessel onto a cerebral aneurysm by surface parameterization and used an anisotropic nonlinear spring model based on the material directions to construct the weakened wall, estimating its material strength and anisotropy by comparing the original surface and the deformed mesh (Zhang et al., 2013). The use of such an equivalent wall thickness appeared to yield a more accurate prediction of the aneurysm rupture site. However, in the case of mechanical simulations of aortic aneurysms, the assessment of wall thickness is still an open issue (Gasser, 2016). The assumption of uniform wall strength and thickness in FE models predicting aneurysm rupture seems to provide better results than the use of a variable wall thickness (Martufi et al., 2015). In fact, most of the structural simulations for the analysis of the deployment of endovascular devices and the consequent interaction with the arterial wall have assumed either an elastic wall with uniform thickness (Altnji et al., 2015; Perrin et al., 2015) or a wall represented as a rigid surface (Auricchio et al., 2013a; Cosentino et al., 2015). The inclusion of calcifications and accurate modeling of mechanical nonhomogeneity due to atherosclerotic degeneration of the arterial wall still imply manual segmentation (Auricchio et al., 2013b) and are limited to a small population of patients (Wang et al., 2017). Readers interested in these topics are referred to (Zhang et al., 2016), where extensive information is reported about geometric modeling and mesh generation from scanned images in the biomedical field.

5.2.3 The Specific Issue of Boundary Conditions

The mechanical loading experienced by endovascular devices implanted into the cardiovascular system can be complex, potentially impairing the performance and mechanical durability of these devices. Although the cyclic radial expansion of arteries, due to the pulsatile nature of the luminal blood pressure, has been the main focus of cardiovascular device durability in the past (Pelton et al., 2008), the importance of other loading components, such as arterial stretching, shortening, bending, twisting, and kinking, which are induced not only by the cardiac and respiration cycles (Ullery et al., 2015) but also by musculoskeletal movements, for example, leg bending (MacTaggart et al., 2014), swallowing, and neck twisting (Robertson et al., 2008), is now acknowledged. These considerations are particularly important for specific vascular districts such as the superficial femoral arteries (SFAs) or popliteal arteries, which are close to important musculoskeletal joints (i.e., hip and knee) and are, at the same time, bounded by muscular tissue. Indeed, SFA biomechanics has recently been investigated using advanced medical imaging (Cheng et al., 2006) and in ex vivo experiments (Poulson et al., 2017), with the objectives to assess the loading imposed onto the implanted stents (Choi et al., 2009) by directly enforcing the measured arterial kinematics (Conti et al., 2017) or to calibrate the arterial model parameters (Petrini et al., 2016). The situation is further complicated by the age dependency of the arterial motion (Kamenskiy et al., 2015) and tortuosity (Thomas et al., 2005). Moreover, biomechanical asymmetry is widely diffused in the body, as demonstrated by the in vivo measurement of the renal artery deformations (Suh et al., 2013). Finally, the presence of implanted devices can dramatically change the dynamic vascular environment (Hirotsu et al., 2017; Nauta et al., 2017), inducing a stiffening of the whole arterial district (de Beaufort et al., 2017a, 2017b). These observations suggest that the sole preoperative data are not enough to inform on the whole range of loading that the device will experience. Therefore, it is evident that the assessment of dedicated boundary conditions in the biomechanical analysis of endovascular devices is fundamental and calls for patient-site-specific investigation. In this respect, there is a knowledge gap that needs to be filled, from both academia and industry, with the aim to design, benchmark, and manufacture long-lasting implanted endovascular devices such as stents and endografts.

5.2.4 Example of Device Modeling: Shape-Memory-Alloy–Based Stent Simulations

Thanks to its unique mechanical features such as pseudoelasticity, Nitinol, the most well-known and used SMA, made of the combination of nickel and titanium, has allowed the design of many innovative applications in the biomedical field (Auricchio et al., 2015a). Among others, cardiovascular self-expanding stents represent the most successful use of Nitinol; they have a high commercial value and call for engineering tools supporting the design of novel devices. To this aim, during the device design stage, it is of paramount importance to accurately predict the complex behavior of such SMA under various loading conditions, using dedicated constitutive modeling. The pioneering study of Witcher in 1997 used structural FEA to estimate the mechanical behavior of Boston Scientific's Symphony stent under in vivo loading conditions. Several simplistic assumptions included a von Mises yield elastoplastic constitutive law to model Nitinol and a pressure load on the stent portion that resembled the in vivo loading conditions, that is, neglecting the arterial wall. In 2000, Rebelo and Perry adopted the constitutive model by Auricchio and Taylor (1997) and by Auricchio et al. (1997) based on the concept of generalized plasticity (Lubliner and Auricchio, 1996) to take pseudoelasticity into account in the FEA simulation of Nitinol stent self-expansion. In 2002, Perry and colleagues extended the study to analyze stent fatigue resistance, which was further investigated in 2003 by Pelton and colleagues, who combined displacement-controlled fatigue experimental tests on laser-cut stent-like devices with nonlinear FEA to compute strains. Furthermore, in 2004, Auricchio and Petrini proposed a robust SMA constitutive model. This model was able to reproduce both pseudoelastic effect and shape-memory effect and was particularly well suited for the simulation of real industrial applications, such as the design of medical stents (Petrini et al., 2005). In 2006, Thériault and colleagues discussed the development of a Nitinol stent that could smoothly expand in the arterial wall by the creep effect of a polymeric cover. In 2008, Kim et al. discussed the mechanical modeling of self-expandable braided stents, proposing an FE model coupled with a preprocessing program for the 3D geometrical modeling of the braided structure. In 2010, Auricchio et al. reviewed the properties of the SMA 3D model described in Auricchio and Petrini (2004), calibrating the model parameters with respect to experimental data and showing its application to the simulation of pseudoelastic Nitinol stent deployment in a simplified atherosclerotic artery model. In 2011, Rebelo and colleagues presented a study in which some common assumptions made in the FEA simulation of Nitinol devices were tested. In 2012, Garcia and colleagues used FEA to perform a parametric analysis of a commercial stent model and estimate the influence of geometrical variables on the stent radial expansion force. Other recent studies have targeted stent design optimization using FEA. For instance, Hsiao and Yin (2013) proposed to shift the highly concentrated stresses/strains away from the stent crown and redistribute them along the stress-free bar arm by tapering the strut width. Alaimo et al. (2017) conformed such a design approach by extending the approach proposed by Azaouzi and colleagues (2013) to a multiobjective optimization framework.

5.2.5 Modeling of Carotid Artery Stenting

The endovascular treatment of carotid stenosis represents one of the main fields of vascular surgery. It has a substantial economic impact, as the global neurovascular intervention market is expected to surpass $2.5 billion by 2018. Such an impact drives the continuous development of novel devices (Schofer et al., 2015) and stimulates biomechanical studies that address the use of structural FEA to design or optimize the design of carotid stents. The first study in this direction was carried out in 2007 by Wu et al., who simulated the implantation of a Nitinol stent in a geometrical idealization of the carotid bifurcation, accounting for the delivery sheath. Following the study of Wu et al., in 2011, Auricchio et al. used structural FEA to evaluate the performance of three different self-expanding stent designs in the same carotid artery model, based on computed angiography tomographic images, toward a quantitative assessment of the relationship between a given carotid stent design and a given patient-specific carotid artery anatomy. The same computational framework was subsequently validated in vitro (Conti et al., 2011) and used to assess the impact of stent scaffolding (Auricchio et al., 2012), as well as the impact of plaque morphology and anisotropic behavior in the arterial modeling (Auricchio et al., 2013b). More recently, Iannaccone et al. (2014) investigated the role of plaque shape and composition on the carotid arterial wall stress after stenting, using structural FE simulations and generalized atherosclerotic carotid geometries, including a damage model to quantify the injury of the vessel. An example of the computational framework aiming at simulating the carotid stent deployment in a patient-specific model derived from medical images is illustrated in Figure 5.1.

5.2.6 Modeling of Transcatheter Aortic Valve Implantation

In the last decade, computational tools have been increasingly used for the simulation of TAVI. The reason is twofold: on the one hand, from the medical point of view, TAVI is turning out to be not only a valuable minimally invasive technique for inoperable patients but also a promising solution in high- or intermediate-risk patients (Smith et al., 2011), and on the other hand, from the engineering point of view, computational tools and simulation technologies are becoming more and more powerful, allowing for the realistic virtual reproduction of real, even complex, procedures in a short time. Similarly to other cardiovascular computational models, in order to satisfy accuracy and reliability requirements, TAVI models have to take into account the patient-specific anatomical details, the characteristics of the patient's arteries (through appropriate constitutive models), the boundary conditions, and the loads governing the prosthesis expansion, as well as those generated by the procedure acting on the anatomical structures. Since the first publication by Dwyer et al. (2009) aiming at characterizing the blood ejection force able to induce a prosthesis migration, several other works that have used patient-specific data have

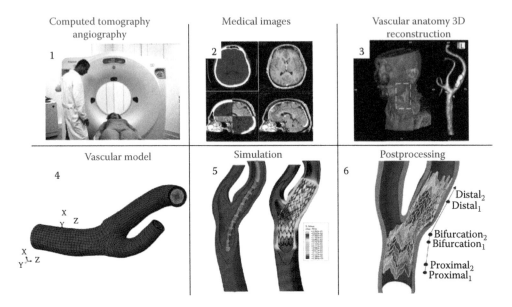

Figure 5.1   Illustrative representation of the steps to be performed for the patient-specific simulation of an endovascular procedure (in this case, carotid artery stenting). Starting from medical images routinely used in clinical practice, an accurate 3D model of the vascular anatomy can be created and transformed into a computational domain suitable for analysis. By combining the vascular model with a given prosthesis model, it is possible to predict the postimplant vessel/prosthesis configuration and compute, through dedicated postprocessing, clinically relevant measures, which would be almost impossible to quantify in vitro or in vivo.

been published. The first study using patient data (from a 68-year-old male) was proposed by Sirois et al. (2011).

The procedure of TAVI is quite complex, and its main steps can be summarized in (a) device crimping, (b) positioning, and (c) expansion. In addition, each of the previously listed steps involves nontrivial physical phenomena, as the strong crimping of a complex-shape device made of materials exhibiting nonlinear behavior or the expansion of the same device that interacts with native tissues and calcifications. For this reason, many authors have focused their work on specific aspects of the entire TAVI procedure. Wang et al. (2012b), for example, focused only on the deployment of a balloon-expandable device within a patient-specific aortic root reconstructed from medical images. Similarly, Gunning et al. (2014) analyzed, in a patient-specific case, the bioprosthetic leaflet deformation due to the deployment of a self-expanding valve. For simplicity, some authors considered only the stent for their numerical investigations: Schievano et al. (2010) and Capelli et al. (2010) proposed an FEA-based methodology to provide information and help clinicians during the planning of percutaneous pulmonary valve implantation. In these works, the implantation site has been simplified using rigid elements, and, at the same time, the presence of the valve has been neglected. Many other studies have focused on the leaflets, while neglecting the stent: for example, Smuts et al. (2011) developed new concepts for different percutaneous aortic leaflet geometries by means of FEA, while Sun et al. (2010) investigated the implications of asymmetric transcatheter prosthesis deployment on a bioprosthetic valve. Capelli et al. (2012) performed patient-specific analyses to explore the feasibility of TAVI in morphologies that were borderline cases for a minimally invasive approach. Tzamtzis et al. (2013) compared the radial force produced by a self-expandable vale (i.e., the Medtronic CoreValve®) and a balloon-expandable one (i.e., the Edwards SAPIEN® valve). The radial force of a self-expanding valve was also investigated by Gessat et al. (2014), who developed an innovative method for extracting this piece of information from images of an implanted device. It is also worth mentioning the works by Auricchio et al. (2014) and Morganti et al. (2014, 2016) that proposed a step-by-step strategy to simulate the entire implantation procedure (from crimping to expansion) of both balloon- and self-expandable prosthetic valves (Figure 5.2).

The developed simulation frameworks, based on patient-specific imaging data, allow for the prediction of useful clinical parameters and advance computational tools as a promising support in the decision-making process. In particular, through predictive simulations, it is possible to become aware of findings that may be correlated with possible procedure complications. For example, the action of the metallic frame of the stent on the native calcified aortic root wall can be evaluated by computing the von Mises aortic wall stresses induced by stent expansion. On the one hand, higher stress values can be related to higher force of adherence between the stent and the aortic wall, and on the other hand, high-stress patterns concentrated in the annular region can indicate a major risk of aortic rupture. In addition to the magnitude of the force induced by the device on the aortic wall, the grade of prosthesis apposition and, consequently, a measure of how well the device is anchored could be evaluated by measuring the contact surface area between the stent and the aortic root. At the same time, structural FEA can be used to quantitatively evaluate the area of perivalvular orifices, which can be assumed to be proportional to the amount of retrograde perivalvular blood flow (i.e., perivalvular leakage). Moreover, the native morphology of the aortic root and, in particular, the quantity and position of calcifications, may induce a noncircular shape into the implanted device, which can have an impact on the valve performance and can be studied by FEA (Morganti et al., 2014, 2016). From the simulation of valve closure, the postoperative device performance can finally be predicted based on the amount of valve coaptation (Figure 5.3).

5.2.7 Beyond Classical Finite Element Methods: Isogeometric Analysis

Finite element analysis represents by far the most used simulation tool for the prediction of the structural behavior of cardiovascular tissues and devices. Yet, the research community is continuously working to advance classical FEA or to even develop completely new concepts that would improve the current situation in terms

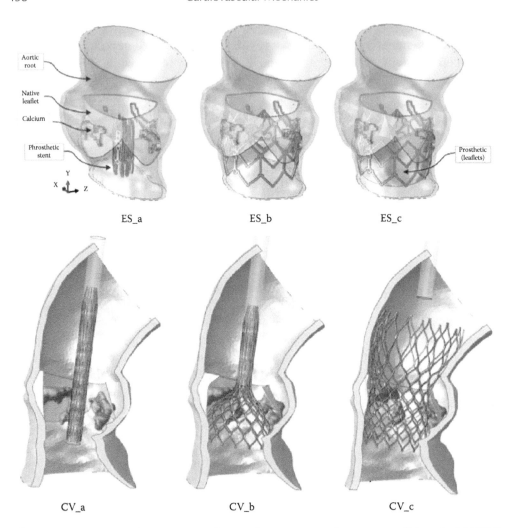

Figure 5.2 Transcatheter aortic valve implantation simulation steps: Edwards SAPIEN XT stent positioning (ES_a), device expansion (ES_b), and postimplant valve performance (ES_c). Medtronic CoreValve stent positioning (CV_a), device opening (CV_b), and final configuration of implanted device (CV_c).

of simulation speed and accuracy. A complete survey of alternative approaches is beyond the scope of this chapter, and we limit the discussion here to IGA (see Cottrell et al., 2009), certainly one of the most celebrated (relatively) new options to enhance FEA performance.

Isogeometric analysis was introduced in 2005 by Hughes and coworkers, with the main goal of bridging the gap between computer-aided design (CAD) and the FEM-based engineering analysis process. Its basic paradigm consists of adopting the same basis functions used for geometry representations in CAD systems, such as

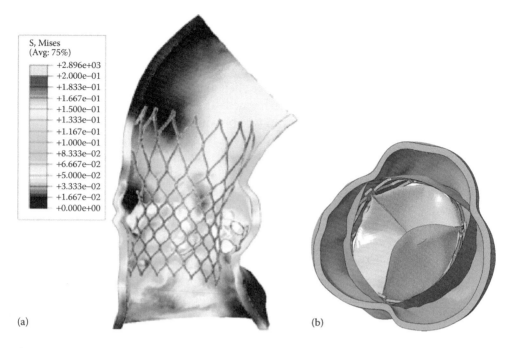

S, Mises
(Avg: 75%)
+2.896e+03
+2.000e−01
+1.833e−01
+1.667e−01
+1.500e−01
+1.333e−01
+1.167e−01
+1.000e−01
+8.333e−02
+6.667e−02
+5.000e−02
+3.333e−02
+1.667e−02
+0.000e+00

(a)   (b)

Figure 5.3   Example of simulation results: (a) von Mises stress pattern on the aortic root, induced by the CoreValve device implantation, and (b) Edwards SAPIEN XT postimplant performance in terms of prosthetic leaflet coaptation.

NURBS (e.g., for the approximation of field variables), in an isoparametric fashion. This leads to a cost-saving simplification of the typically expensive mesh generation and refinement processes required by standard FEA; this was the original motivation for IGA. Moreover, thanks to the high-regularity properties of its basis functions, IGA has shown a better accuracy per degree of freedom and an enhanced robustness compared with standard FEA in a number of applications. Solids and structures are prime examples (see, e.g., Cottrell et al., 2006; Cottrell et al., 2007; Elguedj et al., 2008; Lipton et al., 2010; Schillinger et al., 2012; Caseiro et al., 2015) and also include effective beam, plate, and shell elements (see, e.g., Kiendl et al., 2009; Benson et al., 2010; Echter et al., 2013; Kiendl et al., 2015). Isogeometric analysis has also been successful in fluid mechanics and fluid–structure interaction (see, e.g., Bazilevs et al., 2007; Akkerman et al., 2008; Gomez et al., 2010; Hsu and Bazilevs, 2012; Hsu et al., 2015) and has opened the door to geometrically flexible discretizations of higher-order partial differential equations (PDEs) in primal form (see, e.g., Auricchio et al., 2007; Gomez et al., 2008; Kiendl et al., 2016). Thanks to its more-than-promising results, IGA has attracted a lot of attention and is now regarded as one of the most prominent research areas in modern computational mechanics. Within this context, we focus here on two recent applications that show the potential of IGA for structural biomechanical simulations: aortic valves and SMA stents.

The first study is related to the explicit dynamics simulation of the closure of a patient-specific aortic valve, which has been performed via IGA and commercial FEA code LS-DYNA (Morganti et al., 2015). The complex geometrical model was built starting from medical images by means of conforming multi-patch untrimmed NURBS, and nonlinear shell analyses involving large deformations and contact were successfully performed. The mesh was refined until a good approximation of the leaflet coaptation was obtained. Despite the lack of optimization of the adopted IGA implementation, the IGA simulation was two orders of magnitude faster than that performed with what is considered the fastest shell FE on the market.

Qualitatively similar results were also obtained in the context of the nonlinear static analysis of SMA stent structures by means of 3D solid elements (Auricchio et al., 2015b). Such simulations include large deformations, complex inelastic constitutive laws, and buckling. While it is known that standard low-order FEA may fail to correctly reproduce the underlying physics of the problem unless using extremely fine meshes, IGA was able to produce correct results with (relatively) coarse meshes. In addition, for the same accuracy, the computational time with IGA was more than one order of magnitude faster than that with FEA.

5.3 Simulating Fluids in Cardiovascular Mechanics

The nature of blood as a fluid was already elucidated in the literature (Pedley, 1980; Galdi et al., 2008; Formaggia et al., 2009a; Nichols et al., 2011) and in Chapter 4. Here, we recall the basic features relevant to the selection of a specific mathematical and computational model.

Blood is a complex suspension of several particles, including red cells, blood cells, and platelets, in an aqueous solution (plasma). This nature clearly affects the physical behavior of blood as a liquid and, eventually, the selection of a mathematical model for blood flow. A decisive, extrinsic aspect in this is the domain where blood flows, which is significantly heterogeneous, ranging from one large vessel, the aorta, to a huge number of small capillaries. The relative size of the vessel compared with the size of the particles convected by the bloodstream is critical in selecting an appropriate mathematical description of the rheology, that is, the constitutive law describing the internal actions of the fluid as a continuum. In fact, a continuum description of blood flow in the capillaries may be inappropriate, as opposed to particle modeling, since the cells in the plasma have dimensions comparable to the size of the vessels. The region of interest of the vascular system is also important regarding flow regime. While in large and medium-sized vessels, blood flow features a significant unsteadiness or, more precisely, pulsatility (Nichols et al., 2011), with a prevalence of convective forces, the small vessels and the capillary bed typically feature quasisteady dynamics, dominated by viscous forces. In the latter case, flow is clearly laminar, whereas in large vessels, physical disturbances due to the convective forces may be observed. While in some animals, blood flow may feature turbulent dynamics, in human beings, the timing of a strong acceleration (lasting one third of the heartbeat) during the so-called systole, followed by a relatively quiet phase called diastole (when the heart valve is closed), normally prevents the transition to turbulence, which occurs only under pathological conditions.

In this chapter, we will specifically focus on blood flow in large and medium arteries, which are generally the sites of the most important vascular pathologies. However, numerical aspects of computational hemodynamics that go beyond the specific realm of large arteries will also be covered. Blood will be considered as:

1. Incompressible, so that density ρ is constant.
2. Newtonian, so that the rheology is simply described by a linear relation between the strain and stress tensors. The proportionality coefficient μ (dynamic viscosity) is a constant.
3. Pulsatile, so that inertial forces are accounted for.
4. Laminar, so that no specific modeling of turbulence is required. The numerical treatment of turbulence will be covered briefly, though, as this is crucial for some vascular districts.

These are the usual modeling-simplifying assumptions used for the description of blood flow in large arteries, and they lead to the celebrated system of the incompressible Navier–Stokes equations (NSEs) that are at the core of computational hemodynamics in three dimensions.

Denoting by the velocity vector by $u(x,t)$ and the pressure field by $p(x,t)$, both as functions of the space vector variables x and time t, the incompressible NSEs in a region of interest Ω, like the one illustrated in Figure 5.4, read

$$\begin{cases} \rho\big(\partial_t u+(u\cdot\nabla)u\big)-\mu\nabla\cdot\big(\nabla u+\nabla u^{\mathrm{T}}\big)+\nabla p = f \\ \nabla\cdot u = 0 \end{cases}, \tag{5.1}$$

for $x\in\Omega$ and $t>0$, where f is a (generic) forcing term (e.g., gravity).

Here, the first equation represents the momentum conservation for a Newtonian fluid and the second one follows from the mass conservation.

The equations describing blood dynamics need to be completed by initial conditions on velocity (the only unknown under time derivative) and by conditions to prescribe on the boundary of Ω that we will denote by Γ. These conditions represent the mutual influence of the external tissues and the upstream or downstream circulation on the blood. Generically, the initial conditions are prescribed in the form

$$u(x,0)=u_0(x) \quad \forall x\in\Omega,$$

where $u_0(x)$ is assumed to be given. However, it is difficult to retrieve an accurate knowledge of the velocity field in the entire domain of interest from current measurement devices. It is a good simulation practice to prescribe an arbitrary velocity

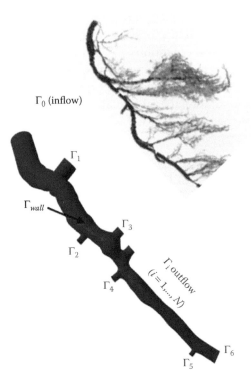

Γ_0 (inflow)

Γ_1

Γ_{wall}

Γ_3

Γ_2

Γ_i outflow
$(i = 1,..., N)$

Γ_4

Γ_6

Γ_5

Figure 5.4 Representation of a typical domain in computational hemodynamics (a coronary artery). The different portions of the boundary are highlighted.

field and then exploit the periodicity of the blood flow, as well as simulate a certain number of heart beats. Typically, after 3–10 heartbeats, depending on the vascular district under consideration, the influence of the initial condition on the numerical solution is significantly lost.

The issue of the boundary conditions is much more delicate, as these conditions have a major impact on the computed solution. Unfortunately, in most cases, a complete data set to prescribe boundary conditions is not available in practice, and the appropriate identification of numerical strategies to fill the gap between the mathematical theory of the NSE and simulation practice is still a subject of ongoing research.

5.3.1 Boundary Conditions: Theory and Practice

Generally speaking, from the mathematical point of view, the boundary conditions mostly occurring in the simulation of blood flow are of two types:

- Velocity conditions, that is, the prescription of the velocity field $v(x,t)$ at every point of the boundary

$$u(x,t) = v(x,t) \text{ for } \in \Gamma \tag{5.2}$$

- Traction conditions, that is, conditions prescribing the normal component of the stress tensor occurring in the momentum equation, in the form

$$p\boldsymbol{n} - \nu\left(\nabla\boldsymbol{u} + \nabla^T\boldsymbol{u}\right)\cdot\boldsymbol{n} = \boldsymbol{d} \tag{5.3}$$

where $\boldsymbol{d}$ is given

Both of them are vector conditions, enforcing three scalar functions at each boundary point. They are mathematically "correct." By this, we mean that they correctly complete the NSEs set, and under some additional assumptions about the regularity of domain Ω and about the initial conditions, it is possible to prove that the problem has a unique solution (the problem is said to be well posed) (Temam, 1984, 1995). Mathematically speaking, velocity conditions are usually called "Dirichlet" conditions, while traction data are called "Neumann" conditions.

Unfortunately, in the simulation of blood flow in real problems, these conditions can be barely prescribed, because data $\boldsymbol{v}$ and $\boldsymbol{d}$ are often not available or measurable, and they cannot be derived from physical arguments. In fact, in most cases, the known data are insufficient to make the problem well posed, and the boundary conditions are said to be "defective." The numerical treatment of defective conditions is currently the subject of active research, as the accurate selection of methodologies for their prescription is critical for the reliability of the numerical modeling. To be more concrete, let us consider the example of the flow rate. The flow rate through a boundary section Γ is technically defined as

$$Q(t) = \rho\int_\Gamma \boldsymbol{u}(\boldsymbol{x},t)\cdot\boldsymbol{n}\,d\boldsymbol{x}. \tag{5.4}$$

This is an integral condition over an entire portion of boundary Γ, available from measurements. It is clearly "defective," as it does not provide pointwise data at each point of the boundary. Another practical case is the prescription of the pressure $p_m(t)$ retrieved from some measurements and prescribed over Γ in the form of

$$p(\boldsymbol{x}\in\Gamma,t) = p_m(t) \tag{5.5}$$

In this case, we have one scalar condition prescribed over the boundary, instead of the vector condition required at each point, $\boldsymbol{x}\in\Gamma$.

There are several practical ways for bridging the gap in an engineering and mathematically consistent way. We will present now a short summary of some possible approaches for the prescription of the flow rate. The reader interested in this topic is referred to (Quarteroni et al., 2016, Formaggia et al., 2009b) and the references therein. As the flow rate $Q(t)$ is a defective condition, one way to provide additional data is through the velocity profile $\boldsymbol{v}(\boldsymbol{x},t)$. An engineering approach consists of the introduction of an arbitrary, yet reasonable velocity profile $\boldsymbol{v}_a(\boldsymbol{x},t)$, such that

$$\rho\int_\Gamma \boldsymbol{v}_a(\boldsymbol{x},t)\cdot\boldsymbol{n}\,d\boldsymbol{x} = Q(t).$$

In most cases, this profile is the parabolic function of the Poiseuille–Hagen solution or of a Womersley profile when Γ has a circular shape. In some circumstances, a flat velocity profile is a more reasonable option (e.g., at the entrance of the ascending aorta). The main advantage of this approach relies on its easiness, as it can be directly applied with standard CFD solvers. The main drawback is the arbitrary selection of a profile that may significantly impact the solution in the region of interest. In fact, to mitigate any effect on the solution, an artificial elongation of the region of interest called flow extension is applied to the computational domain. This is intended to position the prescription of the arbitrary profile farther away from the region of interest, so as to ultimately alleviate the impact of the arbitrary choice on the numerical solution. This approach, partially justified by the theory developed in (Veneziani and Vergara, 2007), stating that the arbitrariness of the velocity profile exponentially decays within the volume of interest, is extremely popular, even if the accurate construction of flow extensions is not necessarily a trivial step, in particular when working on a large volume of patients, as in clinical trials. Other, mathematically sounder approaches are possible. In particular, we recall here two alternative methods.

1. The Lagrange multiplier approach (Formaggia et al., 2002; Veneziani and Vergara, 2004, 2007): In this case, the flow rate is not regarded as a boundary condition but as a constraint assigned to the NSEs. As such, a Lagrange multiplier approach can be pursued, through the variational formulation of the problem. In this manner, no velocity profile needs to be prescribed a priori; instead, it is the by-product of the Lagrange multiplier calculation. As a benchmark, when either a Poiseuille profile or a Womersley profile is the exact solution of the problem, it is correctly retrieved by this approach. The main drawback of this formulation lies in the additional cost required by the Lagrange multiplier. Approximate effective solution methods have been proposed (Veneziani and Vergara, 2007).
2. The data assimilation approach (Formaggia et al. 2008, 2010): In this case, the condition on the flow rate is used for constructing a minimization procedure. The entire solution of the fluid dynamics is reformulated as the minimization of the mismatch between computations and data, under the constraint of the fluid equations.

The latter approach actually defines a change in perspective about boundary conditions. The aim is not to add constraints to a set of equations but to "assimilate" available data into the mathematical model in such a way that the results of the simulation match the available data (Law et al., 2015; Asch et al., 2016). This requires the identification of variables that need tuning to attain the minimization; they are called "control variables." For instance, we can select the normal stress (or traction) $\tau \equiv p\boldsymbol{n} - \nu\,(\nabla\boldsymbol{u} + \nabla^T\boldsymbol{u})\cdot\boldsymbol{n}$ on Γ as control variable and then solve the problem:

Find $\boldsymbol{\tau}$, such that

$$\left(\rho\int_\Gamma \boldsymbol{u}(\tau)\cdot\boldsymbol{n} - Q\right)^2 \text{ is minimal}$$

under constraint given by Equations (5.1).

This approach has been explored in (Formaggia et al. 2008, 2010), also in the case of fluid–structure interaction problems, with excellent numerical results. In fact, the approach is very general and can be applied to a large array of available data, regardless of their nature or incompleteness. In addition, it enforces the condition in a least-square sense, which is particularly appropriate when measured data are noisy. Although the selection of the control variables is critical to the quality of the results obtained after minimization, it is quite free and can be customized to different problems. The main drawback of this approach is its computational cost. The mathematical processes are akin to those of inverse problems that typically require intense iterative schemes. Approximate solution methods and reduced-order modeling become mandatory.

In more general terms, the prescription of boundary conditions is complicated by the "multiscale" nature of the circulatory system. The conditions of the downstream network may also affect the hemodynamics in the region of interest. This is a physical feature of the circulation that ensures resilience to the functioning of the system in the presence of occlusions or other pathologies. An occlusion is generally compensated for by collateral pathways (that under normal circumstances would be listed as redundant), and, more generally, circulation features baroreceptor reflex and chemoreflex mechanisms that regulate the blood supply from the large vessels according to the needs of the peripheral organs. In such cases, the mathematical model should include the presence of peripheral circulation downstream a region of interest. This can be attained by coupling the 3D Equations (5.1) with surrogate models. A popular strategy is the coupling of the NSEs with lumped parameter models (Formaggia et al., 2009b; Quarteroni et al., 2016) or, more generally, surrogate models. The numerical coupling of full and reduced models raises some methodological challenges, as investigated in the literature (see Quarteroni et al., 2016) and the references therein). In this section, to be concrete, but with no claim of completeness, we will address a popular simplified lumped parameter model that potentially captures the most relevant features of the peripheral circulation, the so-called three-element Windkessel model (3WK).

The name Windkessel comes from the air chamber used by German firemen to convert periodic flow into continuous flow, as happens in the peripheral districts. In particular, the 3WK features three parameters, two representing viscous resistances and one representing the global effects of vessel compliance of the peripheral districts. By exploiting the usual analogy between hydraulic networks and electrical circuits, the model is represented by the schematic reported in Figure 5.5, where R_1 and R_2 represent the viscous terms and C represents the compliance.

With the notation in the figure, the underlying mathematical model reads

$$\dot{P}_p + \frac{P_p}{CR_2} = \frac{Q}{C}, P = R_1 Q + P_p.$$

By integration, and assuming that the solution is known at instant t_0, we obtain

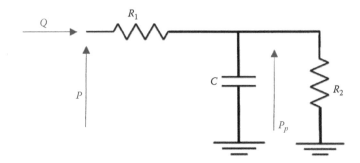

Figure 5.5 Diagram of the 3WK lumped parameter model for peripheral circulation.

$$p_{3WK}(t) = p_{3WK}(t_0)e^{\frac{-t-t_0}{CR_2}} + R_1\left(Q(t) - Q(t_0)e^{\frac{-t-t_0}{CR_2}}\right) + \frac{1}{C}\int_{t_0}^{t}Q(\tau)e^{(\tau-t)/CR_2}\,d\tau.$$

This relation can be used as a condition to prescribe pressure at outlet boundaries and incorporate the presence of the downstream circulation in the form, recalling Equation 5.3,

$$p\boldsymbol{n} - v\left(\nabla\boldsymbol{u} + \nabla^T\boldsymbol{u}\right)\cdot\boldsymbol{n} = p_{3WK}\boldsymbol{n}.$$

Recalling the definition of flow rate, this equation is a condition combining pressure and velocity in a nontrivial manner (Robin condition). In practice, one of the critical aspects when using this type of models is the estimation of parameters R_1, R_2, and C in patient-specific settings. It has been recognized that the reliability of patient-specific simulations strongly lies on the appropriate quantification of these parameters, based on the available data. This is still a subject of active research, and data assimilation techniques such as Kalman-filtering and variational approaches are currently under investigation (see, e.g., Bertoglio et al. 2012, 2014; Romarowski et al., 2017).

5.3.2 A Survey of Numerical Methods for Incompressible Fluids

The incompressible NSEs (Equations 5.1) still represent a mathematical challenge in many respects. Many fundamental theoretical problems are still open for these equations. In practice, the solution to the problem expressed by Equations (5.1), completed by initial and boundary conditions, needs to be obtained by numerical approximation, as analytical methods fail in general. In addition, the numerical solution of these equations is challenging because of their intrinsic features. In cardiovascular problems, the challenge is often compounded by the complexity of the geometries at hand. This subject is one of the pillars of CFDs. As the goal here is not to be exhaustive, the reader is referred to specific textbooks (see, e.g., Ferziger and Peric, 2012). However, we will recall the basic features of the numerical discretization of the problem.

Equations (5.1) constitute a nonlinear system of four PDEs that depend on space and time. The backbone of numerical discretization is to approximate these four equations with a (typically large) algebraic system, as many effective methods for solving algebraic systems of large dimensions are available with modern computers. Ideally, this procedure should be able to combine efficiency (the algebraic system is solved in a reasonable time) and accuracy (the approximation error is under control). Since there are two independent variables, space and time, the discretization is usually performed separately with respect to the two sets, as the differential nature of the problem is different in time and space.

Space discretization can be performed in many ways. Finite differences form the most intuitive method, based on a replacement of the derivatives by incremental quotients, after having discretized the original problem onto a suitable grid of points. These points are usually selected along the Cartesian directions and represent the space of the numerical solution, that is, where the numerical solution is actually computed. The underlying tool for estimating the errors, in this case, is given by the Taylor series expansion of the solution, according to the different Cartesian directions. Despite its simplicity, the method suffers from some drawbacks, in particular due to the lack of a complete rigorous mathematical background (Taylor series expansion can be used if the solution is smooth, which is seldom verified in real problems) and due to the intrinsic "Cartesian" footprint, which makes the treatment of complex geometries challenging.

Another extremely popular approach is the finite volume method, in which the volume of interest is split into many subdomains (or finite volumes) over which the equations are integrated. By an extensive use of the Gauss theorem to reformulate volume to surface integrals, and of quadrature approximations, the system is approximated by a system that determines the average of the solution for each volume. The method features significant simplicity and efficiency. In fact, it is the method of choice in many commercial packages. Nevertheless, the set-up of competitive high-order finite volume schemes may be tricky.

From the mathematical point of view, the solution schemes with the strongest theoretical background belong to the family of the Galerkin methods that include FE methods and spectral methods. These methods directly rely on the so-called weak formulation of the problem, stemming from the application of variational principles (virtual works). They also form the appropriate framework for theoretical analyses dealing with the possible lack of continuity of the solution, as it may occur in some applications. According to these methods, the numerical solution is not obtained by approximating the derivatives (or the integrals of the finite volume formulation) but by postulating a specific shape for the solution, as described by a finite number of parameters. For instance, with linear FEs, the solution is assumed to be piecewise linear over a set of volumes or elements covering the region of interest. Likewise, one can consider piecewise quadratic or even higher-order approximations. The derivative[1] of these functions can be computed to obtain a system of equations for the

---

[1] In fact, the concept of derivative that must be used here is a generalization of the classical definition, and is called generalized or distributional derivative (see, e.g., [Brezzi, Gilardi, 1987]).

parameters describing the approximate solution. The approximation is established in the functional space, where the numerical solution is looked for. Galerkin methods can be analyzed with the tools of functional analysis and approximation theory; these tools lead to a fairly complete picture of the different properties of FEs in terms of accuracy and efficiency (https://femtable.org/). Similarly, spectral methods postulate the solution to be of polynomial form defined at special points (Gaussian nodes) that guarantee high accuracy. Unfortunately, the management of these nodes in real geometries may be troublesome. Spectral elements are a sort of compromise, merging the advantages of spectral methods in a decomposition of local subdomains or macroelements. As a general rule, from the theoretical point of view, the finer the reticulation of the region of interest (the so-called mesh), the more accurate and numerically stable the solution. In practice, under a certain level of refinement, the solution does not sensibly improve, whereas computational costs and sensitivity to rounding errors increase. A good simulation practice is then to identify a mesh, such that the solution does not show significant improvements to refinement (the so-called mesh-independence test). As an example of the fact that research on the development of general methods is still very active, we will mention only IGA, which has already been introduced and discussed in Section 5.2.

For the space discretization of the NSEs, we will focus herein on using the FE method, recalling some key aspects. An extensive study can be found, for example, in Elman et al., (2014) and the bibliography therein. One of the fundamental features of the incompressible NSEs is the saddle-point problem. By this, we mean that the equations are the result of a minimization procedure constrained by the incompressibility. In this respect, pressure is the Lagrange multiplier of the constraint. This circumstance has a primary impact on the numerical discretization by FEs, because the correct formulation of the numerical approximation must obey some constraint on the selection of the trial spaces for velocity and pressure. This constraint is generally called the inf-sup or Babuška-Brezzi condition (1974). From a practical point of view, this condition ensures that the trial space of velocity is "large enough" compared with that of pressure. For instance, a piecewise linear FE approximation for both velocity and pressure is not viable, as the resulting algebraic system is singular. Piecewise quadratic velocities can be coupled to piecewise linear pressures to get a correct numerical approximation. However, this comes at the price of a large algebraic system to solve, with a significant computational burden. A possible workaround is given by numerical stabilization techniques (Hughes et al. 1986), which, however, may affect the accuracy of the solution. The so-called $P2 - P1$ pair (quadratic velocity and linear pressure), also called Taylor-Hood element, is one of the most popular choices in biomedical applications.

The space discretization results in a differential-algebraic system that itself requires a time discretization. This is usually achieved through finite difference schemes, for their simplicity and efficiency; however, space–time FE discretizations are also possible. With finite differences, the time derivative of velocity is replaced by incremental quotients, based on Taylor series expansions, determined at instants, separated by time interval Δt. For simplicity of the presentation, the step size is assumed constant, but it can be automatically adapted to guarantee accuracy during fast transient events and maintain efficiency when the dynamics is slow and less time samples are needed (Veneziani and Villa, 2013).

After time discretization, the system is eventually an algebraic system. Let U^k and P^k be the vectors describing the velocity and the pressure, respectively, in the FE space at time t_k. The algebraic system to be solved for time index k running from 1 to a final step K reads

$$
\begin{bmatrix} A(U^k) & B^T \\ B & 0 \end{bmatrix} \begin{bmatrix} U^k \\ P^k \end{bmatrix} = \begin{bmatrix} f(U^{k-1}) \\ 0 \end{bmatrix}. \tag{5.6}
$$

Matrix A represents the discretization of the momentum equation, while matrix B is the discretization of the divergence operator. Function $f(\cdot)$ represents the action of source terms and boundary conditions. This is an algebraic nonlinear system, and the final step to obtain the numerical solution is a linearization. This can be attained by iterative methods, such as Newton and Picard, that add another level of iterations in the time loop or by extrapolation, that is, by replacing $A(U^k)$ with matrix $A_L = A(U^*)$, where U^* is a time extrapolation of the velocity, based on the previous solutions. The latter is usually preferred in computational hemodynamics for its simplicity and computational efficiency. After linearization, we are left with a linear system in the form

$$
\begin{bmatrix} A_L & B^T \\ B & 0 \end{bmatrix} \begin{bmatrix} U^k \\ P^k \end{bmatrix} = \begin{bmatrix} f(U^{k-1}) \\ 0 \end{bmatrix}. \tag{5.7}
$$

This system is usually large—as required by the fulfillment of the inf-sup condition—and with spectral properties (i.e., eigenvalue distribution) that make the efficient numerical solution quite challenging. In addition, it must be solved at each time step, creating an overall computationally intensive problem. Toward efficient solving, a first necessary requirement is the identification of an appropriate preconditioner, that is, an invertible matrix, P, such that the system $P^{-1}\begin{bmatrix} A_L & B^T \\ B & 0 \end{bmatrix}\begin{bmatrix} U^k \\ P^k \end{bmatrix} = P^{-1}\begin{bmatrix} f(U^{k-1}) \\ 0 \end{bmatrix}$ presents much improved numerical properties for the solution. Unfortunately, in real large-sized problems (featuring on the order of millions of equations), the choice of a good preconditioner is generally not enough for an efficient solution. A possible workaround is then to split the solutions for velocity and pressure and to break down the computational complexity into a sequence of smaller and easier problems. The splitting can be carried out following different approaches; the literature on this topic is huge (Elman et al., 2014). Here, we will simply mention two methods.

1. Chorin–Temam method (split-then-discretize methods): Thanks to a well-known principle of differential vector calculus, called the Hodge decomposition or the Ladyzhenskaya theorem, the velocity solution can be regarded as the divergence-free component of a generic vector. The split is obtained by first computing this vector and then projecting it on the divergence-free space by subtracting the gradient of a scalar field related to the pressure. Overall, the solution is broken down into a standard advection–diffusion–reaction problem and a Poisson problem for the pressure. Each problem can be discretized by standard FE or other methods. The split is approximated only for the presence of the nonlinear convective term and boundary conditions required for the pressure (and not required by the original unsplit problem). An extensive theory on this method and its accuracy have been developed, for example, in Prohl (1997) and Guermond et al. (2006).

2. Algebraic splitting (discretize-then-split method): In this case, the split is the result of an approximate factorization of the matrix of the system into triangular factors:

$$\begin{bmatrix} A_L & B^T \\ B & 0 \end{bmatrix} \approx \begin{bmatrix} A_L & 0 \\ B & S \end{bmatrix} \begin{bmatrix} I & \tilde{B}^T \\ 0 & I \end{bmatrix},$$

where S and $\tilde{B}^T$ have to be properly designed, and I is the identity matrix. In this manner, the original system is naturally split into a sequence of systems, alternatively for velocities and pressures (Perot, 1993; Veneziani and Villa, 2013; Viguerie and Veneziani, 2017). The algebraic splitting approach has a less established theoretical background than the differential one, but it features comparable accuracy and does not have to specify any boundary condition for the pressure, as they are automatically incorporated into the discretization step.

In the specific field of computational hemodynamics, popular strategies rely on splitting methods, either differential or algebraic, the latter being preferred for their versatility regarding boundary conditions.

5.3.3 Turbulence Modeling

Blood generally features a flow regime dominated by pulsatility. High convective terms, measured by the presence of high values of Reynolds number $Re = \rho UL/\mu$, where U is a characteristic velocity of the problem and L is a characteristic length, may develop during the heartbeat, but they typically do not last enough to trigger turbulent dynamics. Still, the presence of highly disturbed flow, as may occur in the ascending aorta, generates numerical instabilities in the approximation process, which are generally addressed with a fine reticulation (direct numerical simulation or DNS). However, in the presence of pathological conditions associated with locally high convective terms, there is an energy cascade from macro- to microscales in the fluid that requires specific modeling. Examples include aortic dissections, where the entry tear between the false lumen and the true lumen causes a strong acceleration of the flow, and the total cavopulmonary connection, a special paediatric surgery that features a cross-shaped connection of vessels (e.g., Mirabella et al., 2013), where the occurrence of colliding streams increases the relative Reynolds number between the incoming flow jets.

Turbulence may be described in different ways, according to the different applications associated with different ranges of the Reynolds number. When an appropriate refinement of the computational grid is not feasible to encompass all the significant microscales involved in the dynamics, the backbone of numerical simulation relies on suitable surrogate modeling of the effects of (unresolved) microscales below the reticulation, up to the medium and large scales, solved by the adopted mesh. Reynolds-averaged Navier–Stokes models (RANS) are suitable for large Reynolds numbers and rely on time-averaged semiempirical procedures. For moderate Reynolds numbers (up to 5000), large-eddy simulations (LES) provide generally more accurate solutions. The surrogate modeling of the unresolved scales can be accomplished by solving an appropriate set of equations. For instance, in the Leray model, the original NSEs are replaced by a more complex (and computationally demanding) system:

$$\begin{cases} \rho\big(\partial_t u + (w \cdot \nabla)u\big) - \mu\nabla \cdot \big(\nabla u + \nabla u^{\mathrm{T}}\big) + \nabla p = f \\ \qquad\qquad \nabla \cdot u = 0 \\ \quad w - \delta^2 \nabla \cdot \big(a(u)\nabla w\big) + \nabla\lambda = u \\ \qquad\qquad \nabla \cdot w = 0 \end{cases} \tag{5.8}$$

where w and λ are auxiliary functions filtering the original set of equations, δ^2 is a parameter empirically selected (called filter radius) as a function of the reticulation size, and $a(\cdot)$ is an empirically design function (called indicator). The rationale for this approach is that the indicator function $a(u)$ is ≈ 0 for low Reynolds numbers and ≈ 1 for high Reynolds numbers, so as to introduce a filtering action on the convective field w occurring in the LES equations. For low Reynolds numbers, $w \approx u$, to be consistent with the original NSEs (Equations 5.1). For high Reynolds numbers, the indicator function stabilizes the numerical solver representing the effect of the high frequencies in the flow. Many different possible indicator functions are available, based on both mathematical arguments (e.g., deconvolution low-pass filtering techniques) and physical arguments (e.g., the Smagorinsky filter) (Bertagna et al., 2016). Since the computation of the indicator function may require the solution of an additional differential problem, the treatment of turbulence introduces additional computational costs; specific methods for the efficient solution of these issues are active research topics.

5.4 Simulating and Reducing Complexity

5.4.1 Fluid–Structure Interaction

A fluid–structure interaction problem in hemodynamics arises when a problem represented by the NSEs (Equations 5.1) is coupled with a structural problem represented by, for example, the equations of (nonlinear) elasticity. In general, the fluid and the solid domains are distinct and are indicated as Ω_f and Ω_s, respectively. The two problems are coupled by interface conditions that prescribe the continuity of the velocities and of the normal stresses existing at the interface Γ

$$
\begin{aligned}
\boldsymbol{u}_f &= \boldsymbol{u}_s \\
\boldsymbol{\sigma}_f \cdot \boldsymbol{n}_f + \boldsymbol{\sigma}_s \cdot \boldsymbol{n}_s &= 0
\end{aligned} \quad \text{on}\,\Gamma, \tag{5.9}
$$

where $\boldsymbol{\sigma}_f$ and $\boldsymbol{\sigma}_s$ are the fluid and solid stress tensors, respectively. When numerically solving these problems, several additional challenges arise beyond the solution of the individual components (fluid and structure). These challenges are diverse, as, in practice, different conditions of interaction are encountered between fluid and structure. In cardiovascular flows, there are two main types of interactions that can be addressed with different approaches: (1) the interaction between the vascular wall and the blood flowing in it, and (2) the interaction between the blood and a body floating in it, such as the leaflets of the aortic valve at the entrance of the aorta and the mitral valve or the venous valves, preventing backflow. The two problems present different features and are typically solved by different approaches.

Numerical methods in the fluid–structure interaction field can be categorized in different ways. Monolithic approaches can be distinguished from partitioned (or segregated) approaches. In the first case, the fluid and structural problems are solved simultaneously as a unique problem, resulting in one linear system after all the needed operations of discretization or linearization. This approach suffers from two drawbacks: (i) the coupled problem joins subproblems with different time constants, and this is reflected by the bad conditioning of the numerical approximation, and (ii) the number of degrees of freedom is generally huge, making the linear systems challenging to solve at each time step and demanding of high-performance computing facilities. Both aspects call for appropriate preconditioners. On the other hand, in segregated approaches, a modular formulation is undertaken, and the fluid and structural problems are generally solved sequentially by replacing interface conditions (Equation 5.9) with appropriate boundary conditions for each subproblem. The coupling of the two problems can then be categorized as strong or weak, depending on the way the interface conditions are enforced at each time step. If conditions in Equation 5.9 are fulfilled approximately (as function of the discretization parameters, for instance, the time step Δt), then the coupling is said to be weak, as it is exact only when the discrete problem tends to be the continuous one. If, in the discrete partitioned problems, the enforcement of Equation 5.9 is exact, then the coupling is said to be strong.

Another classification refers to the reticulation used for the two subdomains. Assuming, for instance, that the two problems will be solved sequentially by using FEs, a mesh needs to be introduced for each problem. The method is said to be fitted if the degrees of freedom at the interface are shared by the two solvers. Unfitted methods are those in which the degrees of freedom at the interface do not necessarily coincide; special procedures are needed to transfer information from one mesh to the other.

To be more concrete, the cases of weak and strong coupling are exemplified by means of pseudocode (using variables reflecting the notation used so far). We first present the pseudocode sequence for the case of weak coupling.

In this sequence, the continuity of velocities is used as a boundary condition for the

```
Algorithm 1: Weak Coupling
Initialize: set u_f_onGamma
while (t<=tfinal){
    sigma_f = solveFluid(omega_f,u_f_onGamma)
    EnforceIC(sigma_s_normal=sigma_f_normal);
    u_s_onGamma = solveStructure(omega_s,sigma_s_normal);
    EnforceIC(u_f_onGamma=u_s_onGamma);
    ManageGeometry(omega_s,omega_f)
    t=t+Deltat
}//end while
```

fluid. At the end of the fluid run, information is retrieved about the normal stress that becomes the surface force term on the boundary for the structural problem. Notice that, at each step, some geometry manipulation is needed to manage the transfer between the degrees of freedom of the two solvers (EnforceIC) and the change of configuration in the domains of interest (similar to a change of topology for a contact between two solids—ManageGeometry). It is also evident that the interface conditions are not prescribed exactly, as, clearly in this implementation, the continuity of the normal stress is, in fact, prescribing the normal fluid stress to equate the normal structural stress at the previous time step.

Instead, in the strong-coupling case, we may have the following pseudocode:

```
Algorithm 2: Strong Coupling
Initialize: set u_f_onGamma
while (t<=tfinal){
  Converge=false;
    while (convergence==false){
      sigma_f = solveFluid(omega_f,u_f_onGamma)
      EnforceIC(sigma_s_normal=sigma_f_normal);
      u_s_onGamma = solveStructure(omega_s,sigma_s_normal);
      EnforceIC(u_f_onGamma=u_s_onGamma);
      ManageGeometry(omega_s,omega_f)
      convergence=TestConvergence(
        abs(u_f_onGamma-u_s_onGamma),
        abs(sigma_s_normal-sigma_f_normal));
  } // end while for the convergence
  t=t+Deltat
}//end while of the time loop
```

In this case, at each iteration, the fluid and structure solvers are subiterated to obtain the exact enforcement of Equation 5.9. Clearly, this second approach is computationally more intensive, as we need to subiterate, and each iteration requires solutions from the fluid and structural solvers. The convergence of these iterations needs to be proved using arguments of functional and numerical analyses (e.g., fixed-point theorem). However, we will see that the weak-coupling approach may suffer from instabilities that make it an unviable option.

Another categorization refers to the frame of reference in which the problem is written. Generally speaking, two classical approaches are considered: the Lagrangian approach, where the problems are written in a fixed frame of reference, and the Eulerian approach, where the frame of reference is evolving with the domain of interest, either $\Omega_f(t)$ or $\Omega_s(t)$. Both the frameworks have pros and cons. However, there are other possibilities that can be numerically more effective. This is the case of the arbitrary Lagrangian–Eulerian (ALE) methods that are popular for simulating the interaction between blood and vascular walls. In the immersed boundary (IB) methods, usually preferred for simulating floating bodies in fluids, a mixed Eulerian (fluid)–Lagrangian (structure) approach is preferred.

5.4.1.1 The Arbitrary Lagrangian–Eulerian Method
The formulation of ALE methods dates to the 1980s (Hughes et al., 1981; Donea et al., 1982). The rationale for the method is that, for the vascular wall, it makes sense to analyze the problem in a Lagrangian framework, since its deformations are quite limited. However, for the fluid problem, this may be impossible. In a Lagrangian approach, the nodes of the FE mesh move with the velocity of the fluid. In the presence of flow recirculation (as may happen downstream a stenosis), this rapidly impairs the quality of the mesh. On the other hand, if a structure is analyzed in a Lagrangian frame of reference, it may be convenient to stick to the same reference at the interface between both domains. For instance, in a grid-fitting approach, we can move the interface nodes with the structure. Therefore, the idea is to introduce another frame of reference that is neither purely Lagrangian nor Eulerian: it moves with the structure at the interface, yet it is Eulerian in other portions of the fluid boundary (such as inflows and outflows) to preserve the geometry of $\Omega_f(t)$ in time. This requires to (i) introduce a new displacement field η_g of the grid and its velocity $w_g = \dot{\eta}_g$, and (ii) rewrite the fluid problem with respect to the moving frame of reference featuring velocity w_g. At this point, the displacement field must obey the following constraints:

$$w_g = \dot{\eta}_s \text{ on } \Gamma, \quad w_g = 0 \text{ on } \Gamma_{in} \bigcup \Gamma_{out}. \qquad (5.10)$$

Clearly, these constraints can be satisfied by multiple choices for velocity w_g. Therefore, the selection of w_g is arbitrary and may obey criteria convenient for the numerical solution. For instance, it may be selected so as to minimize grid distortion and guarantee the quality of the FE solution (Donea et al., 1982). A reasonable choice, trading off computational simplicity and all the requirements, is to solve a Laplace problem (harmonic extension)

$$-\Delta w_g = 0 \text{ in } \Omega_f.$$

with Equation 5.10 as boundary conditions. This approach does not necessarily guarantee sufficient quality for the mesh, depending on the flow regimes, and more refined approaches (not discussed here) may be necessary.

To write the NSEs in an arbitrary frame of reference moving with velocity w_g, we resort to the Reynolds transport theorem, correcting the Lagrange derivative for the fluid

$$\left(\partial_t u\right)_{ALE} = \left(\partial_t u\right) + \left(u - w_g\right) \cdot \nabla u,$$

such that the ALE fluid problem then reads

$$\begin{cases} \rho\left(\partial_t u + \left(\left(u - w_g\right) \cdot \nabla\right)u\right) - \mu\nabla \cdot \left(\nabla u + \nabla u^{\mathrm{T}}\right) + \nabla p = f \\ \nabla \cdot u = 0 \end{cases}. \tag{5.11}$$

The numerical analysis of the solution of this coupled problem is clearly nontrivial. We refer the reader to the literature for a comprehensive understanding of the topic (Nobile and Formaggia, 1999; Formaggia and Nobile, 2004; Fernandez and Gerbeau, 2009). Still, key items are reviewed to help the reader understand the main problems encountered with ALE methods.

5.4.1.1.1 The Added-Mass Effect   When using weak coupling for solution, numerical instabilities occur when the mass of the wall is significantly less than that of the fluid (as happens in cardiovascular applications); the instabilities become more evident in long pipes. The reason of this effect was elucidated in a seminal paper (Causin et al. 2005) for a simplified problem. The analysis gave a theoretical foundation to the instabilities, in terms of the eigenvalue analysis of an operator, lumping the added mass of the fluid into a structural problem (hence the name of "added-mass effect") (Fernandez and Gerbeau, 2009). The analysis showed that the instabilities introduced by weak coupling may make the method unsuitable for vascular problems. On the other hand, strong coupling can be made to converge with appropriate numerical methods; however, this happens at the expense of high computational cost. A trade-off is offered by a semi-implicit coupling, where only part of the coupling is performed during subiterations, and the geometry management is done explicitly.

5.4.1.1.2 Different Treatments of the Interface Conditions and Other Splits   In the previous examples of segregated procedures, one of the interface conditions (Equation 5.9) was simply associated with the fluid problem and the other was associated with the structural problem, similarly to what is done in the Dirichlet–Neumann approach for domain decomposition methods. The iterative procedure reads each interface condition as a boundary condition for the associated problem. However, interface conditions (Equation 5.9) can be replaced by their linear combination with arbitrary parameters, so as to provide a new set of interface conditions to enforce. Although the new conditions are equivalent for the continuous problem, they are different in terms of numerical efficiency, as in Robin–Robin domain decomposition techniques (Quarteroni and Valli, 1999). This idea was explored in Badia et al. (2008), and the selection of the coefficients of the linear combination of the interface conditions that optimize numerical performances is investigated in Gerardo Giorda et al. (2010). In addition, other ways to split the fluid and structural problems, and to bypass the added-mass effect, were introduced in Guidoboni et al. (2009).

5.4.1.1.3 The Geometric Conservation Laws   While assessing the accuracy of the solution to moving-domain problems, it is not possible to distinguish between the accuracy of space discretization and that of time, because the space domain is evolving in time, and the way the discretization is performed also has, in general, an impact on the space accuracy. For instance, the numerical differentiation to obtain fluid velocity u_f from the boundary structural displacement η_s impacts the entire accuracy. The concept of geometrical conservation laws was introduced to have a clear assessment of the interplay between time and space accuracies (Lesoinne and Farath, 1996). These laws provide a set of rules to guarantee a certain order of accuracy for the solution as a function of the order of accuracy of the space discretization and of the numerical approximation of the grid motion in time (see, for instance, Nobile and Formaggia 1999, Proposition 3.1).

5.4.1.2 Immersed Approaches
5.4.1.2.1 Immersed Boundaries: Purpose and Concepts   In many applications, the geometric complexity of the cardiovascular system is such that it is difficult to rely on traditional meshing strategies. By traditional meshing, we mean methods for which the entire geometry is built a priori and/or for which the same type of approach is used to adapt the mesh (i.e., by remeshing the entire mesh). For instance, constrained Delaunay tessellation methods (see, e.g., Frey and George, 2008; Cheng et al., 2012) and implicit function meshing (see, e.g., Persson, 2004; Dapogny et al., 2015) fall into this category. In this sense, traditional meshing fits the classical pipeline for numerical simulations: preprocessing and then processing, where preprocessing involves the mesh-generation part.

Immersed approaches are different in that the geometrical features of the problem are handled within the processing part. Conceptually speaking, given the problem domain $\tilde{\Omega} \subset \Omega$, the main idea consists of accurately solving the problem in Ω. For this reason, most immersed approaches are closely related to interface problems, since the first issues to arise are in the vicinity of $\partial\Omega$. Many immersed approaches relate to finite volume and finite difference methods, but herein, we will restrict ourselves to basic Galerkin methods. There exist numerous methods that could be associated with the terminology "immersed approaches," and we will not provide an exhaustive discussion of all these methods. Rather, the interested reader can delve into the references provided in the bibliography.

5.4.1.2.2 Historical Notes on Immersed Methods   Immersed approaches have a long history and could be traced back to (Hyman, 1952) (see, e.g., Glowinski, 2003). To the best of our knowledge, regarding FE methods, the mathematical analysis of an immersed approach may date back to a study by Babuška (1970) on the FE method with discontinuous coefficients. The term "immersed boundary" was first coined by C. Peskin in 1977, with application to blood flow in the heart, and the idea was further developed in the 1980s and is developing until now (Peskin, 2002). The fictitious domain method (FDM), on the other hand, dates to the work by Glowinski et al. (1994).

A typical Galerkin-type boundary-value problem reads:

Find $\tilde{\boldsymbol{u}}_h \in V_h\left(\tilde{\Omega}\right) \subset V\left(\tilde{\Omega}\right)$, such that

1. $\mathrm{a}\left(\tilde{\mathbf{u}}_h, \tilde{\mathbf{v}}_h\right) = \mathrm{b}\left(\tilde{\mathbf{v}}_h\right)$ for all $\tilde{\mathbf{v}}_h \in V_h\left(\tilde{\Omega}\right)$, and
2. $\tilde{\mathbf{u}}_h = \mathbf{g}$ on $\partial\Omega$.

One of the main issues is how to enforce the second equation. Two main categories of immersed approaches may be considered: 1) via basis modifications, that is, by modifying $V_h\left(\tilde{\Omega}\right)$, such that it includes some knowledge of $\mathbf{g}$ and $\partial\Omega$. Methods that fall into this category are the partition of unity method (PUM) and the extended finite element method (XFEM) or local remeshing (LR), and 2) via a variational form modification, that is, by modifying $\mathrm{a}\left(\tilde{\mathbf{u}}_h, \tilde{\mathbf{v}}_h\right)$ or $\mathrm{b}\left(\tilde{\mathbf{v}}_h\right)$, such that it includes some knowledge of $\mathbf{g}$ and $\partial\Omega$. Methods that fall into this category are, for example, the finite element-immersed boundary method (FE-IBM) or the FDM. We will provide a detailed list of references for each discussed method in the subsequent sections. Notice that, in most applications, a solution $\tilde{\mathbf{u}}$ in $\tilde{\Omega}$ will exhibit a singularity near $\partial\Omega$. Establishing an accurate method is challenging and is still an active area of research.

5.4.1.2.3 Functional Space-Based Approaches   The very idea of this class of methods is to explicitly provide information of the IB in the FE space. This can be done by adding new basis functions that are, for example, discontinuous and/or interpolatory on $\partial\Omega$. Local remeshing can be seen as a way to locally modify the discrete FE spaces to accommodate for $\mathbf{g}$ and $\partial\Omega$.

5.4.1.2.4 Basis Modification   Famous methods within this category are the PUM (see, e.g., Melenk and Babuška, 1996) and the XFEM (see, e.g., Sukumar et al., 2001). For fluid–structure interaction problems, an XFEM method was described in Gerstenberger and Wall (2008), and considering an aortic valve problem, the velocity field would be continuous, but the pressure would be discontinuous across the valve. A method in which the pressure would be discontinuous across the valve was also considered (Buscaglia and Ruas, 2013). In this case, in contrast to (Gerstenberger and Wall, 2008), the velocity gradient would be continuous, to the effect that the accuracy would be reduced, but the method would be slightly less costly. Other method that falls in this category is the immersed interface method (see Li, 1998; Lew and Buscaglia, 2008; Bastian and Engwer, 2009, to cite a few). Although these methods allow for a good approximation of the singularity of $\tilde{\mathbf{u}}$, enforcing essential boundary conditions on $\partial\Omega$ is not straightforward; therefore, weak approaches, such as Lagrange multipliers, Nitsche, and penalty approaches are commonly used (see, e.g., Hansbo and Hansbo, 2002; Hansbo et al., 2008 and references therein).

5.4.1.2.5 Local Remeshing Another "simple" approach is to consider an LR. The advantages are that the fields are easily interpolatory at the interface and that few degrees of freedom are added. Considering fluid–structure interaction (FSI) problems, LR has been used in several studies (van Loon et al., 2006; Ilinca and Hetu, 2012; Frei and Richter, 2014; Auricchio et al., 2015c). In van Loon et al. (2006), the mesh was locally modified while enforcing that the elements in the vicinity remained regular, whereas in other works (Frei and Richter, 2014; Auricchio et al., 2015c), anisotropic elements were employed. Anisotropic elements introduced two issues related to conditioning and the satisfaction of an inf-sup condition. Conditioning aspects dealt with in (Frei and Richter, 2014) for two-dimensional (2D) problems, but a 3D extension is nontrivial. In Auricchio et al. (2015c), it was shown that inf-sup issues may arise in two dimensions with discontinuous-pressure mixed elements, but they are very unlikely for most practical applications using continuous-pressure elements. The interested reader can find more details in Auricchio et al. (2016). Conditioning issues also affect the XFEM method (see, e.g., Zunino, 2011). Finally, the finite cell method (FCM) is worth mentioning (Parvizian et al., 2007). In many respects, the FCM is very similar to the PUM/XFEM method (in particular if one sees the XFEM as in Hansbo (2002). The interested reader may also refer to Joulaian et al. (2013), extending concepts to the h-p framework. An extension of the FCM (Rank et al., 2012) has also been proposed within the isogeometric framework (Cottrell et al., 2009).

5.4.1.2.6 Variational Formulation-Based Approaches In contrast to basis modification methods, in approaches based on variational formulations, the discrete functional space is left untouched, which has the main advantage to maintain the same number of degrees of freedom for the problem. In general, the cost of such an approach is a loss of accuracy, as the basis does not capture the singularities near the interface. Of course, such a statement should be taken with a grain of salt, since depending on the context, near-optimal accuracy could be obtained (see, e.g., Boffi et al. 2008, where time dependence of the problem is taken into account to increase the spatial accuracy of the overall method). Herein, we will first present the IBM and then the fictitious boundary method.

The idea of the IBM (see, e.g., Peskin, 2002) is that "immersed" boundaries (or the action of the solid on the fluid) act as an external load, more precisely as a set of Dirac delta functions. Initially, the method was proposed using finite difference schemes, but a variational formulation was proposed in, for example, Boffi and Gastaldi (2003) and Heltai and Costanzo (2012). Setting the problem within a variational formulation greatly simplifies the formulation, since Dirac deltas are naturally handled.

The FDM, proposed by Glowinski and coworkers (see, e.g., (Glowinski, 2003)), was initially set in the variational setting. In this method, the "immersed" boundaries (or the action of the solid on the fluid) are set using Lagrange multipliers (boundary or distributed Lagrange multipliers can be used for thin or thick structures, respectively).

It is possible to reframe the IBM as an FDM, as shown in Auricchio et al. (2015c) and Boffi et al. (2015). The interested reader may find more information and references on this and on the connection between immersed approaches and elliptic interface problems in Auricchio et al. (2014).

Finally, the immersogeometric method (Kamensky et al., 2015) is similar to the FDM with stabilized Lagrange multipliers (via an augmented Lagrangian formulation) and, in this, resembles Nitsche's method after elimination of the Lagrange multipliers. The main contribution of the work is to frame the FDM within the isogeometric method (Cottrell et al., 2009).

5.4.2 Reduced-Order Methods: An Overview

Advanced applications in physics or engineering need an efficient solution of parametrized PDEs, which requires the computation of the solution of (possibly nonlinear) PDEs for several different "scenarios." A solution by traditional methods such as FEs and finite volumes may not always be feasible. Thus, reduced-order models have been studied in an attempt to deliver accurate solutions at lower computational costs (Quarteroni and Rozza, 2013). When the problem is modeled with nonlinear equations, several complexities need to be faced, in order to guarantee efficiency, accuracy, and reliability; this is also true for reduced-order modeling. Among such complexities are the exploration of the parameter space to build efficient reduced bases (RBs), that is, lower-dimensional approximation spaces but still representative ones to capture fine physical features and details (see, e.g., (Constantine, 2015)); the issue of stability, for example, in noncoercive problems; the difficulty to approximate vectorial multifields (i.e., pressure, velocity, and temperature); and the issue of accurate and fast estimation of stability factors (coercivity and inf-sup constants), as recently summarized in Lassila et al. (2013a). In cardiovascular problems, a combination of different ingredients borrowed from the RB approach (such as online Galerkin projection and approximation stability by supremizers to enrich the approximation spaces) with proper orthogonal decomposition (POD) features, allowing one to build accurate reduced spaces without costly procedures and error estimators, can be used with promising results. These combinations have been tested on nonlinear steady viscous flows modeled by NSEs and characterized by physical and geometrical (domain) parameterizations. This avenue offers a valid alternative approach preserving offline–online computational decomposition procedures, approximation stability, and all the properties inherited from POD (such as orthonormalized basis functions for a robust algebraic stability and hierarchical spaces) as well as those passed on from Galerkin projection (orthogonality, best-fit approximation, and square effects). It also opens the additional possibility to develop an a posteriori error analysis based on residuals and stability factors approximation to endow the POD with online error bounds. The reader can refer to Lassila et al. (2013c) for all the methodological details. A brief historical digression about methodologies, aspects, and milestones taken into consideration in the development of this work follows.

Proper orthogonal decomposition was born to provide efficient model order reduction in turbulent viscous flows, preserving the most important energetic features based on modal analysis and singular-value decomposition (see, e.g., Aubry et al., 1988; Aubry, 1991; Berkooz et al., 1993; Cazemier et al., 1998; Holmes et al., 1998; Ravindran, 2000), with several further improvements achieved in subsequent studies and developments (eigenvalues and eigenvector calculations, error estimation, physical parametrization beside time, optimal sampling, etc.); see, for example, several extensions proposed in other studies (Christensen et al., 1999; Iollo et al., 2000; Kunish and Volkwein, 2003; Utturkar et al., 2005; Bergmann and Iollo, 2008; Bergmann et al., 2009; Hay et al., 2009; Weller et al., 2010; Wang et al., 2012a). Also, worth mentioning are the recent works (Bergmann et al., 2013; Caiazzo et al., 2014,) for state-of-the-art-reviews and bibliographies. Let us also mention window POD techniques, to specialize the RBs and achieve a certain level of efficiency in modeling increasingly complex and extended systems (Grinberg et al., 2013). In the recent years, growing attention has been devoted to stabilization techniques for POD (Iollo et al., 2000; Sirisup and Karniadakis, 2005; Akhtar, 2009; Caiazzo et al., 2014) and to the combination of Galerkin strategies with POD (Chapelle et al., 2012, 2013; Amsallem and Farhat, 2013; Baiges et al., 2013), to cite a few recent contributions.

Now, going back more specifically to RB methods, they were proposed for nonlinear viscous flows in the 1980s (Peterson, 1989), and a milestone contribution was provided by Anthony Patera and his group at Massachusetts Institute of Technology and collaborators at Paris VI (Yvon Maday) and, in more recent years, by others (Nguyen et al., 2005; Veroy and Patera, 2005; Quarteroni and Rozza, 2007; Deparis, 2008; Deparis and Rozza, 2009; Manzoni, 2014), with several recent applications (Manzoni et al., 2012a; Lassila et al. 2013b). Starting from the linear saddle-point problem representing the Stokes system, several studies were carried out to guarantee the stabilization of the reduced parametrized solution for the global approximation, with pressure recovery and algebraic aspects (the extension of these aspects to Navier–Stokes nonlinear flows solved by RB method has been straightforward, as in Rozza (2006)). The former aspect (approximation stability) was taken care of by supremizer enrichment to guarantee the existence of an equivalent parametrized inf-sup constant and the fulfillment of a related equivalent Brezzi condition. It was clear, since the first numerical tests, that a combination of stable global approximated solutions was not always giving a stable solution, especially with geometrical parametrization (also in the linear case). Several options exist for this stabilization, in order to propose efficient, stable, and accurate methodologies (Rozza and Veroy, 2007, p. 200; Gerner and Veroy, 2012; Rozza et al., 2013) and to keep a stable and accurate approximation for the scalar pressure as well. A certain importance is given to flows in parametrized domains for which supremizer enrichment is crucial (Manzoni et al., 2012b). This approach is different from those proposed previously in POD methods with stabilization during the basis calculations (offline) and during the (online) reduced-order methods (e.g., using Stream Upwind Petrov-Galerkin (SUPG) method) (Caiazzo et al., 2014). The latter aspect (algebraic stability) was focused on orthonormalization procedures of Gram–Schmidt (Rozza and Veroy, 2007). More recently, a third stability aspect, based on supremizers, has been introduced and studied for the enrichment of primal, dual, and control reduced spaces for optimal flow control problems in a saddle-point formulation (Negri et al., 2015).

The RB framework is a very useful tool to improve the performance of the approximation stability of flows in the already-attractive and versatile POD setting, especially in parametrized domains. In this way, POD benefits from a previously developed robust framework for the stabilization of viscous flows with computed pressure. At the same time, POD can provide an alternative to costly algorithms in systems where the error bounds are not yet available, and POD implementations are more easily accessible (e.g., in already-developed libraries/codes). The goal is to have several options and possibilities to combine reduced-order ingredients to be able to address important computational needs with the best possible compromise in terms of accuracy, cost, performance, and fulfillment of additional constraints, such as error bounds.

The combination of POD and RB tools is not new. For example, one can mention the POD–greedy synergy approaches for unsteady problems (Haasdonk and Ohlberger, 2008; Nguyen et al., 2009), where the time evolution is captured by POD, while physical and/or geometrical parameters are managed by greedy techniques. Recent works in cardiovascular modeling and simulations with reduced-order methods have been devoted to fluid–structure interactions (see (Lassila et al., 2012; Wang et al., 2012a; Bertagna and Veneziani, 2014; Ballarin, 2015; Ballarin et al., 2016b, 2016c; Ballarin and Rozza, 2016)), stability of flows and bifurcations (see Pitton et al., 2017; Pitton and Rozza, 2017), and optimization and control (e.g., see Manzoni et al., 2012c, Lassila et al., 2013a, 2013b).

Last but not least, two other reduction techniques are worth mentioning: the proper generalized decomposition (PGD, see (Chinesta et al., 2016)) and the hierarchical model reduction (HIMOD) for flows (see (Baroli et al., 2016)). A recent collection of articles about up-to-date research in reduced-order methods is available in Benner et al. (2017).

5.4.3 Reduced-Order Methods: General Formulation

In this section, we aim to introduce the RB approximation for parametrized PDEs, focusing on the POD–Galerkin approach. The need for an efficient resolution method for parametrized PDEs arises in very different contexts (e.g., see Milani et al., 2008; Rozza et al., 2008, 2013; Boyaval et al., 2009; Dedè, 2010; Lassila et al., 2014) and is specifically relevant to cardiovascular applications, from shape optimization and control problems (e.g., see Manzoni et al., 2012c; Lassila et al., 2013a, 2013b) to fast blood simulations (e.g., see Ballarin et al., 2016a; Ballarin et al., 2016c; Manzoni et al., 2012a) and fluid–structure interactions in hemodynamics (see Lassila, 2012; Ballarin and Rozza, 2016; Ballarin et al., 2016b). This field of application is characterized by models governed by parametrized PDEs, possibly nonlinear. Computationally, cardiovascular models in hemodynamics can be very demanding. This is due, on the one hand, to the PDEs governing blood flow (nonlinear NSEs, which need stabilization techniques to give reliable results) and, on the other hand, to the parametrization setting, which can be both physical and geometrical. To face these issues, reduced-order methods can be attractive and versatile (an application of a stabilized reduced-order method to NSEs is discussed in Ballarin et al. (2015)). While classical numerical methods, such as the FE method, do not lend themselves to efficient solutions, reduced-order approaches seem promising to solve many cardiovascular problems in an accurate and reliable fashion. In this section, we propose a POD–Galerkin approach as a strategy to efficiently handle such systems. The method is based on a POD procedure, followed by a Galerkin projection onto the reduced space obtained. It has already been exploited, with promising results in cardiovascular applications (see, e.g., Ballarin et al., 2016a; Ballarin and Rozza, 2016). The general idea of reduced-order techniques and the POD–Galerkin method are introduced in the following subsection.

5.4.3.1 Overview

In order to understand how reduced-order methods work (see Hesthaven et al., 2015; Quarteroni et al., 2015), let us introduce the solution manifold, defined by $M = \{u(\mu) : \mu \in \mathbb{P}\}$. In other words, the solution manifold is the set of the solutions $u(\mu)$ of the parametrized PDE under the variation of parameter μ in the space of the parameters. As in the continuous case, we can define the approximated solution manifold, which is the set of the full-order (i.e., FEs) solution manifold under the variation of μ, that is, $\mathcal{M}_h = \{u_h(\mu) : \mu \in \mathbb{P}\}$. The reduced-order methods aim to build a reduced solution space by exploiting specific (say N) values of parameter μ, to describe the approximated solution manifold in a reliable and fast manner. Then, the reduced system is solved in a lower-dimensional framework compared with the full-order one.

Let H indicate the dimension of the full-order space. The RB approximation is based on two different stages:

1. The offline stage is a (potentially) costly phase, where the solution manifold is explored to build a reduced space capable of describing any particular solution with sufficient accuracy. Computationally, one must solve N problems with H degrees of freedom.
2. The online stage consists of a Galerkin projection onto the RB space, for a particular parameter value. The computational cost of this phase is independent of N.

The online stage is performed every time simulation for a new value of parameter μ is needed. The RB approach is efficient when the online stage is fast to perform: this is possibly true when N is much smaller than H. A reduced space, consisting of linear combinations of the full-order solutions, evaluated in properly chosen N values of parameter μ, is

$$V_N = \operatorname{span}\{u_h(\mu_n) : n = 1, \dots, N\}.$$

There are essentially two classical approaches to build the reduced spaces: one is the so-called greedy algorithm (see Section 3.2.2 in Hesthaven et al. 2015) and the other is POD.

The greedy strategy is an iterative procedure that adds a basis function at each step to improve the reduced approximation. It requires the resolution of N full-order problems. To apply a greedy algorithm, an a posteriori error estimation based on residuals must be available. At each iteration of the process, the parameter of evaluation of the true solution is chosen as the one that maximizes this error estimation (for all the technical details, see Boyaval et al., 2009). In the following text, we will focus instead on POD, which is an attractive and efficient strategy to follow as a sampling procedure. While the greedy algorithm is based on the computation of error estimations that are not always available in some systems, error estimations are not needed to perform a POD reduction.

5.4.3.2 Proper Orthogonal Decomposition

To apply POD, a discrete and finite-dimensional subset of the parameter space is needed. For this specific set of parameters, one can define the discrete approximated manifold

$$\mathcal{M}_h\left(\mathbb{P}_h\right)=\left\{u_h\left(\mu\right):\mu\in\mathbb{P}_h\right\},$$

of cardinality M. When the discretization of the parameter space is fine enough, the discrete approximated solution manifold properly describes the approximated solution manifold $\mathcal{M}_h(\mathbb{P}_h)\sim M_h$.

The POD algorithm is based on two processes:

1. Sampling the discrete parameter space to compute the truth solutions at the chosen parameters
2. Discarding the redundant information

From an algebraic point of view, the N space resulting from the POD algorithm is built through the resolution of an eigenvalue–eigenvector problem on the correlation matrix of the full-order solutions evaluated in M specific parameters. Let us consider the set of the solutions evaluated in these specific values of the parameters:

$$\left\{u_h\left(\mu_m\right):m=1,...,M\right\}.$$

Then, let us define the real-valued correlation matrix as:

$$C_{mq}=\frac{1}{M}\left(u_h\left(\mu_m\right),\mathrm{u}_h\left(\mu_q\right)\right)_V,$$

where V is the solution space and $1\leq m$ and $q\leq M$. Then, the POD approach aims at solving the N-largest eigenvalue–eigenvector problem:

$$Cv_n=\lambda_n v_n,$$

with $1 \leq n \leq N$. The eigenvector has been taken with unitary norm. Giving a descending order to the eigenvalues, the reduced space is built as:

$$V_N = \mathrm{span}\{\xi_1, ..., \xi_N\},$$

where the orthogonal basis is given by:

$$\xi_n = \frac{1}{\sqrt{M}} \sum_{m=1}^{M} (v_n)_m \, u_h(\mu_m),$$

with $1 \leq n \leq N$.

The reduced space construction is performed during the offline stage.

5.4.3.3 Overall Problem Formulation

Let P(μ) be our parameterized PDE problem, with μ physical and/or geometrical parameter in the parameter space. Let Ω be a 2D/3D physical domain and V be a suitable Hilbert space endowed with the norm

$$(v,v) = (v)^2.$$

Let us consider the parameterized V-continuous functionals

$$f(\mu): V \to \mathbb{R},$$

and the parameterized V-bilinear form

$$a(\mu): V \times V \to \mathbb{R}.$$

The parametrized weak formulation of the problem reads: given μ, find $u(\mu)$ in V, such that:

$$a(u(\mu), v; \mu) = f(v; \mu),$$

for all v in V. Under the assumption of coercivity of $a(\mu)$, the Lax–Milgram theorem guarantees the existence and uniqueness of solution $u(\mu)$.

5.4.3.4 Truth Approximation

Let us consider the H-dimensional space $V_h \subset V$. The discrete version of problem P(μ) reads: given μ, find $u_h(\mu)$ in V_h, such that

$$a(u_h(\mu), v; \mu) = f(v; \mu),$$

for all v in V_h. If the dimension H of the discretized space is high, then the problem can be computationally costly. If Lax–Milgram theorem is verified for the continuous version of P(μ), then it also holds for the discretized version, which ensures the existence and uniqueness of $u_h(\mu)$. In the following text, we will refer to the discretized solution as the full-order solution or truth solution. The approach described is the so-called Galerkin projection method onto the discretized space V_h.

5.4.3.5 Affine Decomposition

To ensure the efficiency of the reduced-order methods, the so-called affine decomposition has to be verified. This assumption is essential to guarantee an adequate offline–online procedure, as described in the following text. The bilinear form $a(\mu)$ and the linear form $f(\mu)$ are assumed to be affine in parameter μ, that is, there exist Q_a and Q_f, such that for all the values of μ, the forms can be rewritten as:

$$a(w,v:\mu) = \sum_{q=1}^{Q_a} \Theta_a^q(\mu) a_q(w,v), \qquad \forall w,v \in V$$

and

$$f(v;\mu) = \sum_{q=1}^{Q_f} \Theta_f^q(\mu) f^q(v), \qquad \forall v \in V.$$

In other words, it is assumed that the form of the elliptic problem considered could be written as the finite sum of μ-dependent scalar quantities and μ-independent forms. This assumption allows for the division of the reduction strategy into two stages, offline and online, which will be formally described in the next section.

In some physical systems, the affine assumption is not fulfilled, and then, one must compensate for it through some numerical strategies and techniques. For instance, the empirical interpolation method (EIM, see Barrault et al., 2004) makes it possible to recover the affine structure of the problem and guarantee the efficiency of the reduced-order methods.

5.4.3.6 Reduced-Order Approximation and the Offline–Online Procedure

Let us assume that we have already built the reduced space verifying $V_N \subset V_h \subset V$. Exploiting this new approximated space, let us introduce the reduced problem in a Galerkin projection formulation onto the RB spaces. It is a new approximated problem, and it reads: given μ, find the reduced solution $u_N(\mu)$ in V_N, such that

$$a(u_N(\mu),v;\mu) = f(v;\mu),$$

for all v in V_N. We will refer to this reduced formulation as the reduced problem.

Applying an orthonormalization technique (e.g., POD) to the inner product defined by V, the reduced space can be defined as:

$$V_N = \text{span}\{\zeta_1,\ldots,\zeta_N\}.$$

In this new framework, the reduced solution in terms of the new orthonormalized RB is defined as:

$$u_N(\mu) = \sum_{j=1}^{N} u_N^j(\mu)\zeta_j.$$

Substituting the latter expression in the reduced problem and choosing the basis functions as test functions, the following algebraic reduced system holds:

$$\sum_{j=1}^{N} a(\zeta_j,\zeta_i;\mu)u_N^j(\mu) = f(\zeta_i;\mu), \qquad i = 1,...,N.$$

Usually, the system has a low dimension, but its formulation is linked to the FE approximation space in the basis functions. If one assembles the RB forms for every value of the parameter, the evaluation process will remain computationally expensive. However, thanks to the affine assumption, the assembling process can be decoupled into the offline and online stages, to efficiently solve the system for each new value of the parameter. Specifically, the system is rewritten as:

$$\sum_{j=1}^{N}\sum_{q=1}^{Q_a}\Theta_a^q(\mu)a_q(\zeta_j,\zeta_i)u_N^j(\mu) = \sum_{q=1}^{Q_f}\Theta_f^q(\mu)f^q(\zeta_i), \qquad i = 1,...,N.$$

Under this assumption, it is clear that an RB approximation could be efficiently performed in two different stages: a μ-independent costly offline phase and a real-time μ-dependent online phase. The first procedure is needed only once, while the second process is applied at every new evaluation of μ. In the offline stage, the reduced space is built and orthonormalized. After this preliminary phase, all the μ-independent quantities are assembled and stored. In the online stage, the structures and forms evaluated and stored in the previous step are exploited in order to build the reduced system, and the reduced parametrized solution is computed by a Galerkin projection onto the reduced space. This division of the assembly process allows the user to obtain results quickly and to run multiple simulations in a low-dimensional and computational time-/space-saving framework.

5.5 Conclusion and Perspectives

Mathematical and numerical modeling in cardiovascular mechanics has been a thrilling journey of human creativity and ingenuity, dating back to the work of L. Euler, with relevant contributions of important scientists of today, such as T.J.R. Hughes and C. Peskin. The predictive nature of mathematical and computational models has enhanced the process of understanding the normal and pathophysiological dynamics of the cardiovascular system, as well as the design of devices and therapeutic tools. A solid mathematical and engineering background plays a critical role in the solution of the challenging problems arising in structural hemodynamics and in addressing today's emerging challenges. The efficiency in solving fluid–structure interaction problems, for instance, has experienced terrific improvements over the last 20 years, and complex interactions between the vascular wall and the blood flow can now be elucidated in complex geometries within reasonable times. The combination of new computing architectures and new numerical methodologies has been decisive. Computational investigations are already integral parts of medical research and are also increasingly benefiting the routine in clinical trials and surgical planning. After the revolution introduced by imaging devices in the twentieth century, which enabled clinicians to look "inside" and not just "at" the patients, mathematical and numerical models may further extend the perspective to explore the future and the past of the patients—the "future" in performing reliable simulations of surgery or interventions and the "past" in laying the groundwork for large-scale comparisons among patients with similar clinical situations. Mathematicians, biomedical engineers, and clinicians are teaming up in this revolutionary experience, whose final users are the healthcare system and society, in general. This process has not only triggered new research and new investigations that are useful in other contexts as well but also enabled new professionals and job opportunities, as the experience of HeartFlow demonstrates. In this chapter, we simply provided introductory notions helpful for the presentation of this complex and fascinating—intrinsically multidisciplinary—world. To complete the revolution brought about by computational mechanics, a strong translational effort is still required. The definition of protocols for "best simulation practice," combined with recommendations for "best clinical practice," raises new challenges, ranging from (1) the efficiency of the numerical solution over large numbers of patients, where reduced-order models based on the online–offline paradigm are expected to play a significant role; (2) the storage and retrieval of data, where cloud infrastructures are critical; and (3) the reliability of quantitative analyses, even when the models are affected by significant uncertainty, calling for extensive data assimilation and uncertainty-quantification procedures. Only a strong interdisciplinary effort can successfully meet this challenge, in an integrated effort that will impact not only scientific research but also the cultural background of clinical sciences by progressively moving toward more established "quantitative medicine."

References

Akhtar, I., A.H. Nayfeh, and C.J. Ribbens, On the stability and extension of reduced-order Galerkin models in incompressible flows, *Theoretical and Computational Fluid Dynamics*, 23(3), 213–237, 2009.

Akkerman, I., Y. Bazilevs, V.M. Calo, T.J.R. Hughes, and S. Hulshoff, The role of continuity in residualbased variational multiscale modeling of turbulence, *Computational Mechanics*, 41, 371–378, 2008.

Alaimo, G., F. Auricchio, M. Conti, and M. Zingales, Multi-objective optimization of nitinol stent design, *Medical Engineering & Physics*, 47, 13–24, 2017.

Altnji, H.E., B. Bou-Saïd, and H. Walter-Le Berre, Morphological and stent design risk factors to prevent migration phenomena for a thoracic aneurysm: A numerical analysis, *Medical Engineering & Physics*, 37(1), 23–33, 2015.

Amsallem, D. and C. Farhat, On the stability of reduced-order linearized computational fluid dynamics models based on POD and Galerkin projection: Descriptor versus non-descriptor forms, in *Reduced Order Methods for Modeling and Computational Reduction*, vol. 9, A. Quarteroni and G. Rozza (Eds.). Milano, Italy: Springer, MS&A Series, 2013, pp. 215–233.

Antiga, L., M. Piccinelli, L. Botti, B. Ene-Iordache, A. Remuzzi, and D.A. Steinman, An image-based modeling framework for patient-specific computational hemodynamics, *Medical & Biological Engineering & Computing*, 46(11), 1097, 2008.

Asch, M., M. Bocquet, and M. Nodet, *Data Assimilation: Methods, Algorithms, and Applications*. Philadelphia, PA: Society for Industrial and Applied Mathematics, 2016.

Aubry, N., On the hidden beauty of the proper orthogonal decomposition, *Theoretical Computational Fluid Dynamics*, 2(5), 339–352, 1991.

Aubry, N., P. Holmes, J. Lumley, and E. Stone, The dynamics of coherent structures in the wall region of a turbulent boundary layer, *Journal of Fluid Mechanics*, 192(115), 173355, 1988.

Auricchio, F., L. Beirão da Veiga, A. Buffa, C. Lovadina, A. Reali, and G. Sangalli, A fully "locking-free" isogeometric approach for plane linear elasticity problems: A stream function formulation, *Computer Methods in Applied Mechanics and Engineering*, 197, 160–172, 2007.

Auricchio, F., E. Boatti, and M. Conti, SMA biomedical applications, in *Shape Memory Alloy Engineering for Aerospace, Structural and Biomedical Applications*, L. Lecce and A. Concilio (Eds.). Oxford, UK: Butterworth-Heinemann, 2015a.

Auricchio, F., D. Boffi, L. Gastaldi, A. Lefieux, and A. Reali, A study on unfitted 1d finite element methods, *Computers and Mathematics with Applications*, 68, 2080–2102, 2014.

Auricchio, F., M. Conti, M. De Beule, G. De Santis, and B. Verhegghe, Carotid artery stenting simulation: From patient-specific images to finite element analysis, *Medical Engineering & Physics*, 33(3), 281–289, 2011.

Auricchio, F., M. Conti, A. Ferrara, S. Morganti, and A. Reali, Patient-specific finite element analysis of carotid artery stenting: A focus on vessel modelling, *International Journal for Numerical Methods in Biomedical Engineering*, 29(6), 645–664, 2013a.

Auricchio, F., M. Conti, M. Ferraro, and A. Reali, Evaluation of carotid stent scaffolding through patient-specific finite element analysis, *International Journal for Numerical Methods in Biomedical Engineering*, 28(10), 1043–1055, 2012.

Auricchio, F., M. Conti, M. Ferraro, S. Morganti, A. Reali, and R. Taylor, Innovative and efficient stent flexibility simulations based on isogeometric analysis, *Computer Methods in Applied Mechanics and Engineering*, 295, 347–361, 2015b.

Auricchio, F., M. Conti, S. Marconi, A., Reali, J.L. Tolenaar, and S. Trimarchi, Patient-specific aortic endografting simulation: From diagnosis to prediction, *Computers in Biology and Medicine*, 43(4), 386–394, 2013b.

Auricchio, F., M. Conti, S. Morganti, and A. Reali, Shape memory alloy: From constitutive modeling to finite element analysis of stent deployment, *CMES - Computer Modeling in Engineering and Sciences*, 57(3), 225–243, 2010.

Auricchio, F., A. Lefieux, A. Reali, and A. Veneziani, A locally anisotropic fluid-structure interaction remeshing strategy for thin structures with application to a hinged rigid leaflet, *International Journal for Numerical Methods in Engineering*, 107(2), 155–180, 2015c.

Auricchio, F., A. Lefieux, and A. Reali, *On the Use of Anisotropic Triangles with Mixed Finite Elements: Application to an "Immersed" Approach for Incompressible Flow Problems*, pp. 195–236. Cham, Switzerland: Springer International Publishing, 2016.

Auricchio, F., M. Conti, S. Morganti, and A. Reali, Simulation of transcatheter aortic valve implantation: A patient-specific finite element approach, *Computer Methods in Biomechanics and Biomedical Engineering*, 17(12), 1347–1357, 2014.

Auricchio, F., and L. Petrini, A three-dimensional model describing stress-temperature induced solid phase transformations: Solution algorithm and boundary value problems, *International Journal for Numerical Methods in Engineering*, 61(6), 807–836, 2004.

Auricchio, F., and R. Taylor, Shape-memory alloys: Modelling and numerical simulations of the finite-strain superelastic behavior, *Computer Methods in Applied Mechanics and Engineering*, 143(1–2), 175–194, 1997.

Auricchio, F., R. Taylor, and J. Lubliner, Shape-memory alloys: Macromodelling and numerical simulations of the superelastic behavior, *Computer Methods in Applied Mechanics and Engineering*, 146(3–4), 281–312, 1997.

Azaouzi, M., N. Lebaal, A. Makradi, and S. Belouettar, Optimization based simulation of self-expanding Nitinol stent, *Materials and Design*, 50, 917–928, 2013.

Babuška, I., The finite element method for elliptic equations with discontinuous coefficients, *Computing*, 5, 207–213, 1970.

Badia, S., F. Nobile, and C. Vergara, Fluid–structure partitioned procedures based on Robin transmission conditions, *Journal of Computational Physics*, 227(14), 7027–7051, 2008.

Baiges, J., R. Codina, and S. Idelsohn, Explicit reduced-order models for the stabilized finite element approximation of the incompressible Navier-Stokes equations, *International Journal of Numerical Methods in Fluids*, 72(12), 1219–1243, 2013.

Ballarin, F., A. Manzoni, A. Quarteroni, and G. Rozza, Supremizer stabilization of POD–Galerkin approximation of parametrized steady incompressible Navier–Stokes equations, *International Journal of Numerical Methods in Engineering*, 102(5), 1136–1161, 2015.

Ballarin, F., E. Faggiano, A. Manzoni, A. Quarteroni, G. Rozza, S. Ippolito, C. Antona, and R. Scrofani, Numerical modeling of hemodynamics scenarios of patient-specific coronary artery bypass grafts. *Biomechanics and Modeling in Mechanobiology*, 16(4), 1373–1399, 2017.

Ballarin, F., G. Rozza, and Y. Maday, Reduced-order semi-implicit schemes for fluid-structure interaction problems, Special Volume MoRePaS, Preprint SISSA 36/2016/MATE, 2016b.

Ballarin, F., E. Faggiano, S. Ippolito, A. Manzoni, A. Quarteroni, G. Rozza, and R. Scrofani, Fast simulations of patient-specific haemodynamics of coronary artery bypass grafts based on a POD-Galerkin method and a vascular shape parametrization, *Journal of Computational Physics*, 315, 609–628, 2016c.

Ballarin, F. and G. Rozza, POD–Galerkin monolithic reduced order models for parametrized fluid-structure interaction problems, *International Journal of Numerical Methods in Fluids*, 82, 1010–1034, 2016.

Baroli, D., C.M. Cova, S. Perotto, L. Sala, and A. Veneziani, Hi-POD solution of parametrized fluid dynamics problems: Preliminary results, *MoRePas III, in Proceeding*, 2016.

Barrault, M., Y. Maday, N.C. Nguyen, and A.T. Patera, An empirical interpolation method: Application to efficient reduced-basis discretization of partial differential equations, *Comptes Rendus Mathématique*, 339(9), 667–672, 2004.

Bastian, P. and C. Engwer, An unfitted element method using discontinuous Galerkin, *International Journal for Numerical Methods in Engineering*, 79, 1557–1576, 2009.

Bazilevs, Y., V.M. Calo, J.A. Cottrell, T.J.R. Hughes, A. Reali, and G. Scovazzi, Variational multiscale residual-based turbulence modeling for large eddy simulation of incompressible flows, *Computer Methods in Applied Mechanics and Engineering*, 197, 173–201, 2007.

de Beaufort, H.W.L., M. Coda, M. Conti, T.M.J. van Bakel, F.J.H. Nauta, E. Lanzarone, F.L. Moll, J.A. van Herwaarden, F. Auricchio, and S. Trimarchi, Changes in aortic pulse wave velocity of four thoracic aortic stent grafts in an ex vivo porcine model, *PLoS One*, 12(10), e0186080, 2017a.

de Beaufort, H.W., M. Conti, A.V. Kamman, F.J. Nauta, E. Lanzarone, F.L. Moll, J.A. van Herwaarden, F. Auricchio, and S. Trimarchi, Stent-graft deployment increases aortic stiffness in an ex vivo porcine model, *Annals of Vascular Surgery*, 43, 302–308, 2017b.

Benner, P., M. Ohlberger, A. Patera, G. Rozza, and K. Urban (Eds.), *Model Reduction of Parametrized Systems*, vol. 17. Cham, Switzerland: Springer, MS&A, 2017.

Benson, D.J., Y. Bazilevs, M.C. Hsu, and T.J.R. Hughes, Isogeometric shell analysis: The Reissner-Mindlin shell, *Computer Methods in Applied Mechanics and Engineering*, 199, 276–289, 2010.

Bergmann, M., C.H. Bruneau, and A. Iollo, Enablers for robust POD models, *Journal of Computational Physics*, 228(2), 516–538, 2009.

Bergmann, M., T. Colin, A. Iollo, D. Lombardi, A. Saut, and H. Telib, Reduced order models at work in aeronautics and medicine, in *Reduced Order Methods for Modeling and Computational Reduction*, vol. 9, A. Quarteroni and G. Rozza (Eds.). Milano, Italy: Springer, MS&A, 2013, pp. 305–332.

Berkooz, G., P. Holmes, and J.L. Lumley, The proper orthogonal decomposition in the analysis of turbulent flows, *Annual Review of Fluid Mechanics*, 25(1), 539–575, 1993.

Bertagna, L., A. Quaini, and A., Veneziani, Deconvolution-based nonlinear filtering for incompressible flows at moderately large Reynolds numbers, *International Journal for Numerical Methods in Fluids*, 81(8), 463–488, 2016.

Bertagna, L. and A. Veneziani, A model reduction approach for the variational estimation of vascular compliance by solving an inverse fluid-structure interaction problem, *Inverse Problems*, 30(5), 055006, 2014.

Bertoglio, C., D. Barber, N. Gaddum, I. Valverde, M. Rutten, P. Beerbaum, P. Moireau, R. Hose, and J.F. Gerbeau, Identification of artery wall stiffness: In vitro validation and in vivo results of a data assimilation procedure applied to a 3D fluid–structure interaction model, *Journal of Biomechanics*, 47(5), 1027–1034, 2014.

Bertoglio, C., P. Moireau, and J.F. Gerbeau, Sequential parameter estimation for fluid–structure problems: Application to hemodynamics, *International Journal for Numerical Methods in Biomedical Engineering*, 28(4), 434–455, 2012.

Boffi, D. and L. Gastaldi, A finite element approach for the immersed boundary method, *Computers & Structures*, 81(8), 491–501, 2003.

Boffi, D., L. Gastaldi, L. Heltai, and C. Peskin, On the hyper-elastic formulation of the immersed boundary method, *Computer Methods in Applied Mechanics and Engineering*, 197, 2210–2231, 2008.

Bols, J., L. Taelman, G. De Santis, J. Degroote, B. Verhegghe, P. Segers, and J. Vierendeels, Unstructured hexahedral mesh generation of complex vascular trees using a multi-block grid-based approach, *Computer Methods in Biomechanics and Biomedical Engineering*, 19(6), 663–672, 2016.

Boyaval, S., C. Le Bris, Y. Maday, N.C. Nguyen, and A. Patera, A reduced basis approach for variational problems with stochastic parameters: Application to heat conduction with variable Robin coefficient, *Computer Methods in Applied Mechanics and Engineering*, 198(41), 3187–3206, 2009.

Brezzi, F., On the existence, uniqueness and approximation of saddle-point problems arising from Lagrangian multipliers, *Revue française d'automatique, informatique, recherche opérationnelle. Analyse numérique*, 8(R2), 129–151, 1974.

Brezzi, F. and G. Gilardi, Part 1: Chapter 2, Functional spaces, Chapter 3, Partial differential equations, in *Finite Element Handbook*, H. Kardestuncer and D.H. Norrie (Eds.). New York: McGraw-Hill, 1987.

Buscaglia, G. and V. Ruas, Finite element methods for the Stokes system with interface pressure discontinuities, *IMA Journal of Numerical Analysis*, 35, 220–238, 2015.

Caiazzo, A., T. Iliescu, V. John, and S. Schyschlowa, A numerical investigation of velocity-pressure reduced order models for incompressible flows, *Journal of Computational Physics*, 259, 598–616, 2014.

Capelli, C., A.M. Taylor, F. Migliavacca, P. Bonhoeffer, and S. Schievano, Patient-specific reconstructed anatomies and computer simulations are fundamental for selecting medical device treatment: Application to a new percutaneous pulmonary valve, *Philosophical Transactions of the Royal Society*, 368, 3027–3038, 2010.

Capelli, C., G.M. Bosi, E. Cerri, J. Nordmeyer, T. Odenwald, P. Bonhoeffer, F. Migliavacca, A.M. Taylor, and S. Schievano, Patient-specific simulations of transcatheter aortic valve stent implantation, *Medical & Biological Engineering & Computing*, 50(2), 183–192, 2012.

Caseiro, J., R. Valente, A. Reali, J. Kiendl, F. Auricchio, and R. Alves de Sousa, Assumed natural strain NURBS-based solid-shell element for the analysis of large deformation elasto-plastic thin-shell structures, *Computer Methods in Applied Mechanics and Engineering*, 284, 861–880, 2015.

Causin, P., J.F. Gerbeau, and F. Nobile, Added-mass effect in the design of partitioned algorithms for fluid–structure problems, *Computer Methods in Applied Mechanics and Engineering*, 194(42), 4506–4527, 2005.

Cazemier, W., R.W.C.P. Verstappen, and A.E.P. Veldman, Proper orthogonal decomposition and low-dimensional models for driven cavity flows, *Physics of Fluids*, 10(7), 1685–1699, 1998.

Chapelle, D., A. Gariah, and J. Sainte-Marie, Galerkin approximation with proper orthogonal decomposition: New error estimates and illustrative examples, *ESAIM Mathematical Modelling and Numerical Analysis*, 46, 731–757, 2012.

Chapelle, D., A. Gariah, P. Moireau, and J. Sainte-Marie, A Galerkin strategy with proper orthogonal decomposition for parameter-dependent problems – Analysis, assessments and applications to parameter estimation, *ESAIM Mathematical Modelling and Numerical Analysis*, 47(6), 1821–1843, 2013.

Cheng, S.-W., T. Dey, and J. Shewchuk, *Delaunay Mesh Generation*. Boca Raton, FL: CRC Press, 2012.

Cheng, C.P., N.M. Wilson, R.L. Hallett, R.J. Herfkens, and C.A. Taylor, In vivo MR angiographic quantification of axial and twisting deformations of the superficial femoral artery resulting from maximum hip and knee flexion, *Journal of Vascular and Interventional Radiology*, 17(6), 979–987, 2006.

Chinesta, F., A. Huerta, G. Rozza, and K. Willcox, Model reduction methods in *Encyclopedia of Computational Mechanics*. John Wiley & Sons, Hoboken, NJ, 2017.

Choi, G., C.P. Cheng, N.M. Wilson, and C.A. Taylor, Methods for quantifying three-dimensional deformation of arteries due to pulsatile and nonpulsatile forces: Implications for the design of stents and stent grafts, *Annals of Biomedical Engineering*, 37(1), 14–33, 2009.

Christensen, E.A., M. Brøns, and J.N. Sørensen, Evaluation of proper orthogonal decomposition–based decomposition techniques applied to parameter-dependent nonturbulent flows, *SIAM Journal on Scientific Computing*, 21(4), 1419–1434, 1999.

Conti, M., D.V. Loo, F. Auricchio, M.D. Beule, G.D. Santis, B. Verhegghe, S. Pirrelli, and A. Odero, Impact of carotid stent cell design on vessel scaffolding: A case study comparing experimental investigation and numerical simulations, *Journal of Endovascular Therapy*, 18(3), 397–406.

Conti, M., M. Marconi, G. Campanile, A. Reali, D. Adami, R. Berchiolli, and F. Auricchio, Patient-specific finite element analysis of popliteal stenting, *Meccanica*, 52(3), 633–644, 2017.

Constantine, P.G., *Active Subspaces: Emerging Ideas for Dimension Reduction in Parameter Studies*. Philadelphia, PA: SIAM, 2015.

Cosentino, D., C. Capelli, G. Derrick, S. Khambadkone, V. Muthurangu, A.M. Taylor, and S. Schievano, Patient-specific computational models to support interventional procedures: A case study of complex aortic re-coarctation, *EuroIntervention*, 11(5), 669–672, 2015.

Cottrell, J.A., T.J.R. Hughes, and Y. Bazilevs, *Isogeometric Analysis: Toward Integration of CAD and FEA*. Chichester, UK: Wiley, 2009.

Cottrell, J.A., A. Reali, Y. Bazilevs, and T.J.R. Hughes, Isogeometric analysis of structural vibrations, *Computer Methods in Applied Mechanics and Engineering*, 195, 5257–5296, 2006.

Cottrell, J.A., T.J.R. Hughes, and A. Reali, Studies of refinement and continuity in isogeometric structural analysis, *Computer Methods in Applied Mechanics and Engineering*, 196, 4160–4183, 2007.

Dapogny, C., C. Dobrzynski, and P. Frey, Three-dimensional adaptive domain remeshing, implicit domain meshing, and applications to free and moving boundary problems, *Journal of Computational Physics*, 1, 358–378, 2014.

Dedè, L., Reduced basis method and a posteriori error estimation for parametrized linear-quadratic optimal control problems, *SIAM Journal on Scientific Computing*, 32(2), 997–1019, 2010.

Deparis, S., Reduced basis error bound computation of parameter-dependent Navier-Stokes equations by the natural norm approach, *SIAM Journal on Numerical Analysis*, 46(4), 2039–2067, 2008.

Deparis, S. and G. Rozza, Reduced basis method for multi-parameter-dependent steady Navier-Stokes equations: Applications to natural convection in a cavity, *Journal of Computational Physics*, 228(12), 4359–4378, 2009.

De Santis, G., M. De Beule, K. Van Canneyt, P. Segers, P. Verdonck, and B. Verhegghe, Full-hexahedral structured meshing for image-based computational vascular modelling, *Medical Engineering & Physics*, 33(10), 1318–1325, 2011.

Donea, J., S. Giuliani, and J.P. Halleux, An arbitrary Lagrangian-Eulerian finite element method for transient dynamic fluid-structure interactions, *Computer Methods in Applied Mechanics and Engineering*, 33(1–3), 689–723, 1982.

Dwyer, H.A., P.B. Matthews, A. Azadani, N. Jaussaud, L. Ge, T.S. Guy, and E.E. Tseng, Computational fluid dynamics simulation of transcatheter aortic valve degeneration, *Interactive Cardiovascular and Thoracic Surgery*, 9(2), 301–308, 2009.

Echter, R., B. Oesterle, and M. Bischoff, A hierarchic family of isogeometric shell finite elements, *Computer Methods in Applied Mechanics and Engineering*, 254, 170–180, 2013.

Elguedj, T., Y. Bazilevs, V.M. Calo, and T.J.R. Hughes, B-bar and F-bar projection methods for nearly incompressible linear and non-linear elasticity and plasticity using higher-order NURBS elements, *Computer Methods in Applied Mechanics and Engineering*, 197, 2732–2762, 2008.

Elman, H.C., D.J. Silvester, and A.J. Wathen, Finite elements and fast iterative solvers: With applications in incompressible fluid dynamics, in *Numerical Mathematics & Scientific Computation*. Oxford, UK: Oxford University Press, 2014.

Fernández, M.A., Coupling schemes for incompressible fluid-structure interaction: Implicit, semi-implicit and explicit, *SeMA Journal*, 55(1), 59–108, 2011.

Fernández, M.A. and J.F. Gerbeau, Algorithms for fluid-structure interaction problems, in *Cardiovascular Mathematics*, L. Formaggia, A. Quarteroni, and A. Veneziani (Eds.). Berlin, Germany: Springer, 2009, pp. 307–346.

Ferziger, J.H. and M. Peric, *Computational Methods for Fluid Dynamics*. Berlin, Germany: Springer Science & Business Media, 2012.

Formaggia, L., F. Nobile, A. Quarteroni, and A. Veneziani, Multiscale modelling of the circulatory system: A preliminary analysis, *Computing and Visualization in Science*, 2(2–3), 75–83, 1999.

Formaggia, L., J.F. Gerbeau, F. Nobile, and A. Quarteroni, Numerical treatment of defective boundary conditions for the Navier--Stokes equations, *SIAM Journal on Numerical Analysis*, 40(1), 376–401, 2002.

Formaggia, L. and F. Nobile, Stability analysis of second-order time accurate schemes for ALE–FEM, *Computer Methods in Applied Mechanics and Engineering*, 193(39), 4097–4116, 2004.

Formaggia, L., A. Veneziani, and C. Vergara, A new approach to numerical solution of defective boundary value problems in incompressible fluid dynamics, *SIAM Journal on Numerical Analysis*, 46(6), 2769–2794, 2008.

Formaggia, L., A. Quarteroni, and A. Veneziani, Multiscale models of the vascular system, in *Cardiovascular Mathematics*, L. Formaggia, A. Quarteroni, and A. Veneziani (Eds.). Berlin, Germany: Springer, 2009a, pp. 395–446.

Formaggia, L., A. Quarteroni, and A. Veneziani (Eds.), *Cardiovascular Mathematics: Modeling and Simulation of the Circulatory System*, vol. 1. Berlin, Germany: Springer Science & Business Media, 2009b.

Formaggia, L., A. Veneziani, and C. Vergara, Flow rate boundary problems for an incompressible fluid in deformable domains: Formulations and solution methods, *Computer Methods in Applied Mechanics and Engineering*, 199(9), 677–688, 2010.

Frei, S. and R. Richter, A locally modified parametric finite element method for interface problems, *SIAM Journal on Numerical Analysis*, 52(5), 2315–2334, 2014.

Frey, P. and P.-L. George, *Mesh Generation*. London, UK: Wiley, 2008.

Galdi, G.P., R. Rannacher, A.M. Robertson, and S. Turek, *Hemodynamical Flows*. New Delhi, India: Delhi Book Store, 2008.

Garcia, A., E. Pena, and M. Martinez, Influence of geometrical parameters on radial force during self-expanding stent deployment. Application for a variable radial stiffness stent. *Journal of the Mechanical Behavior of Biomedical Materials*, 10, 166–175, 2012.

Gasser, T.C., Biomechanical rupture risk assessment: A consistent and objective decision-making tool for abdominal aortic aneurysm patients, *AORTA Journal*, 4(2), 42, 2016.

Gaur, S., C.A. Taylor, J.M. Jensen, H.E. Bøtker, E.H. Christiansen, A.K. Kaltoft, N.R. Holm et al., FFR derived from coronary CT angiography in nonculprit lesions of patients with recent STEMI, *JACC: Cardiovascular Imaging*, 10(4), 424–433, 2017.

Gerardo-Giorda, L., F. Nobile, and C. Vergara, Analysis and optimization of Robin–Robin partitioned procedures in fluid-structure interaction problems, *SIAM Journal on Numerical Analysis*, 48(6), 2091–2116, 2010.

Gerner, A. and K. Veroy, Certified reduced basis methods for parametrized saddle point problems, *SIAM Journal on Scientific Computing*, 34(5), A2812–A2836, 2012.

Gerstenberger, A. and W. Wall, An eXtended Finite Element Method/Lagrange multiplier based approach for fluid-structure interaction, *Computer Methods in Applied Mechanics and Engineering*, 197, 1699–1714, 2008.

Gessat, M., et al., Image-based mechanical analysis of stent deformation: Concept and exemplary implementation for aortic valve stents, *IEEE Transactions on Biomedical Engineering*, 61(1), 4–15, 2014.

Glowinski, R., *Handbook of Numerical Analysis: Numerical Methods for Fluids (Part 3)*, vol. 9, ch. VIII. Amsterdam, the Netherlands: North-Holland, 2003.

Glowinski, R., T. Pan, and J. Perieux, A fictitious domain method for external incompressible viscous flow modeled by Navier-Stokes equations, *Computer Methods in Applied Mechanics and Engineering*, 112, 133–148, 1994.

Gomez, H., V.M. Calo, Y. Bazilevs, and T.J.R. Hughes, Isogeometric analysis of the Cahn-Hilliard phase-field model, *Computer Methods in Applied Mechanics and Engineering*, 197(49–50), 4333–4352, 2008.

Gomez, H., T.J.R. Hughes, X. Nogueira, and V.M. Calo, Isogeometric analysis of the isothermal Navier-Stokes-Korteweg equations, *Computer Methods in Applied Mechanics and Engineering*, 199, 1828–1840, 2010.

Guermond, J.L., P. Minev, and J. Shen, An overview of projection methods for incompressible flows, *Computer Methods in Applied Mechanics and Engineering*, 195(44), 6011–6045, 2006.

Guidoboni, G., R. Glowinski, N. Cavallini, and S. Canic, Stable loosely-coupled-type algorithm for fluid–structure interaction in blood flow, *Journal of Computational Physics*, 228(18), 6916–6937, 2009.

Grinberg, L., M. Deng, A. Yakhot, and G. Karniadakis, Window proper orthogonal decomposition: Application to continuum and atomistic data, in *Reduced Order Methods for Modeling and Computational Reduction*, vol. 9, A. Quarteroni and G. Rozza (Eds.). Milano, Italy: Springer, MS&A Series, 2013, pp. 275–304.

Gunning, P.S., T.J. Vaughan, and L.M. McNamara, Simulation of self expanding transcatheter aortic valve in a realistic aortic root: Implications of deployment geometry on leaflet deformation, *Annals of Biomedical Engineering*, 42(9), 1989–2001, 2014.

Haasdonk, B. and M. Ohlberger, Reduced basis method for finite volume approximations of parametrized linear evolution equations, *ESAIM Mathematical Modelling and Numerical Analysis*, 42(2), 277–302, 2008.

Hansbo, A. and P. Hansbo, An unfitted finite element method, based on Nitsche's method, for elliptic interface problems, *Computer Methods in Applied Mechanics and Engineering*, 191, 5537–5552, 2002.

Hansbo, P., C. Lovadina, I. Perugia, and G. Sangalli, A Lagrange multiplier method for the finite element solution of elliptic interface problems using non-matching meshes, *Numerische Mathematik*, 100, 91–115, 2008.

Hay, A., J.T. Borggaard, and D. Pelletier, Local improvements to reduced-order models using sensitivity analysis of the proper orthogonal decomposition, *Journal of Fluid Mechanics*, 629, 41–72, 2009.

Heltai, L. and F. Costanzo, Variational implementation of immersed finite element methods, *Computer Methods in Applied Mechanics and Engineering*, 229(Supplement C), 110–127, 2012.

Hesthaven, J.S., G. Rozza, and B. Stamm, *Certified Reduced Basis Methods for Parametrized Partial Differential Equations*, SpringerBriefs in Mathematics. Milano, Italy: Springer, 2015.

Hirotsu, K.E., G.Y. Suh, J.T. Lee, M.D. Dake, D. Fleischmann, and C.P. Cheng, Changes in geometry and cardiac deformation of the thoracic aorta after TEVAR, *Annals of Vascular Surgery*, 41, 21–22, 2017.

Holmes, P., J.L. Lumley, and G. Berkooz, *Turbulence, Coherent Structures, Dynamical Systems and Symmetry*. Cambridge, UK: Cambridge University Press, 1998.

Hsiao, H.-M. and M.-T. Yin, An intriguing design concept to enhance the pulsatile fatigue life of self-expanding stents, *Biomedical Microdevices*, 16(1), 133–144, 2014.

Hughes, T.J.R., J.A. Cottrell, and Y. Bazilevs, Isogeometric analysis: CAD, finite elements, NURBS, exact geometry and mesh refinement, *Computer Methods in Applied Mechanics and Engineering*, 194, 4135–4195, 2005.

Hughes, T.J., W.K. Liu, and T.K. Zimmermann, Lagrangian-Eulerian finite element formulation for incompressible viscous flows, *Computer Methods in Applied Mechanics and Engineering*, 29(3), 329–349, 1981.

Hughes, T.J., L.P. Franca, and M. Balestra, A new finite element formulation for computational fluid dynamics: V. Circumventing the Babuška-Brezzi condition: A stable Petrov-Galerkin formulation of the Stokes problem accommodating equal-order interpolations, *Computer Methods in Applied Mechanics and Engineering*, 59(1), 85–99, 1986.

Hsu, M.-C. and Y. Bazilevs, Fluid-structure interaction modeling of wind turbines: Simulating the full machine, *Computational Mechanics*, 50, 821–833, 2012.

Hsu, M.-C., D. Kamensky, F. Xu, J. Kiendl, C. Wang, M. Wu, J. Mineroff, A. Reali, Y. Bazilevs, and M. Sacks, Dynamic and fluid-structure interaction simulations of bioprosthetic heart valves using parametric design with t-splines and fung-type material models, *Computational Mechanics*, 55, 1211–1225, 2015.

Hyman, M., Non-iterative numerical solution of boundary-value problems, *Applied Scientific Research, Section B*, 2, 325–351, 1952.

Iannaccone, F., N. Debusschere, S. De Bock, M. De Beule, D. Van Loo, F. Vermassen, P. Segers, and B. Verhegghe, The influence of vascular anatomy on carotid artery stenting: A parametric study for damage assessment, *Journal of Biomechanics*, 47(4), 890–898, 2014.

Ilinca, F. and J.-F. Hetu, Numerical simulation of fluid–solid interaction using an immersed boundary finite element method, *Computers & Fluids*, 59, 31–43, 2012.

Iollo, A., S. Lanteri, and J.A. Désidéri, Stability properties of POD-Galerkin approximations for the compressible Navier-Stokes equations, *Theoretical and Computational Fluid Dynamics*, 13(6), 377–396, 2000.

Lipton, S., J.A. Evans, Y. Bazilevs, T. Elguedj, and T.J.R. Hughes, Robustness of isogeometric structural discretizations under severe mesh distortion, *Computer Methods in Applied Mechanics and Engineering*, 199, 357–373, 2010.

de Jaegere, P., G. De Santis, R. Rodriguez-Olivares, J. Bosmans, N. Bruining, T. Dezutter, Z. Rahhab, N. El Faquir, V. Collas, B. Bosmans, and B. Verhegghe, Patient-specific computer modeling to predict aortic regurgitation after transcatheter aortic valve replacement, *JACC: Cardiovascular Interventions*, 9(5), 508–512, 2016.

Johnson, E., Y. Zhang, and K. Shimada, Estimating an equivalent wall-thickness of a cerebral aneurysm through surface parameterization and a non-linear spring system, *International Journal for Numerical Methods in Biomedical Engineering*, 27(7), 1054–1072, 2011.

Joulaian, M. and A. Düster, Local enrichment of the finite cell method for problems with material interfaces, *Computational Mechanics*, 52(4), 741–762, 2013.

Kamenskiy, A.V., I.I. Pipinos, Y.A. Dzenis, N.Y. Phillips, A.S. Desyatova, J. Kitson, R. Bowen, and J.N. MacTaggart, Effects of age on the physiological and mechanical characteristics of human femoropopliteal arteries, *Acta Biomaterialia*, 11, 304–313, 2015.

Kamensky, D., M.-C. Hsu, D. Schillinger, J.A. Evans, A. Aggarwal, Y. Bazilevs, M.S. Sacks, and T.J.R. Hughes, An immersogeometric variational framework for fluid–structure interaction: Application to bioprosthetic heart valves, *Computer Methods in Applied Mechanics and Engineering*, 284, 1005–1053, 2015.

Kiendl, J., K.-U. Bletzinger, J. Linhard, and R. Wuchner, Isogeometric shell analysis with Kirchhoff-Love elements, *Computer Methods in Applied Mechanics and Engineering*, 198, 3902–3914, 2009.

Kiendl, J., M. Ambati, L. De Lorenzis, H. Gomez, and A. Reali, Phase-field description of brittle fracture in plates and shells, *Computer Methods in Applied Mechanics and Engineering*, 312, 374–394, 2016.

Kiendl, J., M.-C. Hsu, M.C. Wu, A. Reali, Isogeometric Kirchhoff–Love shell formulations for general hyperelastic materials, *Computer Methods in Applied Mechanics and Engineering*, 291, 280–303, 2015.

Kim, J., T. Kang, and W.-R. Yu, Mechanical modeling of self-expandable stent fabricated using braiding technology, *Journal of Biomechanics*, 41(15), 3202–3212, 2008.

Kunisch, K. and S. Volkwein, Galerkin proper orthogonal decomposition methods for a general equation in fluid dynamics, *SIAM Journal on Numerical Analysis*, 40(2), 492–515, 2003.

Lassila, T., A. Quarteroni, and G. Rozza, A reduced basis model with parametric coupling for fluid-structure interaction problems, *SIAM Journal on Scientific Computing*, 34(2), A1187–A1213, 2012.

Lassila, T., A. Manzoni, A. Quarteroni, and G. Rozza, A reduced computational and geometrical framework for inverse problems in haemodynamics, *International Journal for Numerical Methods in Biomedical Engineering*, 29(7), 741–776, 2013a.

Lassila, T., A. Manzoni, A. Quarteroni, and G. Rozza, Boundary control and shape optimization for the robust design of bypass anastomoses under uncertainty, *ESAIM Mathematical Modelling and Numerical Analysis*, 47(4), 1107–1131, 2013b.

Lassila, T., A. Manzoni, A. Quarteroni, and G. Rozza, Model order reduction in fluid dynamics: Challenges and perspectives, in *Reduced Order Methods for Modeling and Computational Reduction*, vol. 9, A. Quarteroni and G. Rozza (Eds.). Milano, Italy: Springer, MS&A Series, 2013c, pp. 235–274.

Lassila, T., A. Manzoni, A. Quarteroni, and G. Rozza, Model order reduction in fluid dynamics: Challenges and perspectives, in *Reduced Order Methods for Modeling and Computational Reduction*, A. Quarteroni and G. Rozza (Eds.). Springer, New York, 2014, pp. 235–273.

Law, K., A. Stuart, and K. Zygalakis, *Data Assimilation: A Mathematical Introduction*, vol. 62. Cham, Switerland: Springer, 2015.

Lew, A. and G. Buscaglia, A discontinuous-galerkin-based immersed boundary method, *International Journal for Numerical Methods in Engineering*, 76, 427–454, 2008.

Lesoinne, M. and C. Farhat, Geometric conservation laws for flow problems with moving boundaries and deformable meshes, and their impact on aeroelastic computations, *Computer Methods in Applied Mechanics and Engineering*, 134(1–2), 71–90, 1996.

Li, Z., The immersed interface method using a finite element formulation, *Applied Numerical Mathematics*, 27, 253–267, 1998.

van Loon, R., P. Anderson, and F. van de Vosse, A fluid-structure interaction method with solid-rigid contact for heart valve dynamics, *Journal of Computational Physics*, 217, 806–823, 2006.

Lubliner, J. and F. Auricchio, Generalized plasticity and shape-memory alloys, *International Journal of Solids and Structures*, 33(7), 991–1003, 1996.

MacTaggart, J.N., N.Y. Phillips, C.S. Lomneth, I.I. Pipinos, R. Bowen, B.T. Baxter, J. Johanning, G.M. Longo, A.S. Desyatova, M.J. Moulton, and Y.A. Dzenis, Three-dimensional bending, torsion and axial compression of the femoropopliteal artery during limb flexion, *Journal of Biomechanics*, 47(10), 2249–2256, 2014.

Manzoni, A., A. Quarteroni, and G. Rozza, Model reduction techniques for fast blood flow simulation in parametrized geometries, *International Journal for Numerical Methods in Biomedical Engineering*, 28(6–7), 604–625, 2012a.

Manzoni, A., A. Quarteroni, and G. Rozza, Shape optimization for viscous flows by reduced basis methods and free-form deformation, *International Journal for Numerical Methods in Fluids*, 70(5), 646–670, 2012b.

Manzoni, A., A. Quarteroni, and G. Rozza, Shape optimization of cardiovascular geometries by reduced basis methods and free-form deformation techniques, *International Journal for Numerical Methods in Fluids*, 70(5), 646–670, 2012c.

Manzoni, A., An efficient computational framework for reduced basis approximation and a posteriori error estimation of parametrized Navier-Stokes flows, *ESAIM Mathematical Modelling and Numerical Analysis*, 48, 1199–1226, 2014.

Martufi, G., A. Satriano, R.D. Moore, D.A. Vorp, and E.S. Di Martino, Local quantification of wall thickness and intraluminal thrombus offer insight into the mechanical properties of the aneurysmal aorta, *Annals of Biomedical Engineering*, 43(8), 1759–1771, 2015.

Melenk, J. and I. Babuska, The partition of unity finite element method: Basic theory and applications, *Computer Methods in Applied Mechanics and Engineering*, 139, 289–314, 1996.

Milani, R., A. Quarteroni, and G. Rozza, Reduced basis method for linear elasticity problems with many parameters, *Computer Methods in Applied Mechanics and Engineering*, 197(51), 4812–4829, 2008.

Mirabella, L., C.M. Haggerty, T. Passerini, M. Piccinelli, A.J. Powell, P.J. Del Nido, A. Veneziani, and A.P. Yoganathan, Treatment planning for a TCPC test case: A numerical investigation under rigid and moving wall assumptions, *International Journal for Numerical Methods in Biomedical Engineering*, 29(2), 197–216, 2013.

Morganti, S., F. Auricchio, D.J. Benson, F.I. Gambarin, S. Hartmann, T.J.R. Hughes, and A. Reali, Patient-specific isogeometric structural analysis of aortic valve closure, *Computer Methods in Applied Mechanics and Engineering*, 284, 508–520, 2015.

Morganti, S., M. Conti, M. Aiello, A. Valentini, A. Mazzola, A. Reali, and F. Auricchio, Simulation of transcatheter aortic valve implantation through patient-specific finite element analysis: Two clinical cases, *Journal of Biomechanics*, 47(11), 2547–2555, 2014.

Morganti, S., N. Brambilla, A.S. Petronio, A. Reali, F. Bedogni, and F. Auricchio, Prediction of patient-specific post-operative outcomes of TAVI procedure: The impact of the positioning strategy on valve performance, *Journal of Biomechanics*, 49(12), 2513–2519, 2016.

Morlacchi, S. and F. Migliavacca, Modeling stented coronary arteries: Where we are, where to go, *Annals of Biomedical Engineering*, 41(7), 1428–1444, 2013.

Nauta, F.J., G.H. van Bogerijen, C. Trentin, M. Conti, F. Auricchio, F.L. Moll, J.A. van Herwaarden, and S. Trimarchi, Impact of thoracic endovascular aortic repair on pulsatile circumferential and longitudinal strain in patients with aneurysm, *Journal of Endovascular Therapy*, 24(2), 281–289, 2017.

Negri, F., A. Manzoni, and G. Rozza, Certified reduced basis method for parametrized optimal control problems governed by the Stokes equations, *Computers & Mathematics with Applications*, 69, 319–336, 2015.

Nguyen, N.C., K. Veroy, and A.T. Patera, Certified real-time solution of parametrized partial differential equations, in *Handbook of Materials Modeling*, Yip, S. (Ed.). New York: Springer, 2005, pp. 1523–1558.

Nguyen, N.C., G. Rozza, and A.T. Patera, Reduced basis approximation and a posteriori error estimation for the time-dependent viscous Burgers equation, *Calcolo*, 46(3), 157–185, 2009.

Nichols, W., M. O'Rourke, and C. Vlachopoulos (Eds.). *McDonald's Blood Flow in Arteries: Theoretical, Experimental and Clinical Principles*. Boca Raton, FL: CRC Press, 2011.

Nobile, F. and L. Formaggia, A stability analysis for the arbitrary lagrangian: Eulerian formulation with finite elements, *East-West Journal of Numerical Mathematics*, 7, 105–132, 1999.

Parvizian, J., A. Düster, and E. Rank, Finite cell method, *Computational Mechanics*, 41(1), 121–133, 2007.

Pdeley, T., *The Fluid Mechanics of Large Blood Vessels*. Cambridge, UK: Cambridge University Press, 1980.

Pelton, A., X.-Y. Gong, and T. Duerig, Fatigue testing of diamond-shaped specimens, in *Medical Device Materials - Proceedings of the Materials and Processes for Medical Devices Conference 2003*, S. Shrivastava (Ed.). Anaheim, CA, pp. 199–204, 2003.

Pelton, A.R., V. Schroeder, M.R. Mitchell, X.Y. Gong, M. Barney, and S.W. Robertson, Fatigue and durability of Nitinol stents, *Journal of the Mechanical Behavior of Biomedical Materials*, 1(2), 153–164, 2008.

Perot, J.B., An analysis of the fractional step method, *Journal of Computational Physics*, 108(1), 51–58, 1993.

Perrin, D., P. Badel, L. Orgéas, C. Geindreau, A. Dumenil, J.N. Albertini, and S. Avril, Patient-specific numerical simulation of stent-graft deployment: Validation on three clinical cases, *Journal of Biomechanics*, 48(10), 1868–1875, 2015.

Perry, M., S. Oktay, and J. Muskivitch, Finite element analysis and fatigue of stents, *Minimally Invasive Therapy and Allied Technologies*, 11(4), 165–171, 2002.

Persson, P.-O., Mesh generation for implicit geometries. PhD thesis, Massachusetts Institute of Technology, 2004.

Peskin, C., Numerical analysis of blood flow in the heart, *Journal of Computational Physics*, 25, 220–252, 1977.

Peskin, C.S., The immersed boundary method, *Acta Numerica*, 11, 1–39, 2002.

Peterson, J.S., The reduced basis method for incompressible viscous flow calculations, *SIAM Journal on Scientific and Statistical Computing*, 10, 777–786, 1989.

Petrini, L., F. Migliavacca, P. Massarotti, S. Schievano, G. Dubini, and F. Auricchio, Computational studies of shape memory alloy behavior in biomedical applications, *Journal of Biomechanical Engineering*, 127(4), 716–725, 2005.

Petrini, L., A. Trotta, E. Dordoni, F. Migliavacca, G. Dubini, P.V. Lawford, J.N. Gosai, D.M. Ryan, D. Testi, and G. Pennati, A computational approach for the prediction of fatigue behaviour in peripheral stents: Application to a clinical case, *Annals of Biomedical Engineering*, 44(2), 536–547, 2016.

Pitton, G., A. Quaini, and G. Rozza, Computational reduction strategies for the detection of steady bifurcations in incompressible fluid-dynamics: Applications to Coanda effect in cardiology, *Journal of Computational Physics*, 344, 534–557, 2017.

Pitton, G. and G. Rozza, On the application of reduced basis methods to bifurcation problems in incompressible fluid dynamics, *Journal of Scientific Computing*, 2017. doi:10.1007/s10915-017-0419-6.

Poulson, W., A. Kamenskiy, A. Seas, P. Deegan, C. Lomneth, and J. MacTaggart, Limb flexion-induced axial compression and bending in human femoropopliteal artery segments, *Journal of Vascular Surgery*, 67(2), 607–613, 2018.

Prohl, A., *Projection and Quasi-compressibility Methods for Solving the Incompressible Navier-Stokes Equations*. Stuttgart, Germany: Teubner, 1997.

Quarteroni, A., A. Manzoni, and F. Negri, *Reduced Basis Methods for Partial Differential Equations: An Introduction*, vol. 92. Springer, New York, 2015.

Quarteroni, A. and G. Rozza, Numerical solution of parametrized Navier-Stokes equations by reduced basis methods, *Numerical Methods for Partial Differential Equations*, 23(4), 923–948, 2007.

Quarteroni, A. and G. Rozza (Eds), *Reduced Order Methods for Modeling and Computational Reduction*, vol. 9. Milano, Italy: Springer, MS&A Series, 2013.

Quarteroni, A. and A. Valli, *Domain Decomposition Methods for Partial Differential Equations* (No. CMCS-BOOK-2009-019). Oxford, UK: Oxford University Press, 1999.

Quarteroni, A., A. Veneziani, and C. Vergara, Geometric multiscale modeling of the cardiovascular system, between theory and practice, *Computer Methods in Applied Mechanics and Engineering*, 302, 193–252, 2016.

Rank, E., M. Ruess, S. Kollmannsberger, D. Schillinger, and A. Düster, Geometric modeling, isogeometric analysis and the finite cell method, *Computer Methods in Applied Mechanics and Engineering*, 249, 104–115, 2012.

Ravindran, S.S., A reduced-order approach for optimal control of fluids using proper orthogonal decomposition, *International Journal for Numerical Methods in Fluids*, 34, 425–448, 2000.

Rebelo, N. and M. Perry, Finite element analysis for the design of Nitinol medical devices, *Minimally Invasive Therapy and Allied Technologies*, 9(2), 75–80, 2000.

Rebelo, N., R. Radford, A. Zipse, M. Schlun, and G. Dreher, On modeling assumptions in finite element analysis of stents, *Journal of Medical Devices, Transactions of the ASME*, 5(3), 031007, 2011.

Robertson, S.W., C.P. Cheng, and M.K. Razavi, Biomechanical response of stented carotid arteries to swallowing and neck motion, *Journal of Endovascular Therapy*, 15(6), 663–671, 2008.

Rozza, G., D.B.C. Huynh, and A.T. Patera, Reduced basis approximation and a posteriori error estimation for affinely parametrized elliptic coercive partial differential equations to transport and continuum mechanics. *Archives of Computational Methods in Engineering*, 15(3), 229–275, 2008.

Rozza, G., D.B.P. Huynh, and A. Manzoni, Reduced basis approximation and a posteriori error estimation for Stokes flows in parametrized geometries: Roles of the inf-sup stability constants, *Numerische Mathematik*, 125(1), 115–152, 2013.

Rozza, G., Real-time reduced basis solutions for Navier-Stokes equations: Optimization of parametrized bypass configurations, *ECCOMAS CFD in Proceedings on CFD*, Deft University of Technology, The Netherlands, 2006.

Rozza, G. and K. Veroy, On the stability of reduced basis methods for Stokes equations in parametrized domains, *Computer Methods in Applied Mechanics and Engineering*, 196(7), 1244–1260, 2007.

Schievano, S., A.M. Taylor, C. Capelli, P. Lurz, J. Nordmeyer, F. Migliavacca, and P. Bonhoeffer, Patient specific finite element analysis results in more accurate prediction of stent fractures: Application to percutaneous pulmonary valve implantation, *Journal of Biomechanics*, 43(4), 687–693, 2010.

Schillinger, D., L. Dede, M.A. Scott, J.A. Evans, M.J. Borden, E. Rank, and T.J.R. Hughes, An isogeometric design-through-analysis methodology based on adaptive hierarchical refinement of NURBS, immersed boundary methods, and T-spline CAD surfaces, *Computer Methods in Applied Mechanics and Engineering*, 249–250, 116–150, 2012.

Schofer, J., P. Musiałek, K. Bijuklic, R. Kolvenbach, M. Trystula, Z. Siudak, and H. Sievert, A prospective, multicenter study of a novel mesh-covered carotid stent: The CGuard CARENET trial (Carotid Embolic Protection Using MicroNet). *JACC: Cardiovascular Interventions*, 8(9), 1229–1234, 2015.

Sirisup, S. and G.E. Karniadakis, Stability and accuracy of periodic flow solutions obtained by a POD-penalty method, *Journal of Physics D*, 202(3), 218–237, 2005.

Sirois, E., Q. Wang, and W. Sun, Fluid simulation of a transcatheter aortic valve deployment into a patient-specific aortic root, *Cardiovascular Engineering and Technology*, 2(3), 186–195, 2011.

Smith, C.R., Transcatheter versus surgical aortic-valve replacement in high-risk patients, *New England Journal of Medicine*, 364(23), 2187–2198, 2011.

Smuts, A.N., D.C. Blaine, C. Scheffer, H. Weich, A.F. Doubell, and K.H. Dellimore. Application of finite element analysis to the design of tissue leaflets for a percutaneous aortic valve, *Journal of the Mechanical Behavior of Biomedical Materials*, 4(1), 85–98, 2011.

Sukumar, N., D.L. Chopp, N. Moes, and T. Belytschko, Modeling holes and inclusions by level sets in the extended finite-element method, *Computer Methods in Applied Mechanics and Engineering*, 190, 6183–6200, 2001.

Sun, W., K. Li, and E. Sirois, Simulated elliptical bioprosthetic valve deformation: Implications for asymmetric transcatheter valve deployment, *Journal of Biomechanics*, 43(16), 3085–3090, 2010.

Suh, G.Y., G. Choi, M.T. Draney, R.J. Herfkens, R.L. Dalman, and C.P. Cheng, Respiratory-induced 3D deformations of the renal arteries quantified with geometric modeling during inspiration and expiration breath-holds of magnetic resonance angiography, *Journal of Magnetic Resonance Imaging*, 38(6), 1325–1332, 2013.

Taylor, C.A., T.A. Fonte, and J.K. Min, Computational fluid dynamics applied to cardiac computed tomography for noninvasive quantification of fractional flow reserve, *Journal of the American College of Cardiology*, 61(22), 2233–2241, 2013.

Thériault, P., P. Terriault, V. Brailovski, and R. Gallo, Finite element modeling of a progressively expanding shape memory stent, *Journal of Biomechanics*, 39(15), 2837–2844, 2006.

Temam, R., *Navier-Stokes Equations*, vol. 2, pp. xii+-526. Amsterdam, the Netherlands: North-Holland, 1984.

Temam, R., *Navier–Stokes Equations and Nonlinear Functional Analysis*. Philadelphia, PA: Society for Industrial and Applied Mathematics, 1995.

Thomas, J.B., L. Antiga, S.L. Che, J.S. Milner, D.A.H. Steinman, J.D. Spence, B.K. Rutt, and D.A. Steinman, Variation in the carotid bifurcation geometry of young versus older adults, *Stroke*, 36(11), 2450–2456, 2005.

Townsend, N., M. Nichols, P. Scarborough, and M. Rayner, Cardiovascular disease in Europe-epidemiological update 2015, *European Heart Journal*, 36(40), 2696–2705, 2015.

Tzamtzis, S., J. Viquerat, J. Yap, M.J. Mullen, and G. Burriesci, Numerical analysis of the radial force produced by the Medtronic-CoreValve and Edwards-SAPIEN after transcatheter aortic valve implantation (TAVI), *Medical Engineering & Physics*, 35(1), 125–130, 2013.

Ullery, B.W., G.Y. Suh, J.T. Lee, B. Liu, R. Stineman, R.L. Dalman, and C.P. Cheng, Geometry and respiratory-induced deformation of abdominal branch vessels and stents after complex endovascular aneurysm repair, *Journal of Vascular Surgery*, 61(4), 875–885, 2015.

Utturkar, Y., B. Zhang, and W. Shyy, Reduced-order description of fluid flow with moving boundaries by proper orthogonal decomposition, *International Journal of Heat and Fluid Flow*, 26(2), 276–288, 2005.

Veneziani, A. and C. Vergara, Flow rate defective boundary conditions in haemodynamics simulations, *International Journal for Numerical Methods in Fluids*, 47(8–9), 803–816, 2005.

Veneziani, A. and C. Vergara, An approximate method for solving incompressible Navier-Stokes problems with flow rate conditions, *Computer Methods in Applied Mechanics and Engineering*, 196(9), 1685–1700, 2007.

Veneziani, A. and C. Vergara, Inverse problems in Cardiovascular Mathematics: Toward patient-specific data assimilation and optimization, *International Journal for Numerical Methods in Biomedical Engineering*, 29(7), 723–725, 2013.

Veneziani, A. and U. Villa, ALADINS: An ALgebraic splitting time ADaptive solver for the Incompressible Navier–Stokes equations, *Journal of Computational Physics*, 238, 359–375, 2013.

Veroy, K. and A.T. Patera, Certified real-time solution of the parametrized steady incompressible Navier-Stokes equations: Rigorous reduced-basis a posteriori error bounds, *International Journal for Numerical Methods in Fluids*, 47(8–9), 773–788, 2005.

Viguerie, A. and A. Veneziani, Inexact algebraic factorization methods for the steady incompressible Navier-Stokes equations at moderate Reynolds numbers, *Computer Methods in Applied Mechanics and Engineering*, to appear, 2017

Wang, Z., I. Akhtar, J. Borggaard, and T. Iliescu, Proper orthogonal decomposition closure models for turbulent flows: A numerical comparison, *Computer Methods in Applied Mechanics and Engineering*, 237–240, 10–26, 2012a.

Wang, Q., G. Canton, J. Guo, X. Guo, T.S. Hatsukami, K.L. Billiar, C. Yuan, Z. Wu, and D. Tang, MRI-based patient-specific human carotid atherosclerotic vessel material property variations in patients, vessel location and long-term follow up, *PLoS One*, 12(7), e0180829, 2017.

Wang, Q., E. Sirois, and W. Sun, Patient-specific modeling of biomechanical interaction in transcatheter aortic valve deployment, *Journal of Biomechanics*, 45(11), 1965–1971, 2012b.

Weller, J., E. Lombardi, M. Bergmann, and A. Iollo, Numerical methods for low-order modeling of fluid flows based on POD, *International Journal for Numerical Methods in Fluids*, 63(2), 249–268, 2010.

Whitcher, F., Simulation of in vivo loading conditions of nitinol vascular stent structures, *Computers and Structures*, 64(5–6), 1005–1011, 1997.

Wu, W., M. Qi, X.P. Liu, D.Z. Yang, and W.Q. Wang, Delivery and release of nitinol stent in carotid artery and their interactions: A finite element analysis, *Journal of Biomechanics*, 40(13), 3034–3040, 2007.

Yushkevich, P.A., J. Piven, H.C. Hazlett, R.G. Smith, S. Ho, J.C. Gee, and G. Gerig, User-guided 3D active contour segmentation of anatomical structures: Significantly improved efficiency and reliability, *Neuroimage*, 31(3), 1116–1128, 2006.

Zhang, Y., Y. Bazilevs, S. Goswami, C.L. Bajaj, and T.J. Hughes, Patient-specific vascular NURBS modeling for isogeometric analysis of blood flow, *Computer Methods in Applied Mechanics and Engineering*, 196(29), 2943–2959, 2007.

Zhang, H., Y. Jiao, E. Johnson, L. Zhan, Y. Zhang, and K. Shimada, Modelling anisotropic material property of cerebral aneurysms for fluid–structure interaction simulation, *Computer Methods in Biomechanics and Biomedical Engineering: Imaging & Visualization*, 1(3), 164–174, 2013.

Zhang, Y.J., *Geometric Modeling and Mesh Generation from Scanned Images*, vol. 6. Boca Raton, FL: CRC Press, 2016.

Zunino, P., L. Cattaneo, and C.M. Colciago, An unfitted interface penalty method for the numerical approximation of contrast problems, *Applied Numerical Mathematics*, 61, 1059–1076, 2011.

6

Aortic and Arterial Mechanics

S. Avril

Contents

6.1 Introduction

Knowledge of the mechanical properties of the aorta is essential, as important concerns regarding the treatment of aortic pathologies, such as atherosclerosis, aneurysms, and dissections, are fundamentally mechanobiological. A comprehensive review is presented in the current chapter. As the function of arteries is to carry blood to the peripheral organs, the main biomechanical properties of interest are elasticity and rupture properties. Regarding elastic properties, an essential parameter remains the physiological linearized elastic modulus in the circumferential direction; however, sophisticated constitutive equations, including hyperelasticity, are available to model the complex coupled roles played by collagen, elastin, and smooth muscle cells (SMCs) in the mechanics of the aorta. Regarding rupture properties, tensile strengths in the axial and circumferential directions are on the order of 1.5 MPa in the thoracic aorta, and the radial strength, which is important regarding dissections, is about 0.1 MPa. All these properties may vary spatially and change with the adaptation of the aortic wall to different conditions through growth and remodeling. The progression of diseases, such as aneurysms and atherosclerosis, also manifests with alterations of these material properties. After presenting how the mechanical properties of elastic arteries, including the aorta, can be measured and how they can be used in models to predict the biomechanical response of these models under different circumstances, a section will focus on the biomechanics of the ascending thoracic aorta. The chapter will end with current challenges regarding predictive numerical simulations for personalized medicine.

6.2 Mechanical Properties of Arteries

6.2.1 Mechanical Function of Arteries

6.2.1.1 Arterial Pressure and Wall Stress

Arteries are in charge of carrying blood to the peripheral organs. The blood pressure P exerts a force perpendicular to the luminal surface of the artery, which causes its distension. It is compensated by radial and circumferential wall tensions that oppose distension. Assuming a perfectly cylindrical shape, the resulting circumferential stress σ_{circ} can be estimated by Laplace's law, considering the wall as a thin, long circular tube of radius r and thickness t. There are several expressions of Laplace's law, such as $\sigma_{circ} = Pr/h$ [1], according to which the circumferential stress is directly related to the pressure and to the geometry of the wall. It is also accepted that modifications of the circumferential stress lead to a remodeling of the wall and changes in its structure. In particular, these changes include thickening of the wall (hypertrophy of the smooth muscle) when mechanical stress is increased; conversely, the changes include wall atrophy when mechanical stress is decreased [2].

However, let us note that this estimate by Laplace's law gives only an average value. It neglects the influence of the microstructure of the wall and does not make it possible to evaluate the transmural variations of the circumferential stress. In addition, blood pressure is not constant but varies during the cardiac cycle. In particular, the pulse pressure plays an important role in the remodeling of large arteries [3].

Figure 6.1 shows two successive cycles of arterial pressure. There is a rise in pressure during systolic ejection, followed by a peak and then a decrease in pressure during ventricular diastole. The measured systolic blood pressure (SBP) is the maximum value at the peak. The dicrotic notch corresponds to the closure of the aortic valve and is followed by a drop in diastolic pressure. The measured diastolic blood pressure (DBP) is the minimum value of the curve. These characteristic values of blood pressure can be measured with an automatic or manual sphygmomanometer with stethoscope. The pressure can also be recorded continuously over several cycles, either by means of a catheter inserted in the artery or by a noninvasive technique, such as applanation tonometry, when the access is possible (for instance, common carotid arteries). Finally, it should be emphasized that the arterial pressure curve is not the same, according to the location of the artery analyzed in the vascular tree. It depends on the size and elasticity of the artery in question. Normal blood pressure values in humans are between 100 and 140 mmHg for SBP and between 60 and 90 mmHg for DBP. The mean arterial pressure (MAP) corresponds to the area under the pressure curve. It is closer to DBP than to SBP and is assumed to be nearly constant throughout the arterial tree in the supine position, at least until blood reaches the resistance arterioles.

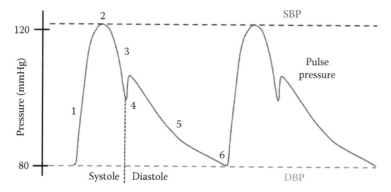

Figure 6.1   Schematic representation of two successive cycles of arterial pressure.

6.2.1.2 Arterial Compliance

The heart acts as a pulsatile pump that propels blood into the vascular system during its contraction (systole). Part of the blood ejected during systole is stored during distension of the aorta and the proximal arteries. The function of the large elastic arteries is to relay the contraction of the heart when it enters its relaxation phase (diastole), thanks to their compliance. After closing the aortic valve, the aorta and the proximal arteries retract elastically and restore the volume of blood stored. This is the Windkessel effect, by which blood pressure is maintained and blood flow is increased in diastole, which ensure a continuous and nonpulsatile flow in the peripheral arteries and the capillaries. This function of diastolic relay of the cardiac contraction is directly related to the elastic properties of the large arteries, which are conferred on them by the large quantity of elastic fibers and type III collagen in the media [1,2].

The compliance of an artery can be measured experimentally from the pressure–volume relationships. Indeed, arterial compliance is defined as the ratio between the increase in luminal volume and the increase in pressure that induces it: it corresponds to the slope of the pressure–volume curve. In addition, arterial distensibility is defined as the relative variation of volume with respect to the pressure variation. It is, therefore, a relationship between compliance and luminal volume.

Since the pressure–volume relationship is not linear for an artery, compliance and distensibility vary with the pressure level. The higher the pressure, the more the stress on collagen fibers and the greater the resistance to distension. Thus, compliance and distensibility decrease as pressure increases. It should be noted that these two parameters are often measured by studying a cross-section of the artery, with the assumption that the artery does not change in length. Cross-sectional studies can be carried out by using external ultrasound probes for superficial arteries, such as common carotid and femoral arteries and the radial or brachial arteries, or by magnetic resonance imaging (MRI) for the aorta [4].

6.2.1.3 Pulse Wave

The impact produced by the blood on the walls of the aorta during cardiac ejection generates a pressure wave called a pulse wave, which propagates along the arterial tree from the aorta to the peripheral arteries. It causes a radial deformation of the arterial wall, which enables diastolic relay of the cardiac contraction. The pulse wave velocity (PWV) is considered a parameter that represents arterial stiffness. Indeed, the Moens–Korteweg relationship relates the PWV to the geometrical and mechanical characteristics of the artery when it is considered a thin-walled isotropic tube of infinite length:

$$VOP = \sqrt{\frac{E_{inc}h}{2\rho r}}, \tag{6.1}$$

where E_{inc} is the incremental Young's modulus of the arterial wall, h is its thickness, r is its radius, and ρ is the density of the blood. The stiffer the artery (i.e., the higher its modulus of elasticity), the higher the PWV. For a healthy middle-aged individual, PWV generally ranges between 4 and 10 m/s.

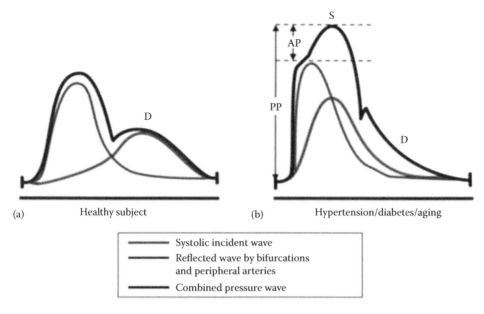

Figure 6.2 Schematic of arterial pressure waveforms and calculation of augmentation index. (a) Pulse waveforms in healthy compliant vasculature; rebound wave reflection occurs during diastole (D). (b) With hypertension, diabetes, or aging, the pulse wave reflection occurs earlier. (Adapted from Kum, F., and Karalliedde, J., *Integr. Blood Press. Contr.*, 3, 63, 2010.)

When the incident pressure wave encounters bifurcations or peripheral resistance arteries, it is partially reflected. The reflected wave propagates backward and is added to the incident wave. The reflected wave has an important impact on the shape and amplitude of the pressure profiles and explains their variations along the arterial tree. Indeed, in the peripheral arteries located closer to reflection sites, the reflected wave returns more quickly than in other arteries. The reflected wave adds to the incident wave earlier in the cardiac cycle by increasing SBP, while it mainly affects DBP for elastic arteries near the heart (Figure 6.2). In the same way, in the elderly or patients suffering from vascular pathologies and in those whose arteries are more rigid, the SBP is increased by the reflected wave. This phenomenon can be quantified by the increase index, defined as the ratio between the pressure increase and the pulse pressure, the pressure increase being the difference between the first and second systolic peaks [4].

6.2.2 Nonlinear Elasticity

The mechanical properties of an artery depend on its geometry and on the proportions of its various microconstituents, described in Chapter 1. Smooth muscle cells control the vasomotion of the arteries, which relates to the active mechanical properties of the arteries, while the passive mechanical properties of the arteries are determined by the extracellular matrix (ECM), in particular the elastin and collagen fibers. The elastic arteries of large caliber, in which we are interested in this chapter, contain more elastic fibers than muscular fibers. They, therefore, exhibit a small vasomotricity, and their passive properties are preponderant in the characterization of their mechanical behavior. The active properties related to the muscular tone of the arterial wall will be discussed in Section 6.2.7.

Elastin fibers are highly elastic and resist to distension forces generated by blood pressure. Collagen fibers are much more rigid and almost inextensible and prevent the distension of the artery. However, they are arranged in the wall, so as to be stressed only under high distension levels. They are recruited gradually when the pressure increases and are only truly stretched for high pressures, that is, greater than about 125 mmHg in healthy situations. Thus, the arteries exhibit a highly nonlinear pressure–diameter response with characteristic stiffness under high pressure.

Individual contributions of elastin and collagen fibers to the overall nonlinear response of arterial tissue were identified by Roach and Burton [6]. The difference in behavior between elastin and collagen was demonstrated by recording the tension-circumference relationships of intact human external iliac arteries and then performing selective enzymatic digestions of collagen and elastin.

It appears that the distension of an artery mainly depends on its elastic fibers at low pressure and on its collagen fibers at high pressure. The initial slope of the stress-strain curves roughly indicates the state of the elastic fibers, while its final slope roughly reflects the state of the collagen.

The arteries, therefore, have a nonlinear elastic behavior that can be modeled by a hyperelastic behavioral relationship, originally developed for elastomers such as rubber. The stress field is obtained by deriving a deformation energy function; several types of this function have been proposed in the literature: exponential, polynomial, and so on. We will return to this in detail in Section 6.3.3.

6.2.3 Incompressibility

Like many soft biological tissues, the arteries are generally considered incompressible. Patel and Vaishnav [7] demonstrated the incompressibility of the arteries experimentally by comparing the resistance of the material with changes in volume. Carew et al. [8] immersed arterial segments in water in a closed chamber and observed a volume change of 0.165% at a pressure of 181 mmHg. They concluded that this result justified the assumption of incompressibility. Finally, Tardy [9] measured in vivo the relative variations in volume per unit length of the radial artery and found values less than 1% under physiological conditions.

6.2.4 Anisotropy

Numerous studies agree that the vascular tissue is anisotropic; that is, its elastic properties are not the same in all directions. The first study documenting the anisotropy of the arteries was carried out by Patel and Fry in 1966 on dog arterial segments [10]. Several studies have subsequently confirmed this result [10–14].

Nevertheless, many authors have modeled arteries by using isotropic constitutive equations. Dobrin and Doyle showed that, by assuming isotropy, the circumferential elastic modulus was overestimated by 17% at a pressure of 80 mmHg [12].

6.2.5 Residual Stresses

Intuitively, the reference state chosen to study an arterial segment corresponds to a state without external loads, that is, without pressure or longitudinal forces. However, this state does not correspond to a state free of constraints. Indeed, residual longitudinal and circumferential stresses remain in the arterial segment. They are nonuniform and result from tissue growth and adaptation to their mechanical environment during development [15]. They are released only when the vessel is severed and removed from its environment.

The existence of residual circumferential and radial stresses has been demonstrated by Vaishnav and Vossoughi [16] and Fung [17]. They observed that by radially cutting an arterial ring, the artery opens by itself by an angle that can be measured by joining the middle of the internal arc at its extremities (Figure 6.3). Therefore, the state "zero stress" can be represented by an open arterial segment. It should be noted that the opening angle varies according to species, the arterial site considered, and its condition. Fung and Liu [18] observed changes in the opening angle after only a few days of pressure increase (high blood pressure, or HBP). Thus, the opening angle appears as a marker of the remodeling of the arterial wall.

It is important to note that residual stresses play a central role in vascular mechanics, because they modify the distribution of stresses in the arterial wall [19]. Indeed, they make it possible to reduce the circumferential stresses toward the intimal portion of the wall, as well as the stress gradient across the wall [20]. This result was illustrated by Delfino et al. [21] by using an isotropic three-dimensional (3D) finite element model of the human carotid bifurcation. Semi-analytical approaches considering the anisotropy of arterial tissue showed the same trend [22,23]. However,

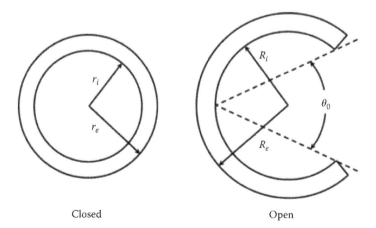

Closed   Open

Figure 6.3   Schematic of the opening angle experiment.

residual stresses, as revealed by sometimes extreme opening angles in the elderly, may lead to increased stresses toward the adventitial portion of the wall [24].

On the other hand, Greenwald et al. [25] showed that the opening angle is not correlated with smooth muscle activation and the collagen content in the wall but is rather associated with elastic fibers. Indeed, treatment of segments of rat aorta with elastase reduced the angle of opening, while collagenase had no effect on the angle of opening. Moreover, the opening angles of the different aortic layers of the wall were different [26].

Azeloglu et al. [8] investigated, both numerically and experimentally, the regulating role of proteoglycans present in the arterial wall. They showed that, with an inhomogeneous distribution of proteoglycans through the wall thickness, the Donnan osmotic pressure would vary through the wall thickness, resulting in an inhomogeneous swelling stress field in the solid matrix, which would significantly affect the opening angle observed experimentally. The residual stress state in arteries has also been shown to be dependent on location and influenced by a host of other factors, a review of which can be found in [6].

6.2.6 Axial Stretch

During excision of an arterial segment, a reduction in length or longitudinal retraction is observed. This phenomenon shows the existence of a longitudinal prestress exerted by the surrounding tissue. Moreover, Han [27] noted that the longitudinal extension does not vary after the radial opening of the vessels and is therefore the same at zero stress. In vivo, because of the presence of perivascular tissues, arteries retain a fixed length, which does not vary with pressure. Van Loon [28] showed that, in dog arteries, the axial force–length curves obtained in vitro for different pressure levels intersected at a single point. The length at this point corresponds to a constant axial force, regardless of pressure. In turn, this makes it possible to estimate the longitudinal extension in vivo, defined as the ratio between the length of the arterial segment in vivo and the length of the arterial segment in the reference state without constraint [29].

6.2.7 Vascular Contraction

A unique feature of many soft tissues is their ability to contract via actin–myosin interactions within specialized cells called myocytes. Examples include the cardiac muscle of the heart, the skeletal muscle of the arms and legs, and the smooth muscle, which is found in many tissues, including the airways, arteries, and uterus. A famous equation in muscle mechanics was postulated in 1938 by A.V. Hill to describe the force-velocity relationship. This relationship, like many subsequent ones, focuses on one-dimensional (1D) behavior of the myocyte or muscle along its axis; data typically come from tests on muscle fibers or strips or, in some cases, rings taken from arteries or airways. Although much has been learned, much remains to be discovered, particularly with respect to the multiaxial behavior. The interested reader is referred to Fung [17].

6.2.8 Vascular Adaptation

Vascular adaptation refers to the cell-mediated mechanical effects of growth, atrophy, remodeling, and healing. Like all tissues and organs, the vasculature undergoes many changes during normal development and aging, as well as in disease and injury. Morphological, histological, and biomechanical changes stem from growth and remodeling that follow maturation. Under normal conditions, the mature arterial wall is fairly stable: turnover of endothelial cells is on the order of 0.02% per day, except in regions of complex flow (e.g., near a bifurcation), where it may be as high as a few percentages per day, whereas turnover of SMCs is about 0.06% per day. The half-life of collagen is on the order of weeks to months, whereas the half-life of elastin is comparable to the life span of the organism [30]. Normal tissue maintenance is thus accomplished via slow, steady processes by which constituents are turned over in a balanced manner, the deposition of proteins being balanced by degradation. The natural tendency toward stability of normal biological states is called *homeostasis*. In response to persistent nonhomeostatic stimuli, such as altered needs of distal tissues due to consistent exercise or inactivity, local alterations in hemodynamic loads, local changes in the expression of growth factors or vasoactive substances, microgravity, and surgery, the rates of turnover of various constituents can increase dramatically and the arterial wall can quickly undergo significant modification via unbalanced cellular activity: via hyperplasia, hypertrophy, apoptosis, and migration of cells, as well as via unequal synthesis and degradation of the ECM. The biomechanical theory for modeling these effects will be briefly explained in Section 6.3.5.

6.2.9 Alterations of Mechanical Properties in Aging and Vascular Pathologies

There are many different types of arterial pathologies, and together, they represent one of the leading causes of death in the world. Myocardial infarction and stroke affect 120,000 and 150,000 people, respectively, per year in France. Stroke is the leading cause of disability in adults worldwide, the second leading cause of dementia (after Alzheimer's disease), and the third leading cause of death in industrialized countries (after heart disease and cancer). Myocardial infarction is mainly triggered by the obstruction of an artery feeding the heart, and stroke is mainly triggered by the obstruction of an artery feeding the brain. Eventually, this leads to ischemia, defined as the metabolic demand being unmet, leading to tissue suffering and ultimate necrosis. Ischemia is most often triggered by the rupture of an atheroma plaque, a lipid deposit that forms on the inner wall of the arteries with age and under the influence of various risk factors (sex, heredity, food, physical inactivity, smoking, etc.). When an atheroma plaque ruptures, a clot typically forms; this may cause thrombosis by obstructing blood flow through an artery. The clot may also migrate or form upstream (e.g., in the heart chambers).

High blood pressure is a major risk factor for various cardiovascular pathologies, including atherosclerosis, stroke, and aneurysms.

Vascular pathologies are generally associated with remodeling of the affected arterial wall. Therefore, the structural and functional modifications of the wall result in changes in mechanical properties. The evaluation and understanding of these changes in mechanical behavior are used to guide therapeutic solutions and prevent cardiovascular events.

In the following section, we briefly present the evolution of the arterial structure due to aging and two important pathologies: abdominal aortic aneurysm (AAA) and hypertension.

6.2.9.1 Vascular Aging
Aging is accompanied by significant changes in the cellular and extracellular components of the arterial wall. It has often been confused with atherosclerosis, because atherosclerosis is also strongly influenced by age. However, in contrast to atherosclerosis, which is a localized disease and results in a reduction in arterial lumen (stenosis), aging is a diffuse physiological process that leads to enlargement of arterial lumen [31]. This enlargement often occurs with an increase in blood pressure (without known causal relationship) and thus an increase in circumferential wall stress. The internal and external arterial diameters increase during aging and the wall thickens, with an important hypertrophy of the intima. The length of the arteries also increases with age, and arterial tortuosities may appear [32].

From a histological point of view, there is an evolution of the composition of the ECM during development, maturation, and aging. The elastic fibers are gradually altered; they disorganize and appear finer and fragmented. The amount of collagen in the media increases with age, while the elastin content remains stable. Thus, the collagen-to-elastin ratio increases, which leads to stiffer arteries [33].

6.2.9.2 Hypertension
Hypertension or HBP is the most common cardiovascular disease, affecting a quarter of the global population. It is defined by an SBP greater than 140 mmHg and a DBP greater than 90 mmHg. The short-term response of a large artery to an increase in pressure consists of a distension of the arterial wall and a decrease in its thickness. The circumferential wall stress is then increased. To normalize the circumferential stress, adaptive phenomena take place in the medium term. An increase in the internal diameter and thickening of the media are observed, mainly by hypertrophy and hyperplasia of SMCs and by an increase in the synthesis of collagen, elastin, and proteoglycans [34,35]. This type of remodeling has been observed both in experimental studies in animal models and in clinical studies [36]. Interestingly, despite the increase in elastin and collagen content, their relative mass densities and elastin-to-collagen volume ratios are not altered [37]. Peripheral resistance arteries may exhibit variable levels of hypertrophy and remodeling [38]. Remodeling contributes to an increase in peripheral vascular resistance, generally associated with hypertension. This increase in resistance leads to an increase in pulse pressure, which, in turn, is an arterial remodeling trigger that leads to enlargement and thickening of the large arteries [3]. Therefore, the remodeling induced by initial HBP is amplified; this maintains HBP, thus forming a vicious circle [39].

Hypertension is a factor in the development of atherosclerosis [40] and aortic aneurysms [41]. This is related to multiple aspects, including increased wall stress and increased transmural diffusion. High blood pressure is the main preventable risk factor for AAA and is treatable by appropriate management.

6.2.9.3 Abdominal Aortic Aneurysms

An aneurysm is defined as a localized and permanent dilatation of more than 50% of the initial diameter of an artery, with loss of parallelism of the edges. The aorta is a common site for the development of aneurysms, including the ascending, descending, and abdominal regions. Ninety percent of the AAAs are located between the renal arteries and the iliac bifurcation. The dilatation of the aorta gradually weakens the wall, which can then rupture and cause massive internal bleeding in more than 65% of cases. Other complications include arterial thrombosis and embolism. Abdominal aortic aneurysm is the third leading cause of cardiovascular mortality in developed countries and ranks as the thirteenth most common cause of death in the United States [42]. Owing to an aging population, increased prevalence of hypertension, increased smoking, screening programs, and improved diagnostic tools, the incidence of AAA has continued to grow during the last decades. Abdominal aortic aneurysm more frequently affects men older than 60 years. The prevalence after the age of 60 years is 4%–8% in men and 1%–3% in women [41–44].

The majority of AAAs are asymptomatic and go unnoticed because of their slow development. Approximately one third of AAAs are detected in routine medical examinations by detection of pulsatile abdominal wall. Most of the time, the other two thirds are accidentally discovered during medical imaging tests performed for other pathologies. Conventional diagnostic and surveillance techniques include abdominal ultrasound, a technique of choice, because it is very sensitive; computed tomography (CT); and MRI [45]. The growth rate of AAA is highly variable. When detected, AAA requires regular monitoring of diameter. Indeed, some aneurysms evolve very slowly and never reach the rupture point, while others may develop rapidly and reach a high-risk status.

The exact causes of AAA are not yet well known. Nevertheless, several risk factors are involved in their occurrence:

- HBP [41]
- Smoking or smoking history [46]
- Family history, suggesting genetic factors [47]
- Age, sex [41], and ethnicity (much lower prevalence in Asian populations) [48]
- Atherosclerosis [49]
- Obesity [50]

The development of AAA is determined by the destruction of the aortic media due to the alteration of the proteins of the ECM in the aortic wall and the loss of SMCs. One of the most important histological features of the aneurysm [51] is the decrease in the concentration of elastic fibers during the growth of AAA, up to rupture. Compared with healthy abdominal aorta, a loss of up to 90% of elastin can be observed in AAA, with the remaining amount being mostly fragmented. The rarefaction of elastin seems to be one of the first step in the formation of AAA [52]. Collagen is also involved in the pathophysiology of AAA. Unlike elastin, the concentration of collagen does not decrease during the progression of AAA but tends to increase to compensate for the loss of elastin. The synthesis of collagen is increased in the adventitia, which thickens by the formation of perivascular fibrosis. This strengthening provides the mechanical strength that compensates for the destruction of the media and its loss of functionality. Nevertheless, despite compensatory synthesis, the collagen appears altered, with loss of functionality, realignment towards the circumferential direction, and an increase in the degree of crosslinking, which alters the aortic distensibility. Finally, degradation of collagen appears to be the ultimate cause of rupture [52].

Inflammation is a major characteristic of AAA, affecting mainly the external part of the media and the adventitia. The AAA wall has a characteristic inflammatory infiltrate composed of macrophages, T and B lymphocytes, neutrophils, and mast cells. These cells lead to the release of proinflammatory cytokines and proteases, responsible for the degradation of ECM proteins.

To the scarcity of the ECM in the media, we must add the reduction of the density of the SMCs. Indeed, the number of SMCs in the AAA wall is reduced by 74% compared with the normal aorta. Moreover, the remaining SMCs predominantly have an advanced apoptotic state [53]. However, medial SMCs are an important source of elastin and collagen synthesis and play a protective role against inflammation and proteolysis [54]. Therefore, loss of SMCs could be a major factor in the progression of AAA by unbalancing the remodeling of the ECM.

Finally, in approximately 75% of the patients, the wall of the AAA is covered with an intraluminal thrombus (ILT), which consists of coagulation of a dense network of fibrin trapping red blood cells, platelets, blood proteins, and cellular debris. It generally has an inhomogeneous structure, with a thin, rigid, highly biologically active layer, while the medial and abluminal layers are less rigid and resistant, because they are affected by progressive fibrinolysis [55]. Many studies have suggested that thrombus may play a protective role for the wall of the aneurysm by reducing and modifying the distribution of wall stresses [56–58]. However, several studies have also clearly demonstrated that the thrombus does not reduce the pressure on the aneurysmal wall [59,60]. In addition, the thrombus presents an important source of proteolytic and inflammatory factors. Comparative histological studies have shown that the thrombus-coated aneurysm wall is thinner and more inflammatory and contains less elastin and SMCs [61]. The size of the thrombus is also associated with faster AAA growth. Thus, embrittlement of the wall under the effect of the thrombus might be predominant as compared with the protection by reduction of the wall stresses [62] or strains [60].

Current widespread clinical thinking is that AAA rupture is best predicted by monitoring its maximum diameter; specifically, the risk of rupture is highest when the aneurysm reaches 5 or 5.5 cm in diameter. Such clinical assessment methods to evaluate AAA rupture potential are unreliable [63–65]. In general, an enlarging AAA is accompanied by both an increase in wall stress and a decrease in wall strength, and both these parameters are critical and need to be taken into account, as the event of AAA rupture occurs when the former exceeds the latter. For these reasons, much attention has been focused over the years on the biomechanics of AAA, particularly with regard to wall stress assessment [65]. Laplace's law has been erroneously applied, but it is not reliable for the analyses of the complexly shaped AAA [63]. Rather, more established and accurate methods such as finite element analysis (FEA) are required. Constitutive models for AAA wall and ILT continue to be developed [66]. These efforts, along with the advent of more accurate imaging techniques, will lead to improved estimates of AAA wall stress and strength distributions in vivo.

6.3 Experimental Techniques to Study Mechanical Behavior of Arteries

Biomechanical properties of excised aortas, especially from animals, have been intensively studied by many researchers over the past decades [67]. Arteries exhibit a highly nonlinear mechanical behavior, which has been investigated from different points of view. As a first approach to arterial biomechanics, the macroscopic response of the arterial wall has been characterized through different uniaxial, biaxial, and tension–inflation tests along different physiologically relevant directions. More recently, experimental set-ups coupling mechanical testing with live microscopy have been developed to decipher the microstructural mechanisms that are behind the nonlinear character of the response.

Experimental studies are necessary to study the alterations in mechanical properties caused by structural and functional changes in pathological arteries. In clinical follow-up, several noninvasive in vivo tests can be performed to control blood pressure, wall remodeling, and compliance. Where excision of samples is possible, further studies may be carried out with in vitro mechanical characterization tests. However, because of the scarcity and difficulty of recovering intact and fresh human tissues, numerous in vitro mechanical tests have been carried out on tissues derived from animal models that attempt to reproduce human pathologies. The results of these experimental tests have permitted the development of theoretical or numerical models. They have also made it possible to identify the material parameters for different types of arteries.

This section presents the main tests commonly performed in vivo during patient follow-up and in vitro on arterial samples.

6.3.1 In Vivo Noninvasive Methods

Aging and changes in arterial mechanical properties can be controlled noninvasively by measuring arterial stiffness, arterial pressure, intima-media thickness, and arterial diameter. Arterial stiffness has received particular attention in the recent years, as it can be considered a tissue biomarker that represents the alterations in the arterial wall and measures the cumulative influence of cardiovascular risk factors over time [4]. Therefore, many methods of measuring arterial stiffness have been developed, and, for some of them, epidemiological studies have demonstrated the predictive value of arterial rigidity for cardiovascular events [68]. They are mainly based on techniques of applanation tonometry, ultrasonography, and MRI.

The measurement of carotid–femoral PWV is considered the clinical reference method for determining aortic stiffness, because it is the simplest, most direct, and most validated method in epidemiology, physiology, and pharmacology. Indeed, the aorta represents the greater part of the path between the carotid and femoral arteries. It is also the first artery at the exit of the heart, and it majorly contributes to the diastolic relay of the cardiac contraction. As a mechanical parameter, PWV does not, of course, take into account the complexity of the mechanical properties of arteries, but it is simple to measure and has shown its effectiveness in the clinical follow-up of patients. Nineteen studies have shown the predictive value of carotid–femoral PWV for cardiovascular events in various populations [68]. Other anatomical sites are also of interest for the measurement of arterial stiffness, in particular the carotid artery, which is frequently a place of atheromatous plaque formation.

6.3.2 In Vitro Tissue Tests

The different techniques that were developed for characterizing the incremental elastic modulus in vivo reveal only a small part of the whole mechanical behavior of the arterial wall. The in vivo incremental elastic modulus is usually sufficient to understand the effects of the arterial compliance on the blood circulation (Windkessel effect), the PWV effect and its changes with age [69,70], and hypertension [71], for instance.

However, it is insufficient for modeling the response of the aortic wall to abnormal forces, such as those applied by a stent or an endograft [72–74], or for determining the strength of the tissue and the risks of aneurysm rupture or dissections [75,76].

More comprehensive characterizations of the arterial wall are necessary, from the stress-free state up to failure, under different combinations of uniaxial and biaxial loadings. These characterizations can be carried out only in vitro on excised specimens. More details about experimental methods will be presented in Chapter 4, but specific methods and related issues pertinent to arteries are discussed in the present chapter.

In vitro tests are performed on arterial samples taken away from their natural environment. Although some mechanical tests may approximate such conditions, they do not generally reproduce the complex in vivo loading conditions, including the influence of perivascular tissues. However, they provide access to information that cannot be obtained in vivo, such as residual stresses and the individual mechanical behavior of the different layers of the wall (intima, media, and adventitia). In addition, it is important to note that no testing standards exist for soft tissues.

6.3.2.1 Uniaxial Tensile Tests
Given the difficulty in collecting intact pathological arteries, the simplest mechanical test to be performed at the tissue scale, and one of the most commonly used, is the uniaxial tensile test. It can be carried out in the circumferential and longitudinal directions, in order to assess the anisotropy of the tissues. The uniaxial tensile test measures the force exerted on the test piece in response to the elongation imposed on it or vice versa. A dog bone sample may be cut in the excised arterial segment, with the circumferential or longitudinal direction as the main axis. The obtained

stress–strain curve may be used to assess the stiffness and other material properties of the tissue, as well as the stress and strain at rupture.

6.3.2.2 Ring Tests
Another simple mechanical test that can be performed on arterial tissues is the ring tensile test, which is particularly suited to the naturally cylindrical shape of the arteries. Two hooks are inserted into an arterial ring and then stretched, and the force exerted on the ring is measured according to its elongation. These tests, used in pharmacology, also make it possible to determine the active mechanical properties related to the contraction of SMCs in response to vasoconstricting agents [77], in the presence or absence of an "intact" endothelium.

6.3.2.3 Biaxial Tensile Tests
To characterize the anisotropic nature of the arterial tissue, it is possible to carry out biaxial traction tests. These tissue characterization tests have been applied to the study of numerous vascular pathologies [1], including HBP and AAA. Concerning the latter pathology, in general, it appears that the aneurysmal tissue is stiffer than the healthy aortic tissue but is more prone to rupture. Moreover, several studies have shown an important heterogeneity of the mechanical properties, depending on the location of the sample. As for the anisotropy of aneurysmal tissue, all studies do not agree: some have found an increased anisotropic character [78–81], while others have shown a tendency toward isotropy [82,83].

6.3.3 In Vitro Arterial Tests (Tension Inflation)

The mechanical properties determined at the scale of the tissue are not sufficient to characterize the overall behavior of arteries, which have complex structures because of their geometry and material heterogeneity. To analyze the mechanical behavior at the scale of the vascular structure, one can carry out extension–inflation tests. These tests are more similar to the loading conditions encountered in vivo and preserve the integrity of the vascular wall and its tubular structure. They typically consist of longitudinally stretching the artery until it reaches an extension close to the in vivo conditions and then pressurizing it to physiological pressure levels. Alternatively, simpler closed-end, free-extension conditions may be applied [84]. It is then possible to obtain the pressure–volume or pressure–diameter relationships, as well as the corresponding longitudinal force values. These relationships can then be used to develop models of mechanical behavior, especially in the hyperelastic case [11,13,85,86]. The tensile–inflation tests evidence a salient feature of the in vivo prestretch: for axial prestretches smaller (or larger) than the in vivo prestretch, the axial reaction force decreases (or increases) when the pressure increases. However, when the axial prestretch is equal to the in vivo prestretch, the axial reaction force does not depend on the applied inner pressure [86,87] and remains constant during pressurization. Similar results exist for isotonic tests, in which the axial force is kept constant but the axial prestretch varies with the applied pressure [11].

6.3.4 Use of Full-Field Measurements

A common limitation to most of the techniques cited previously is the assumption of uniform material properties. This is also a limitation in most of the FEAs in vascular biomechanics. This situation does not result from computational or theoretical limitations but rather from the lack of experimental quantification of actual regional variations in material properties. The existence and potential importance of nonuniform properties are supported by advances in vascular mechanobiology [30], which imply that cells should be expected to build in regional variations in material properties.

To begin to address the need for new methods of quantification of regional material properties in blood vessels having complex geometry, techniques based on digital image correlation (DIC) were introduced [88–93]. They allow for the geometric reconstruction and tracking of surface displacements and thus calculation of strains across local areas or even the entire artery, using the concept of panoramic DIC [92].

Recent progress in inverse methods has permitted to reconstruct regional distributions of material properties from these data in different situations [94,95]. Extensions using in vivo imaging with MRI are also under development [96].

6.3.5 Effect of Environmental and Preservation Conditions

6.3.5.1 Tissue Collection
In vivo arteries are subjected to residual stresses and prestretch, the amount of which depends on the organ and species under consideration. This in vivo stress–strain state originates from the growth and remodeling processes undergone by arteries and allows for achieving a homeostatic stress state that is nearly uniform and equibiaxial across the arterial wall thickness [97]. Consequently, excising and cutting open arterial segments partially release this existing in vivo stress–strain state, but there is no certainty that the load-free configuration corresponds to a stress- or strain-free configuration.

The biological nature and the physiological functions of the arterial tissue render the characterization of the mechanical properties a delicate task: harvesting the tissue implies the death of cells, with different consequences: (1) in vitro characterization investigates only the passive response of the tissue and therefore cannot account for the active role of SMCs in distributing the load across the tissue thickness, and (2) the end of constituent turnover and the progressive degradation of the organic constituents making up the tissue have consequences on the mechanical response of the tissue. In addition, harvesting the tissue implies the relaxation of some of the prestress and prestretch existing in the arterial tissue in vivo, leading to fiber rearrangements in the microstructure, with consequences on the macroscopic mechanical response.

6.3.5.2 Tissue Storage
Owing to the biological nature of arterial tissue, the storage conditions and the temperature of test may have an impact on the in vitro mechanical response of the arterial tissue.

Regarding storage procedures, the arteries are usually harvested during surgery for humans, in freshly sacrificed animals, or shortly after death. After excision, the arterial sample may be stored for 2–3 days in a saline solution at 4°C or kept frozen at −20°C or −80°C [98,99] to prevent the sample from drying up and to avoid accelerated sample degradation. The impact of these different protocols on the mechanical properties was investigated by comparing the uniaxial tensile response of specimen stemming from the same tissue sample but subjected to different preparation protocols. Regarding the temperature of test, one of the following two choices is classically made: either ambient room temperature or physiological temperature. Again, the uniaxial tensile responses relative to different temperatures of tests were compared.

Several studies [100–102] reported no significant variations in the mechanical response after storage, while, in other studies [103–105], the variations in the mechanical behavior encompassed variations in the initial and final stress–strain slopes, as well as changes in the knee point of stress–strain curves and in the ultimate stress. These variations may be explained by some damage experienced by the samples during freezing or refrigerating: formation of ice crystals and bulk water movement [103] can induce fiber cracking, loss of crosslinks, networks disruption, and cell death. These variations may also be explained by the decrease in the collagen content after 48-hour cold storage [104], as well as by the exact procedure followed to freeze the sample. Still, it seems impossible to decide on the directions of variations, since different studies have come to apparently contradictory results. However, it is generally admitted that the mechanical properties of arterial samples are better preserved by freezing than by refrigeration [104,105]. Zemánek et al. [100] studied the influence of the temperature on the mechanical response of the arterial wall and showed that samples were stiffer at ambient temperature than at in vivo temperature, since a temperature increase by 1°C resulted in a 5% stiffness decrease; this finding is in good agreement with [17].

6.3.5.3 Tissue Preconditioning

Another important feature of arterial mechanics is the existence of a transient mechanical response: during the first mechanical cycles, the mechanical response of the arterial wall exhibits an important hysteresis, whereby the loading and unloading paths do not coincide. The hysteresis is reduced after several load cycles; the stabilized mechanical response barely shows any hysteresis. Experimentalists usually get rid of this transient response by performing several preconditioning cycles. The number and amplitude of preconditioning cycles vary in the literature, owing to the absence of standards or guidelines, but the loading path and maximum load generally coincide with the last applied loading. The underlying microstructural mechanisms occurring during preconditioning have not yet been elucidated. They may be related to some viscous effects, since the transient response is also observed after a prolonged stop of the mechanical loading. Interestingly, Zemánek et al. [100] noticed that no preconditioning was necessary for equibiaxial tensile tests of arterial tissue.

6.3.5.4 Effect of Strain Rate

Another much-debated feature is the strain rate dependence of the arterial mechanical response. It is now admitted that at low strain rates, the mechanical response of arteries does not vary with the strain rate [100,106,107]. However, the viscous character of arteries is a much more complex question, since creep and relaxation phenomena should be investigated.

6.3.6 Layer Specificity

Arteries exhibit a layer-specific mechanical response, which depends on the layer morphology. Mechanical tests on the tunica intima were performed by [108,109]: the intima exhibits a stiffer mechanical response when loaded in the longitudinal direction than in the circumferential direction, which is in good agreement with the longitudinal orientation of the fibers of the internal elastic lamina [110]. However, it is generally agreed that the tunica intima barely contributes to the mechanical response of arteries. Regarding the tunica media, the circumferential direction shows a stiffer uniaxial response than the longitudinal direction, which correlates with the preferred circumferential orientation of the fiber networks in the media. By contrast, in the tunica adventitia, the uniaxial mechanical response is stiffer in the longitudinal direction than in the circumferential direction [108,109]. Finally, the larger elastin content in the media than in the adventitia makes the media more compliant, while the adventitia can bear larger loads.

6.4 Constitutive Models of Arteries

As already introduced in Section 6.1, the elastic modulus is the most commonly used mechanical parameter to describe the behavior of elastic materials. It characterizes the linear relationship between the stress (force per unit area) and the strain (ratio between the total deformation to the initial dimension) during a tensile test. If a body is isotropic, its elastic modulus is the same, whatever be the direction of tension, and it is called Young's modulus.

However, the unique microscopic composition of the arterial wall requires anisotropic and nonlinear stress–strain relationships [1,111,112] At low strains, few collagen fibers are straightened and most of them are crimped or curled. The elastic response of elastin dominates the mechanical behavior, and the wall is relatively extensible. At high strains, most of the collagen fibers are straightened and recruited to bear the stress. The mechanical properties of collagen dominate, and the wall is relatively inextensible. Authors have been able to observe the gradual recruitment of collagen fibers [113] and relate it to the stiffening behavior of arteries [111,112].

This very specific structure provides optimal behavior for expansion and contraction of the vessel wall during the cardiac cycle and limits distension of the wall when exposed to extreme pressures.

As aortic tissue is a nonlinear and anisotropic material, it is not possible to obtain a unique value of elastic modulus, as the latter is continuously varying with the different forces applied. The incremental modulus, or the tangent modulus, which is defined as the differentiation of the stress–strain relationship in the circumferential direction, has been proposed to take into consideration the variation of the elastic modulus.

It is usually admitted that within the range of strain variations between diastole and systole, the incremental modulus in the circumferential direction, further denoted by E, remains constant [96,114–116]. The range of strain variations between diastole and systole is sufficiently narrow with regard to the whole range of strain variations, which backs up the linear assumption within this physiological range.

The incremental modulus may be estimated in vivo by using simple equations. A classical approach is based on Laplace's law [62]:

$$E = \Delta p \frac{R/h}{\Delta R/R} = \frac{R/h}{DC} \qquad (6.2)$$

where R is the inner radius of the artery, h is the thickness, Δp is the pressure variation between diastole and systole, ΔR is the radius variation between diastole and systole, and DC is the distensibility. Mean ΔR greater than 10% has been observed in the thoracic aorta [111,112], and the incremental modulus is about 500 kPa.

The age effect was also investigated [69,70]: on an average, incremental moduli was 330 kPa below 35 years of age and 670 kPa above 35 years of age. Isnard et al. [71] compared the incremental moduli of the aortic arch between hypertensive and normal subjects, reporting values of 1071 ± 131 kPa versus 526 ± 0.045 kPa. To our knowledge, the local effects of perivascular tissue and of branches on the elastic properties of the aorta have never been investigated.

Several studies [103,117] have laid emphasis on the dependence of the mechanical response on the sample location along the aortic tree. The aortic stiffness was found to be higher in distal regions than in proximal regions [107,118–120], which correlated with a higher collagen content in the distal aortic regions. This property may be directly related to the difference in mechanical function between proximal and distal regions: proximal regions of the aortic tree directly receive blood from the heart and therefore need to exhibit larger damping properties, which is microstructurally conveyed by larger elastin content and more undulated collagen bundles in the proximal aorta [119].

6.4.1 Nonlinearity

The arterial wall exhibits a highly nonlinear mechanical response, which was already described in the 1880s [121]: while at low applied stresses, arteries are very easily deformed, the arterial response becomes much stiffer at higher applied stresses. This nonlinear response is mostly attributed to the interactions between collagen and elastin in the tissue. By imparting compressive stresses to the collagen [122], the presence of elastin increases the collagen folding, resulting in a more compliant response of the tissue [123], since straightened collagen fibers are much stiffer than elastin fibers. Consequently, degrading elastin leads to vessel enlargement. This results in a mechanical response being softer (i.e., more stretchable) in the lower-stress regime and stiffer in the higher-stress regime [109,124]. Elastin degradation also leads to an earlier recruitment of collagen fibers, which is conducive to the mechanical response being stiffer sooner [119,125]. Collagen degradation leads to the disappearance of the progressive stiffening of the mechanical response, while the initial slope of the stress–strain curves remains unchanged [109].

6.4.2 Hyperelasticity

Taking into account the nonlinear behavior, most continuum models of arteries are hyperelastic. In a nutshell, hyperelasticity expresses the relationship between the strain energy stored in a solid and the deformations undergone by the material. It assumes that the stress depends only on the current strain state and not on the path between initial and final strain states. Although soft tissues typically do not satisfy such assumption, Fung introduced the concept of pseudohyperelasticity, which has rendered hyperelastic models very popular in biomechanics [17]. Functional forms of strain energy density are numerous [23]. Let us introduce the basic mathematical concepts needed to define strain energy density functions.

6.4.2.1 Theory of Finite Deformations

Deformations are mathematically described as functions that map the material particle position vector X (in the reference configuration at a given time t) to the material particle position vector x in the current configuration:

$$x = \phi(X, t) \tag{6.3}$$

$$X = \phi^{-1}(x, t) \tag{6.4}$$

The displacement vector is defined as: $U(X, t) = x - X = \phi(X, t) - X$.

The velocity vector is defined by taking time derivatives of the mapping, as follows:

$$\dot{U}(X, t) = \left[\frac{\partial \phi(X, t)}{\partial t} \right]_X \tag{6.5}$$

It can also be expressed in terms of the spatial description by inserting the inverse mapping:

$$v(x, t) = \dot{U}\left(\phi^{-1}(x, t), t\right) \tag{6.6}$$

The deformation gradient for the transformation is:

$$F(X, t) = \frac{\partial \phi(X, t)}{\partial x} \tag{6.7}$$

The right Cauchy–Green stretch tensor is:

$$C = F^T F \tag{6.8}$$

The left Cauchy–Green stretch tensor is:

$$B = FF^T \tag{6.9}$$

The Green–Lagrange strain tensor is:

$$E = \frac{1}{2}(C - 1) \tag{6.10}$$

where 1 is the identity tensor.

6.4.2.2 Stress Tensors

The first stress tensor that must be introduced is the Cauchy stress tensor σ. It describes the stress state in the deformed body and is defined in the spatial configuration. The traction vector obtained from the application of the surface normal n is called the Cauchy traction vector:

$$t = \sigma.n \tag{6.11}$$

Since it describes the actual stress in the body, the Cauchy stress is called the true stress in engineering.

It is convenient to define the second Piola–Kirchhoff stress tensor S, such as:

$$S = JF^{-1}.\sigma.F^{-T} \tag{6.12}$$

where $J = \det(F)$. The second Piola–Kirchhoff stress tensor is defined in the reference configuration and is the work conjugate of the Green–Lagrange strain tensor E. It also has the attractive property that, like the Cauchy stress tensor, it is symmetric for nonpolar materials.

6.4.2.3 Constitutive Equations

In hyperelasticity, the existence of a strain energy density function W is assumed, from which a constitutive relationship between stress and strain is derived. The total energy that is needed to deform the body is dependent only on the initial and end states and not on the loading path. The strain energy density function can be expressed as a function of the Cauchy–Green right tensor: $W(C)$.

The stress–strain relationship is written as:

$$\sigma = 2J^{-1}F.\frac{\partial W}{\partial C}.F^T \tag{6.13}$$

For isotropic models, W depends only on the first three invariants of C:

$$I_1 = tr(C) \tag{6.14}$$

$$I_2 = \frac{1}{2}\left[\left(tr(C) \right)^2 - tr\left(C^2 \right) \right]$$ (6.15)

$$I_3 = det(C)$$ (6.16)

For an incompressible material, the strain energy density function does not depend on I_3. In this case, the stress is derived according to:

$$\sigma = -p\mathbf{1} + 2\mathbf{F} \cdot \frac{\partial W}{\partial C} \cdot \mathbf{F}^T$$ (6.17)

where p is a Lagrange multiplier enforcing the incompressibility constraint. In problems that can be solved analytically, p is determined using boundary conditions. In numerical implementations, such as using the finite element method, p is a numerically large factor that also enforces the incompressibility constraint but through a penalty method.

Numerous energy functions have been used to describe the mechanical behavior of arteries. For a detailed review, the reader can refer to the book by Humphrey [1]. Despite the large amount of data showing that healthy and aneurysmal arteries are anisotropic [81], many studies still use isotropic mechanical behavior relationships, particularly in numerical finite element models.

Among all the strain energy density functions proposed for arteries, we will distinguish those that have been established through a phenomenological approach, based on experimental data, and those motivated by the arterial microstructure.

The most common strain energy density functions for arteries are described in the following subsections.

6.4.2.3.1 Demiray

$$W = \frac{\beta}{2\alpha}\left(e^{\alpha(I_1 - 3)} - 1 \right)$$ (6.18)

where α and β are material constants.

The Demiray strain energy function can sometimes be completed with a neo-Hookean term:

$$W = \mu_1 \left(I_1 - 3 \right) + \frac{\beta}{2\alpha}\left(e^{\alpha(I_1 - 3)} - 1 \right)$$ (6.19)

6.4.2.3.2 Yeoh

$$W = \sum_n c_n \left(I_1 - 3 \right)^n$$ (6.20)

where c_n are material constants.

6.4.2.3.3 Fung

$$W = \frac{c}{2}\left(e^{c_1 E_{\theta\theta}^2 + c_2 E_{LL}^2 + 2 c_3 E_{\theta\theta} E_{LL}} - 1\right)$$

(6.21)

where c, c_1, c_2, and c_3 are material constants.

6.4.2.3.4 Holzapfel

$$W = \frac{c}{2}(I_1 - 3) + \frac{k_1}{2k_2}\sum_{i=4,6}\left(e^{k_2(I_i - 1)^2} - 1\right)$$

(6.22)

where c, k_1, and k_2 are material constants; $I_4 = M_1.(C.M_1)$; and $I_6 = M_2.(C.M_2)$.
M_1 and M_2 are unit vectors characterizing two preferred directions of fibers in the reference configuration.

This strain energy function models a composite material made of a matrix reinforced with fibers. The parameters c and k_1 are the effective stiffnesses of a matrix and fiber phases, respectively, both having dimensions of force per unit length. The k_2 parameter is a nondimensional parameter that governs the tissue's strain-stiffening response.

6.4.2.3.5 Gasser with Dispersion

$$W = \frac{c}{2}(I_1 - 3) + \frac{k_1}{2k_2}\sum_{i=4,6}\left(e^{k_2\left[\kappa(I_1 - 3) + (1 - 3\kappa)(I_i - 1)^2\right]} - 1\right)$$

(6.23)

where c, k_1, and k_2 are material constants and $\kappa = \int_0^\pi \rho(\theta)\sin^3(\theta)d\theta$.

When $\kappa = 0$, the equation models a composite with all the fibers perfectly aligned in the direction M_1 or M_2, while when $\kappa = 1/3$, the fibers would have no preferential direction (isotropic).

6.4.2.3.6 Humphrey with Four Families of Fibers

$$W = \frac{c}{2}(I_1 - 3) + \sum_{i\in[1,4]}\frac{c_i}{2k_i}\left(e^{k_i(I_i - 1)^2} - 1\right)$$

(6.24)

where c, c_i, and k_i are material constants and $I_i = M_i.(C.M_i)$. M_i is a unit vector characterizing the preferred direction of fibers in the reference configuration. The four preferred directions are the circumferential direction, the axial direction, and two symmetric diagonal directions defined by the angle to the circumferential direction $\mp\theta$.

Except Fung's model, all these models are written in their incompressible versions. They may also be used in compressible versions in which it is common to additively split the strain energy function into a term depending only on the change of volume and another term independent of volume changes [23]. In this case, we introduce

$$\bar{F} = \frac{1}{J^{1/3}} F \qquad (6.25)$$

And then derive $\bar{C}$, $\bar{E}$, and the normalized invariants as well. However, there are known issues with slightly compressible anisotropic formulations when using this approach [126,127].

6.4.2.4 Multilayer Models (Including Residual Stresses)

Most constitutive relations and stress analyses have employed an informal homogenization procedure and treated the wall as a single layer. Such an approach has enabled significant advances, including the discovery of important implications of residual stresses and the development of growth and remodeling models that capture salient aspects of arterial adaptation. Nevertheless, stress analyses that account for the different layers of the arterial wall, notably the media and adventitia in all vessels and also the intima in aging and particular diseases, can provide additional information that is essential, depending on the question of interest. Indeed, given the recent recognition of the differential mechanobiological roles of medial SMCs and adventitial fibroblasts [128], there is a pressing need to better understand the layer-specific differences in the local mechanical environments experienced by these different types of cells.

Several investigators have used a two-layer model (the two layers being the media and the adventitia layers) with Holzapfel's model [23]. Recently, Bellini et al. [129] presented a new approach for modeling layer-specific arterial wall mechanics that was motivated by recent growth and remodeling simulations and based on histologically and clinically measurable data. In particular, in contrast to classical approaches that employed either an intact or a radially cut traction-free configuration as a reference, they used the in vivo homeostatic state as a biologically and clinically relevant reference configuration and built a new bilayered model of the arterial wall. Moreover, they endowed the primary structurally significant constituents—elastic fibers, smooth muscle, and fibrillar collagen—with individual "deposition stretches," which ensured that the in vivo reference configuration was defined by homeostatic stresses. Embracing the material nonuniformity of the wall clearly distinguished between a requisite, computationally convenient reference configuration for the artery and the actual stress-free (i.e., natural) configurations for the individual constituents. This "constrained mixture" approach allowed one to naturally account for tensile stresses in all constituents at physiological and supraphysiological pressures, as well as for the most compressive stresses that necessarily emerge in some constituents at subphysiological pressures. The separate prescription of material properties in the media and adventitia was based primarily on histologic information on individual mass fractions and orientations of constituents. In addition to achieving fits to in vitro biaxial mechanical data that were comparable to prior reports that use classical homogenized models, Bellini's model also allowed one to predict associated traction-free configurations, which can serve as independent validations. Therefore, one advantage of this approach is that it does not require one to prescribe residual stress-related opening angles, which cannot be measured in vivo and cannot be prescribed easily whenever the geometry is not cylindrical. Rather, one merely needs to prescribe point-wise deposition stretches within an assumed homeostatic state, regardless of the overall geometry of the wall. A 3D finite element implementation of this model was recently published [130].

6.4.3 Multiscale Modeling

Although most of the models discussed previously were motivated by the structure of the arterial wall, many are phenomenological in the sense that material parameters have to be calibrated using experimental tests.

True multiscale modeling would consist of entering the mechanical properties of each microconstituent of the arterial wall in a model and deduce the macroscopic properties by using homogenization approaches.

The arterial wall owes its main mechanical characteristics, such as the progressive stiffening and anisotropy, to collagen fibers and their orientations. In most of the available constitutive models, fiber families are characterized by their orientation angles, while their progressive stiffening is modeled through exponential functions of the stretch. The selection of a constitutive behavior implies the choice of a number of collagen fiber families. The determination of their orientations can be done in two ways: either by histologic examination of the tissue [131] or by inverse method, searching for the orientation angles that best fit the macroscopic behavior of the tissue.

Modeling the progressive recruitment of collagen fibers is another important question that needs to be addressed. In the (ex vivo) load-free configuration, microscopic observations evidence crimped fibers with different orientations that the mechanical loading tends to stretch and reorient along the principal strain directions. At high stretches, the collagen fibers are perfectly straight and parallel to each other. However, the physiological load lies between these two extreme situations and poses the question of the collagen fiber engagement under physiological conditions. Different experimental studies have shown that only partial engagement of the collagen fibers is reached at physiological pressure: only 5%–10% of the fibers actively participate in the mechanical behavior of vascular tissues at these pressures. This progressive recruitment is the physical origin of the nonlinear character and progressive stiffening of the response of vascular tissues; it is generally implicitly accounted for by the introduction of exponential functions in the constitutive models (see Section 6.4.3), but in some specific models, a probability distribution function for the engagement strain of the fibers has been introduced [113].

6.4.4 Mechanobiology

Many experiments have shown that the stress field dictates, at least in part, the way in which the microstructure of arteries is organized. This observation led to the concept of functional adaptation, wherein it is thought that arteries functionally adapt to maintain particular mechanical metrics (e.g., stress) near target values. To accomplish this, tissues often develop regionally varying stiffness, strength, and anisotropy. Models of growth and remodeling necessarily involve reaction–diffusion equations. There has been a trend to embed the reaction–diffusion framework within tissue mechanics [3,4]. The primary assumption is that one models volumetric growth through a growth tensor F_g, which describes changes between two fictitious stress-free configurations: the original body is imagined to be fictitiously cut into small stress-free pieces, each of which is allowed to grow separately via F_g, with $det(F_g) = 1$. Because these growths need not be compatible, internal forces are often needed to assemble the grown pieces, via F_a, into a continuous configuration. This, in general, produces residual stresses, which are now known to exist in many soft tissues. The formulation is completed by considering elastic deformations, via F_a, from the intact but residually stressed traction-free configuration to a current configuration that is induced by external mechanical loads.

The initial boundary value problem is solved by introducing a constitutive relation for the stress response to the deformation $F_e F_a$, which is often assumed to be incompressible hyperelastic, as well as a relation for the evolution of the stress-free configuration via F_g. Thus, growth is assumed to occur in stress-free configurations and typically not affect material properties. Although such theory, called the theory of kinematic growth, yields many reasonable predictions, Humphrey and coworkers have suggested that it models consequences of growth and remodeling rather than the processes by which they occur. Growth and remodeling necessarily occur in stressed, nonfictitious stress-free configurations, and they occur via the production, removal, and organization of different constituents; moreover, growth and remodeling need not restore stresses exactly to homeostatic values.

Therefore, Humphrey and coworkers introduced a conceptually different approach to model growth and remodeling, one that is based on tracking the turnover of individual constituents in stressed configurations (the constrained mixture model [6,7]). Recently, Cyron et al. [132] worked on a unified theory between kinematic growth and constrained mixture theory.

6.4.5 Identification of Constitutive Properties

To identify the material parameters corresponding to a given type of artery, the data from the experimental tests must be compared with the chosen mechanical behavior model by solving an *inverse problem*. In the case of conventional uniaxial or biaxial tests at the tissue scale, the experimental data can be translated directly into terms of stress–strain relationships. Therefore, it is sufficient to optimize the parameters of the constitutive model by suing the experimental stress–strain curves and minimizing the difference between the experimental stress and the stress computed by the model at the different deformation levels. Numerical nonlinear fitting methods, such as the least squares method, are used for this purpose.

In the case of more complex tests, two possibilities may arise: if simplifying hypotheses can be made to establish analytical equations of the mechanical problem, then these equations may be solved numerically (by optimization, as before). This is the case, for example, of the inflation–extension test [23]. The same approach can also be used in the case of pressure–diameter data obtained in vivo [133,134]. If the geometry or loading is too complex to express the analytical equations of the mechanical problem, then a finite element model, coupled with an inverse method, may be used. Interestingly, a new approach for the biaxial characterization of in vitro human arteries was recently proposed [88]. It permits the identification of the material constants in Holzapfel's model or Humphrey's model, even with heterogeneous strain and stress distributions in arterial segments. From the full-field experimental data obtained from inflation–extension tests, an inverse approach, called the virtual fields method (VFM), can be used for deriving the material parameters of the tested arterial segment. The results obtained for human thoracic aortas are promising [90,140]. More details about this method can be found in [94] and [135].

6.5 Mechanics of the Ascending Thoracic Aorta

The human ascending thoracic aorta and thoracic arch are segments of an elastic artery, whose mechanical properties play a crucial role in damping the pressure wave that occurs within the vessel and in channeling the blood flow coming from the heart (Figure 6.4).

The main pathologies affecting the ascending thoracic aorta are dissections and aneurysms (dilatations). Ascending thoracic aorta aneurysms (ATAAs) represent

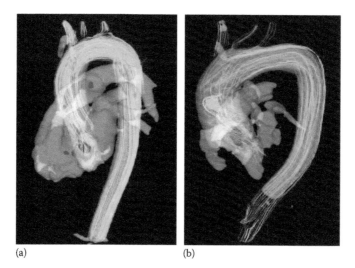

(a)   (b)

Figure 6.4 Comparison of blood flows for heathy ascending thoracic aorta and ATAA. (a) Laminar flow in a healthy young patient. (b) Disturbed hemodynamics in a patient suffering from both ATAA and aortic insufficiency.

one-tenth of aortic aneurysms, but the surgical repair of ascending thoracic aortic pathologies, especially ATAA, and type A dissections is very complex. Conversely to AAA, of which 50%–75% (depending on countries) are now treated by endovascular repair (EVAR) interventions, ATAAs are commonly treated by conventional surgery, with open chest, requiring heart–lung machine. Note that, as treated by conventional surgery, ATAA is a large source of excised tissue, providing many biomechanical samples.

The mechanics of the ascending thoracic aorta is special, not only because of its crucial role in hemodynamics but also because it has to bear the motions of the heart, which constitute a permanent cyclic loading that is found in no other artery [136]. When compared with AAA, the literature on computational biomechanics of aortic dissections is scarce. The few reports that are available highlight the potential of computational modeling, but they also reveal many shortcomings [137]. For all these reasons, we decided to dedicate a specific section to the mechanics of the ascending thoracic aorta and ATAA.

6.5.1 Fracture Mechanics of Ascending Thoracic Aorta Aneurysm

Tensile strengths of the thoracic aorta in the axial and circumferential directions were previously reported in the literature [90,101,138–147]. Mohan and Melvin [148] reported an average ultimate stress of 1.14 MPa in quasistatic biaxial tension and an average ultimate stress of 1.96 MPa in dynamic ($20\ \mathrm{s^{-1}}$) biaxial tension. McLean et al. [146] identified the strength in the radial direction, but this was based on porcine data (0.06 MPa). Sommer et al. [147] showed that porcine tissues may be significantly different from human tissues. Strength was also identified using inflation tests on intact segments [149], yielding an average strength of 2.5 MPa.

Compared with the normal tissue, aneurysmal specimens displayed lower wall thickness and failure strain and higher maximum elastic modulus (MEM) than control specimens but equal failure stress in the majority of regions and directions [144]. The formation of ATAA was associated with stiffening and weakening of the aortic wall [139].

More recently, the anisotropy of the aortic wall was demonstrated by significantly different results for MEM between the circumferential and longitudinal orientations [143]. Interestingly, the aorta is longitudinally stiffer in the greater curvature than in the lower curvature, which can correlate to the physiological movement of the arch [150]. Marked heterogeneity was evident in healthy and aneurysmal aortas (variations between anterior, posterior, and lateral) [141].

Uniaxial tests do not reveal the whole mechanical behavior of the arterial walls, as there exists coupling effects between the axial and circumferential stresses. Biaxial tests have to be carried out for a complete characterization [148]. An interesting procedure for characterizing the biaxial properties of the aorta is the bulge inflation test, combined with DIC, to measure the local strain and stress fields across the specimen and to derive the local constitutive parameters by using an inverse approach [90]. It does not reveal any significant imbalance between the circumferential and axial directions in terms of response, which tends to show that the aneurysm does not present a marked anisotropy in terms of elastic response. This suggests that wall degeneration has led to a more random distribution of the collagen fibers.

Biomechanical studies have also achieved better insight in ATAA rupture or dissection [139,151,152,170–176] and attempted to elucidate the risk profile of the thoracic aorta [13,153]. Recently, our group developed an approach to identify the patient-specific material properties of ATAAs by minimization of the difference between model predictions and gated CT images [114]. Moreover, we characterized the mechanical properties of ATAA on samples collected from patients undergoing surgical repair. We also defined a rupture risk based on the brittleness of the tissue (the rupture criterion is reached when the stretch applied to the tissue is greater than its maximum extensibility or distensibility) and showed a strong correlation between this rupture risk criterion and the physiological elastic modulus of ATAAs estimated from a bulge inflation test [15]. A failure criterion based on in vitro ultimate stretch showed a significant correlation with the aortic membrane stiffness deduced from in vivo distensibility.

The strength of the aortic tissue is generally defined as the maximum stress that the tissue can withstand before failing. However, when the maximum stress ratio between the stress applied to the tissue in vivo and its strength was derived, it was noted that most of the collected ATAA samples were far from rupture. Alternatively, one can define rupture when the stretch applied to the tissue exceeds its maximum extensibility or distensibility. This definition of rupture may be even more physiologically meaningful, as it is reported that aneurysm ruptures or dissections often occur at a time of severe emotional stress or physical exertion [154]. Such situations can induce significant changes in blood volumes in the aorta, making less compliant aneurysms more prone to rupture, as they cannot sustain such volume changes. Based on this analysis, Martin et al. defined a similar criterion, named the diameter risk, which is the ratio between the current diameter of the aneurysm and the rupture diameter [154]. They showed that the diameter risk increased significantly with the physiological elastic modulus of the artery. Indeed, if the aortic wall is stiff, a rather large increase of pressure can be induced by a small increase in blood volume.

One explanation for this phenomenon may be the mechanism of collagen recruitment described by Hill et al. [113]. As collagen recruitment increases with the load, the tangent stiffness of the tissue also increases. Collagen recruitment can be expected to be delayed in the tissue when it still contains a significant fraction of intact elastin. At physiological pressures, when elastin is not fragmented, only a small fraction of collagen contributes to the aortic stiffness, which is relatively small (<1 MPa). Conversely, when elastic lamellae and elastic fibers are highly disrupted, collagen can be expected to be recruited earlier and contribute significantly to the stiffness at physiological pressures, thereby increasing the stiffness (>1 MPa).

This mechanism of higher recruitment of collagen at physiological pressures is in line with the findings of Iliopoulos et al. [114], who showed that the fraction of elastin, but not collagen, decreased in ATAA specimens, displaying lower wall thickness and failure strain and higher peak elastic modulus than control specimens but equal failure stress. Moreover, it is commonly admitted that the elastin fraction decreases with age.

The level of collagen recruitment may be related to the stretch-based rupture criterion, but not the stress-based rupture criterion. Indeed, some specimens showed a relatively large extensibility but ruptured at a relatively small stress. When collagen is recruited, it can withstand stresses until damage initiates, with ruptures at the fiber level, as demonstrated by Weisbecker et al. [109,155]. A dense and crosslinked network of collagen will permit to reach larger stresses before the initiation of damage and eventually ultimate stress.

6.5.2 Fluid Mechanics in Ascending Thoracic Aorta Aneurysm

Perturbed hemodynamics has frequently been reported in ATAA [156–158]. It is a consequence of the altered aortic arch configuration (for instance, shift from type I to type II, as introduced in Figure 6.5), but it is often associated with aortic valve phenotype, which is believed to play a key role in the development and growth of clinically significant aortic dilatations. The bicuspid aortic valve (BAV) lesions are reported to considerably change the distribution and magnitude of the wall shear stress (WSS) along the ATAA. Moreover, recent studies have shown that even in the absence of ATAA, the aortic annulus and root dimensions are significantly larger in patients with BAV aortic insufficiency (AI) than in patients with BAV stenosis [159].

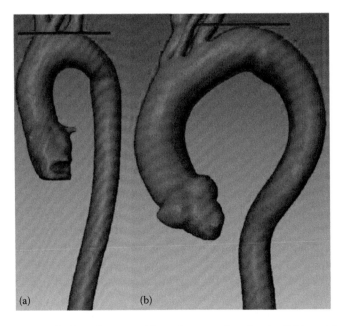

Figure 6.5 Aortic arch classification: (a) in the type I arch, the LSA originates from the top of the (outer) curvature. (b) In the type II arch, the LSA originates from below the outer curvature. (From Nathan, D. P. et al., *Ann. Thorac. Surg.*, 91, 458–463, 2011.)

Our group recently examined the hemodynamics in ATAA with concomitant AI by combining four-dimensional (4D) MRI analyses and computational fluid dynamics (CFD) studies [160]. The objectives of this research were to observe the effect of secondary flow on the ATAA hemodynamics and to understand how the degree of AI may be indicative of possible rupture risk. From the 3D streamlines, flow eccentricity was observed in patients affected by BAV and AI. During systole, flow helicity induced flow impingement against the aneurysmal wall, generating a nonhomeostatic distribution of the WSS, which was found to be higher and more extended than the WSS distribution in TAV (tricuspid aortic valve) patients. This helicity grew during the blood flow deceleration and diastolic phase due to the blood flow regurgitation, resulting in local WSS peaks. The highest time-averaged wall shear stress (TAWSS) was found in these areas. From the velocity field results, recirculation and vortices were found in the ATAA region in TAV patients affected by AI. The jet flow impingement against the aortic wall was found in the region around the bulge, downstream of the area of maximum dilatation. The maximum TAWSS was found in the same region. One patient showed no region of jet flow impingement but developed a bulge on the inner curvature side of the aorta. In summary, the existence of jet flow impingement and the TAWSS magnitude at its location were mostly associated with the orientation of the inlet. This orientation was quantified as the angle between the plane of the inlet cross-section and the transverse plane of the thorax. An angle of about 25 degrees exists in healthy subjects. The angle can go up to 70 degrees in patients who have the largest TAWSS. The angle change comes from the change in aorta morphology during ATAA development. Patients with ATAA commonly have a larger curvature, which may result from a larger increase of the aorta length on the outer curvature side than on the inner curvature side. Different structural properties on the inner and outer curvature sides have already been reported, and these may be associated with the contact between the pulmonary artery and the aorta on the inner curvature side. It should be noted that the ATAA development is associated with a decrease of the aorta axial stretch in mice models of the Marfan syndrome, which results from elastin fragmentation and faster collagen turnover. These effects (elastin loss and axial stretch decrease) are expected to be more pronounced in the areas exposed to larger hemodynamic loading, which would be more favorable to fatigue damage of elastin and aorta remodeling. Moreover, this remodeling (i.e., aorta diameter increase, arch length increase, and aortic unfolding) may lead to functional aortic alterations such as decreased aortic distensibility and increased aortic arch PWV.

It also appeared from our study that no simple relationship exists between wall strength and WSS. Large TAWSS values in the bulging region of aneurysms may even be associated with relatively large strength. In addition, large strength difference between TAV and BAV patients is associated with relatively small peak of WSS and minor TAWSS variations. Actually, if it can be showed that aortic wall remodeling and subsequent morphological changes have an important effect on WSS, the reciprocal is less obvious, as it is still unclear that whether or not WSS-mediated mechanics affect remodeling in the ascending thoracic aorta. Generally, maintenance of arterial caliber in response to increased blood pressure (to restore WSS to normal) tends to involve vessel-level changes in vasoactivity, which is greater in muscular arteries than in elastic arteries. There is still little information on possible basal tone in the human aorta.

Some authors have shown the effect of the type of aortic valve on blood flow in the ascending thoracic aorta [161]. Patient-specific computational fluid dynamics has revealed high WSS and low oscillatory shear index in the greater curvature of BAV aortas, with highly eccentric and helical flow. In patients with aortic valve disease and aortic aneurysm, morbidity or mortality can occur before size criteria for intervention are met. Patient-specific CFD provides noninvasive functional and hemodynamic assessment of the thoracic aorta. With validation, it may enable the development of an individualized approach to diagnosis and management of aortic disease, beyond traditional guidelines.

6.5.3 Mechanics of Dissections

The failure properties of greatest interest to the thoracic aorta are the dissection properties [151,162,163]. From the mechanical point of view, tear and dissection appear if the stresses acting on the wall rise above the ultimate value for the aorta wall tissue [29,151,164]. Pasta et al. [151] performed delamination tests on thoracic aorta tissue samples excised from patients undergoing ATAA repair. They manually created an initial delamination plane (i.e., an intimal tear) and showed a difference in the dissection strength between the circumferential and longitudinal directions. In addition, they effectively measured the separation forces. Some authors also characterized the dissection energy [149]. Reported values, for an abdominal aorta, are less than 10 mJ/cm.

Yet, no direct in vivo measurement of stresses or strength is feasible. Stresses in the aorta wall are due to the concomitant influences of many factors, including the shape of the aorta, the characteristics of the wall material, and the interaction between the fluid and solid domains. Mechanical stress plays a crucial role in the function of the cardiovascular system; therefore, stress analysis is a useful tool for understanding vascular pathophysiology [84].

One of the earlier studies [162], using an idealized geometry, suggested that the longitudinal stress in the wall could be a key cause of circumferentially orientated tears, which have been reported to be the more common orientation.

Nathan et al. [165] used FEA to demonstrate increased wall stress in the human thoracic aorta above the sinotubular junction (STJ) and distal to the left subclavian artery (LSA), where the intimal tears that result in types A and B aortic dissections typically occur. The wall stress above the STJ was greater than that distal to the LSA, consistent with type A dissections being more common than type B dissections. Their findings suggest that localized maxima in peak pressure load-induced wall stresses above the STJ and distal to the LSA ostium may account for the development of types A and B aortic dissections, respectively, which commonly occur at these locations.

They also assessed the possible effects of aortic arch configuration on wall stress in the aortic arch. The patients were classified by location of the LSA with respect to the plane parallel to the outer (greater) curvature of the aortic arch (Figure 6.5).

In the first group (type I aortic arch), the LSA arose from the top, or outer curvature, of the aortic arch. In the second group (type II aortic arch), the LSA arose below the outer (greater) curvature of the aortic arch. This aortic arch classification was based on age-related changes in arch configuration: older patients more often have type II arches [70]. However, the aortic arch configuration had no effect on the distribution of predicted wall stress in the normal human thoracic aorta.

Because mechanical stress in the aortic wall is proportional to blood pressure and vessel diameter, hypertension and aortic dilation are known risk factors for dissections. Wall abnormalities may also promote dissections, but similar alterations have been reported in normal aging, and alone, they may not cause dissections. Interestingly, these factors fail to explain the transverse orientation and the common proximal location of the tear. This is important because aortic dissection will be prevented only when its underlying causes are better identified. Beller et al. [166] proposed that aortic root motion may be an additional risk factor for aortic dissection, determining both the tear location and orientation by increasing the wall stress in a specific manner. Several studies applying cinematography and contrast injections have visualized aortic root motion, wherein the root is displaced downward during systole and returns to its previous position in diastole [167]. Cine–MRI studies in healthy subjects revealed an axial downward motion of 8.9 mm [168] and a clockwise axial twist of 6 degrees during systole [169]. The force driving the aortic annulus motion is the ventricular traction accompanying every heartbeat. This force is transmitted to the aortic root, the ascending aorta, the transverse aortic arch, and the supra-aortic vessels. Thus, the aortic root motion has a direct influence on the deformation of the aorta and on the mechanical stress exerted on the aortic wall.

6.6 Conclusion

This chapter focusing on arterial and aortic mechanics reveals that intense research has been carried out on the measurement of mechanical properties and on how they can be used in computational models to predict the biomechanical response of arteries and the aorta in many different conditions.

However, several aspects need to be improved before computational models can be reliably used in clinical situations for diagnosis purpose or surgical planning. Such aspects include the boundary conditions and the material properties that have to be obtained in a patient-specific manner. These parameters are difficult to obtain in real clinical situations and have been approximated to a large extent in the literature. The rapid development of 4D MRI [160] may permit important progress in these regards in the near future.

The combination of CFD and structural FEAs has led to a better understanding of flow pressure distribution, wall shear stress quantification, and the effect of material properties and geometrical parameters. Computational methods have made patient-specific analyses possible, a feature that is essential to deciphering the special biomechanical conditions at play in a particular ATAA patient. Each patient has his/her own unique anatomy and pathophysiology that affect material properties and boundary conditions, which, in turn, can significantly influence their clinical management.

Unfortunately, CFD/FE methods, while potentially providing crucial information about the pathophysiological mechanics of an aneurysm, can be very time-consuming methods to undertake. This is made worse by the fact that fluid–structure interaction (FSI) approaches are computationally expensive and complex methods for routine use in real-life clinical situations. Therefore, a much simpler interface needs to be developed, wherein the vascular clinician is in a position to assess the prognosis of the patient, evaluate the rupture risk of the aneurysm, and proceed to surgical planning, either with endovascular or conservative treatments, but always in a customized fashion.

Finally, the most important challenge in aortic mechanics is to appropriately characterize and model the structural alterations of arteries. For instance, the growth rate of an ATAA, used as a criterion to justify surgical intervention, is calculated from maximum diameter measurements at two subsequent time points; however, this measure cannot reflect the complex changes in vessel wall morphology and local areas of weakening that underline the strong regional heterogeneity of ATAA. Indeed, ATAA disease is characterized by a strong regional heterogeneity within the thoracic segments in terms of biomechanical properties, atherosclerotic distribution, proteolytic activity, and cell signaling pathways. The current intense research efforts in mechanobiology will hopefully lead to major breakthroughs in this area in the coming years.

References

1. Humphrey, J. D. (2013). *Cardiovascular Solid Mechanics: Cells, Tissues, and Organs.* Springer Science & Business Media, New York.
2. Tedgui, A., Levy, B., and Puytorac, P. D. (1995). Biologie de la paroi arterielle. Aspects normaux et pathologiques. *Annee Biologique*, 34(3), 174–174.
3. Boutouyrie, P., Bussy, C., Lacolley, P., Girerd, X., Laloux, B., and Laurent, S. (1999). Association between local pulse pressure, mean blood pressure, and large-artery remodeling. *Circulation*, 100(13), 1387–1393.
4. Laurent, S., Cockcroft, J., Van Bortel, L., Boutouyrie, P., Giannattasio, C., Hayoz, D., Hayoz, D. et al. (2006). Expert consensus document on arterial stiffness: Methodological issues and clinical applications. *European Heart Journal*, 27(21), 2588–2605.
5. Kum, F., and Karalliedde, J. (2010). Critical appraisal of the differential effects of antihypertensive agents on arterial stiffness. *Integrated Blood Pressure Control*, 3, 63.
6. Roach, M. R., and Burton, A. C. (1957). The reason for the shape of the distensibility curves of arteries. *Canadian Journal of Biochemistry and Physiology*, 35(8), 681–690.
7. Patel, D. J., and Vaishnav, R. N. (1980). *Basic Hemodynamics and Its Role in Disease Processes*. Baltimore, MD: University Park Press.
8. Carew, T. E., Vaishnav, R. N., and Patel, D. J. (1968). Compressibility of the arterial wall. *Circulation Research*, 23(1), 61–68.
9. Tardy, Y., and Meister, J. J. (1993). Noninvasive characterization of the mechanical properties of arteries. *Annals of Biomedical Engineering*, 21(3), 307–308.

10. Patel, D. J., Fry, D. L., and Janicki, J. S. (1966). Longitudinal tethering of arteries in dogs. *Circulation Research*, 19(6), 1011–1021.

11. Cox, R. H. (1975). Anisotropic properties of the canine carotid artery in-vitro. *Journal of Biomechanics*, 8(5), 293–300.

12. Dobrin, P. B., and Doyle, J. M. (1970). Vascular smooth muscle and the anisotropy of dog carotid artery. *Circulation Research*, 27(1), 105–119.

13. Dobrin, P. B. (1986). Biaxial anisotropy of dog carotid artery: Estimation of circumferential elastic modulus. *Journal of Biomechanics*, 19(5), 351–358.

14. Vaishnav, R. N., Young, J. T., Janicki, J. S., and Patel, D. J. (1972). Nonlinear anisotropic elastic properties of the canine aorta. *Biophysical Journal*, 12(8), 1008–1027.

15. Matsumoto, T., Hayashi, K., and Ide, K. (1995). Residual strain and local strain distributions in the rabbit atherosclerotic aorta. *Journal of Biomechanics*, 28(10), 1207–1217.

16. Vaishnav, R. N., and Vossoughi, J. (1987). Residual stress and strain in aortic segments. *Journal of Biomechanics*, 20(3), 235–239.

17. Fung, Y. C. (2013). *Biomechanics: Mechanical Properties of Living Tissues*. Springer Science & Business Media, New York.

18. Fung, Y. C., and Liu, S. Q. (1989). Change of residual strains in arteries due to hypertrophy caused by aortic constriction. *Circulation Research*, 65(5), 1340–1349.

19. Chuong, C. J., and Fung, Y. C. (1986). Residual stress in arteries. In *Frontiers in Biomechanics* (pp. 117–129). New York: Springer.

20. Chaudhry, H. R., Bukiet, B., Davis, A., Ritter, A. B., and Findley, T. (1997). Residual stresses in oscillating thoracic arteries reduce circumferential stresses and stress gradients. *Journal of Biomechanics*, 30(1), 57–62.

21. Delfino, A., Stergiopulos, N., Moore, J. E., and Meister, J. J. (1997). Residual strain effects on the stress field in a thick wall finite element model of the human carotid bifurcation. *Journal of Biomechanics*, 30(8), 777–786.

22. Humphrey, J. D., and Na, S. (2002). Elastodynamics and arterial wall stress. *Annals of Biomedical Engineering*, 30(4), 509–523.

23. Holzapfel, G. A., Gasser, T. C., and Ogden, R. W. (2000). A new constitutive framework for arterial wall mechanics and comparative study of material models. *Journal of Elasticity*, 61, 1–48.

24. Labrosse, M. R., Gerson, E. R., Veinot, J. P., and Beller, C. J. (2013). Mechanical characterization of human aortas from pressurization testing and a paradigm shift for circumferential residual stress. *Journal of the Mechanical Behavior of Biomedical Materials*, 17, 44–55.

25. Rachev, A., Kane, T. P. C., and Meister, J. J. (1997). Experimental investigation of the distribution of residual strains in the artery wall. *Journal of Biomechanical Engineering*, 119(4), 438–444.

26. Holzapfel, G. A., and Ogden, R. W. (2009). Modelling the layer-specific three-dimensional residual stresses in arteries, with an application to the human aorta. *Journal of the Royal Society Interface*, 7(46), 787–799.

27. Han, H. C., and Fung, Y. C. (1995). Longitudinal strain of canine and porcine aortas. *Journal of Biomechanics*, 28(5), 637–641.

28. Van Loon, P. (1976). Length-force and volume-pressure relationships of arteries. *Biorheology*, 14(4), 181–201.

29. Humphrey, J. D., Eberth, J. F., Dye, W. W., and Gleason, R. L. (2009). Fundamental role of axial stress in compensatory adaptations by arteries. *Journal of Biomechanics*, 42, 1–8.

30. Humphrey, J. D. (2008). Vascular adaptation and mechanical homeostasis at tissue, cellular, and sub-cellular levels. *Cell Biochemistry and Biophysics*, 50(2), 53–78.

31. Virmani, R., Avolio, A. P., Mergner, W. J., Robinowitz, M., Herderick, E. E., Cornhill, J. F., Guo, S. Y., Liu, T. H., Ou, D. Y., and O'Rourke, M. (1991). Effect of aging on aortic morphology in populations with high and low prevalence of hypertension and atherosclerosis. Comparison between occidental and Chinese communities. *The American Journal of Pathology*, 139(5), 1119–1129.

32. Del Corso, L., Moruzzo, D., Conte, B., Agelli, M., Romanelli, A. M., Pastine, F., Protti, M., Pentimone, F., and Baggiani, G. (1998). Tortuosity, kinking, and coiling of the carotid artery: Expression of atherosclerosis or aging? *Angiology*, 49(5), 361–371.

33. Levy, B. (2006). Modifications de la paroi artérielle au cours du vieillissement. *La Revue de médecine interne*, 27, S40–S42.

34. Clark, J. M., and Glagov, S. (1985). Transmural organization of the arterial media. The lamellar unit revisited. *Arteriosclerosis, Thrombosis, and Vascular Biology*, 5(1), 19–34.

35. Gibbons, G. H., and Dzau, V. J. (1994). The emerging concept of vascular remodeling. *New England Journal of Medicine*, 330(20), 1431–1438.

36. Hayashi, K., and Naiki, T. (2009). Adaptation and remodeling of vascular wall; biomechanical response to hypertension. *Journal of the Mechanical Behavior of Biomedical Materials*, 2(1), 3–19.

37. Lee, R. M. (1989). *Blood Vessel Changes in Hypertension Structure and Function* (Vol. 2). Boca Raton, FL: CRC Press.

38. Mulvany, M. J. (2012). Small artery remodelling in hypertension. *Basic & Clinical Pharmacology & Toxicology*, 110(1), 49–55.

39. Laurent, S., and Boutouyrie, P. (2015). The structural factor of hypertension. *Circulation Research*, 116(6), 1007–1021.

40. Lehoux, S., Castier, Y., and Tedgui, A. (2006). Molecular mechanisms of the vascular responses to haemodynamic forces. *Journal of Internal Medicine*, 259(4), 381–392.

41. Vardulaki, K. A., Walker, N. M., Day, N. E., Duffy, S. W., Ashton, H. A., and Scott, R. A. P. (2000). Quantifying the risks of hypertension, age, sex and smoking in patients with abdominal aortic aneurysm. *British Journal of Surgery*, 87(2), 195–200.

42. Sakalihasan, N., Limet, R., and Defawe, O. D. (2005). Abdominal aortic aneurysm. *The Lancet*, 365(9470), 1577–1589.

43. Lederle, F. A., Johnson, G. R., Wilson, S. E., Chute, E. P., Hye, R. J., Makaroun, M. S., and Makhoul, R. G. (2000). The aneurysm detection and management study screening program: Validation cohort and final results. *Archives of Internal Medicine*, 160(10), 1425–1430.

44. Lederle, F. A., Johnson, G. R., and Wilson, S. E. (2001). Abdominal aortic aneurysm in women. *Journal of Vascular Surgery*, 34(1), 122–126.

45. Klink, A., Hyafil, F., Rudd, J., Faries, P., Fuster, V., Mallat, Z., Meilhac, O. et al. (2011). Diagnostic and therapeutic strategies for small abdominal aortic aneurysms. *Nature Reviews Cardiology*, 8(6), 338–347.

46. Wilmink, T. B., Quick, C. R., and Day, N. E. (1999). The association between cigarette smoking and abdominal aortic aneurysms. *Journal of Vascular Surgery*, 30(6), 1099–1105.

47. Salem, M. K., Rayt, H. S., Hussey, G., Rafelt, S., Nelson, C. P., Sayers, R. D., Naylor, A. R., and Nasim, A. (2009). Should Asian men be included in abdominal aortic aneurysm screening programmes? *European Journal of Vascular and Endovascular Surgery*, 38(6), 748–749.

48. Larsson, E., Granath, F., Swedenborg, J., and Hultgren, R. (2009). A population-based case-control study of the familial risk of abdominal aortic aneurysm. *Journal of Vascular Surgery*, 49(1), 47–51.

49. Golledge, J., and Norman, P. E. (2010). Atherosclerosis and abdominal aortic aneurysm. *Arteriosclerosis, Thrombosis, and Vascular Biology*, 30(6), 1075–1077

50. Golledge, J., Clancy, P., Jamrozik, K., and Norman, P. E. (2007). Obesity, adipokines, and abdominal aortic aneurysm. *Circulation*, 116(20), 2275–2279.

51. Sakalihasan, N., Heyeres, A., Nusgens, B. V., Limet, R., and Lapiére, C. M. (1993). Modifications of the extracellular matrix of aneurysmal abdominal aortas as a function of their size. *European Journal of Vascular Surgery*, 7(6), 633–637.

52. Dobrin, P. B., and Mrkvicka, R. (1994). Failure of elastin or collagen as possible critical connective tissue alterations underlying aneurysmal dilatation. *Vascular*, 2(4), 484–488.

53. Lopez-Candales, A., Holmes, D. R., Liao, S., Scott, M. J., Wickline, S. A., and Thompson, R. W. (1997). Decreased vascular smooth muscle cell density in medial degeneration of human abdominal aortic aneurysms. *The American Journal of Pathology*, 150(3), 993.

54. Allaire, E., Muscatelli-Groux, B., Mandet, C., Guinault, A. M., Bruneval, P., Desgranges, P., Clowes, A., Melliere, D., and Becquemin, J. P. (2002). Paracrine effect of vascular smooth muscle cells in the prevention of aortic aneurysm formation. *Journal of Vascular Surgery*, 36(5), 1018–1026.

55. Piechota-Polanczyk, A., Jozkowicz, A., Nowak, W., Eilenberg, W., Neumayer, C., Malinski, T., Huk, I., and Brostjan, C. (2014). The abdominal aortic aneurysm and intraluminal thrombus: Current concepts of development and treatment. *Frontiers in Cardiovascular Medicine*, 2, 19.

56. Di Martino, E. S., Bohra, A., Geest, J. P. V., Gupta, N., Makaroun, M. S., and Vorp, D. A. (2006). Biomechanical properties of ruptured versus electively repaired abdominal aortic aneurysm wall tissue. *Journal of Vascular Surgery*, 43(3), 570–576.

57. Mower, W. R., Quiñones, W. J., and Gambhir, S. S. (1997). Effect of intraluminal thrombus on abdominal aortic aneurysm wall stress. *Journal of Vascular Surgery*, 26(4), 602–608.

58. Wang, D. H., Makaroun, M. S., Webster, M. W., and Vorp, D. A. (2002). Effect of intraluminal thrombus on wall stress in patient-specific models of abdominal aortic aneurysm. *Journal of Vascular Surgery*, 36(3), 598–604.

59. Schurink, G. W. H., van Baalen, J. M., Visser, M. J., and van Bockel, J. H. (2000). Thrombus within an aortic aneurysm does not reduce pressure on the aneurysmal wall. *Journal of Vascular Surgery*, 31(3), 501–506.

60. Thubrikar, M. J., Robicsek, F., Labrosse, M., Chervenkoff, V., and Fowler, B. L. (2003). Effect of thrombus on abdominal aortic aneurysm wall dilation and stress. *Journal of Cardiovascular Surgery*, 44(1), 67.

61. Kazi, M., Thyberg, J., Religa, P., Roy, J., Eriksson, P., Hedin, U., and Swedenborg, J. (2003). Influence of intraluminal thrombus on structural and cellular composition of abdominal aortic aneurysm wall. *Journal of Vascular Surgery*, 38(6), 1283–1292.

62. Speelman, L., Schurink, G. W. H., Bosboom, E. M. H., Buth, J., Breeuwer, M., van de Vosse, F. N., and Jacobs, M. H. (2010). The mechanical role of thrombus on the growth rate of an abdominal aortic aneurysm. *Journal of Vascular Surgery*, 51(1), 19–26.

63. Vorp, D. A. (2007). Biomechanics of abdominal aortic aneurysm. *Journal of Biomechanics*, 40(9), 1887–1902.

64. Raghavan, M. L., and Vorp, D. A. (2000). Toward a biomechanical tool to evaluate rupture potential of abdominal aortic aneurysm: Identification of a finite strain constitutive model and evaluation of its applicability. *Journal of Biomechanics*, 33(4), 475–482.

65. Gasser, T. C., Auer, M., Labruto, F., Swedenborg, J., and Roy, J. (2010). Biomechanical rupture risk assessment of abdominal aortic aneurysms: Model complexity versus predictability of finite element simulations. *European Journal of Vascular and Endovascular Surgery*, 40(2), 176–185.

66. McGloughlin, T. M. (Ed.). (2011). *Biomechanics and Mechanobiology of Aneurysms*. Berlin, Germany: Springer.

67. Duprey, A., Khanafer, K., Schlicht, M., Avril, S., Williams, D., and Berguer, R. (2009). Ex vivo characterization of biomechanical behavior of ascending thoracic aortic aneurysm using uniaxial tensile testing. *European Journal of Vascular and Endovascular Surgery*, 39(6), 700–707.

68. Laurent, S., Marais, L., and Boutouyrie, P. (2016). The noninvasive assessment of vascular aging. *Canadian Journal of Cardiology*, 32(5), 669–679.

69. Lénàrd, Z., Studinger, P., Kovàts, Z., Reneman, R., and Kollai, M. (2001). Comparison of aortic arch and carotid sinus distensibility in humans—relation to baroreflex sensitivity. *Autonomic Neuroscience: Basic and Clinical*, 92, 92–99.

70. Morrison, T. M., Choi, G., Zarins, C. K., and Taylor, C. A. (2009). Circumferential and longitudinal cyclic strain of the human thoracic aorta: Age-related changes. *Journal of Vascular Surgery*, 49, 1029–1036.

71. Isnard, R. N., Pannier, B. M., Laurent, S., London, G. M., Diebold, B., and Safar, M. E. (1999). Pulsatile diameter and elastic modulus of the aortic arch in essential hypertension: A noninvasive study. *JACC*, 13(2), 399–405.

72. De Bock, S., Iannaccone, F., De Santis, G., De Beule, M., Van Loo, D., Devos, D., Vermassen, F., Segers, P., and Verhegghe, B. (2012). Virtual evaluation of stent graft deployment: A validated modeling and simulation study. *Journal of the Mechanical Behavior of Biomedical Materials*, 13, 129–139.

73. Demanget, N., Avril, S., Badel, P., Orgéas, L., Geindreau, C., Albertini, J. N., and Favre, J. P. (2012). Computational comparison of the bending behaviour of aortic stent-grafts. *Journal of the Mechanical Behaviors of Biomedical Materials*, 5(1), 272–282.

74. Demanget, N., Latil, P., Orgéas, L., Badel, P., Avril, S., Geindreau, C., Albertini, J. N., and Favre, J. P. (2012). Severe bending of two aortic stent-grafts: An experimental and numerical mechanical analysis. *Annals of Biomedical Engineering*, 40(12), 2674–2686.

75. McGloughlin, T. (2012). *Biomechanics and Mechanobiology of Aneurysms*. Berlin, Germany: Springer.

76. Fillinger, M. (2007). Who should we operate on and how do we decide: Predicting rupture and survival in patients with aortic aneurysm. *Seminars in Vascular Surgery*, 20(2), 121–127.

77. Cox, R. H. (1983). Comparison of arterial wall mechanics using ring and cylindrical segments. *American Journal of Physiology-Heart and Circulatory Physiology*, 244(2), H298–H303.

78. O'Leary, S. A., Healey, D. A., Kavanagh, E. G., Walsh, M. T., McGloughlin, T. M., and Doyle, B. J. (2014). The biaxial biomechanical behavior of abdominal aortic aneurysm tissue. *Annals of Biomedical Engineering*, 42(12), 2440–2450.

79. Pierce, D. M., Maier, F., Weisbecker, H., Viertler, C., Verbrugghe, P., Famaey, N., Fourneau, I., Herijgers, P., and Holzapfel, G. A. (2015). Human thoracic and abdominal aortic aneurysmal tissues: Damage experiments, statistical analysis and constitutive modeling. *Journal of the Mechanical Behavior of Biomedical Materials*, 41, 92–107.

80. Sassani, S. G., Kakisis, J., Tsangaris, S., and Sokolis, D. P. (2015). Layer-dependent wall properties of abdominal aortic aneurysms: Experimental study and material characterization. *Journal of the Mechanical Behavior of Biomedical Materials*, 49, 141–161.

81. Geest, J. P. V., Sacks, M. S., and Vorp, D. A. (2006). The effects of aneurysm on the biaxial mechanical behavior of human abdominal aorta. *Journal of Biomechanics*, 39(7), 1324–1334.

82. Teng, Z., Feng, J., Zhang, Y., Huang, Y., Sutcliffe, M. P., Brown, A. J., Jing, Z., Gillard, J. H., and Lu, Q. (2015). Layer-and direction-specific material properties, extreme extensibility and ultimate material strength of human abdominal aorta and aneurysm: A uniaxial extension study. *Annals of Biomedical Engineering*, 43(11), 2745–2759.

83. Vorp, D. A., Raghavan, M. L., Muluk, S. C., Makaroun, M. S., Steed, D. L., Shapiro, R., and Webster, M. W. (1996). Wall strength and stiffness of aneurysmal and non-aneurysmal abdominal aorta. *Annals of the New York Academy of Sciences*, 800(1), 274–276.

84. Labrosse, M. R., Beller, C. J., Mesana, T., and Veinot, J. P. (2009). Mechanical behavior of human aortas: Experiments, material constants and 3-D finite element modeling including residual stress. *Journal of Biomechanics*, 42, 996–1004.

85. Ferruzzi, J., Vorp, D. A., and Humphrey, J. D. (2010). On constitutive descriptors of the biaxial mechanical behaviour of human abdominal aorta and aneurysms. *Journal of the Royal Society Interface*, 8(56), 435–450.

86. Weizsäcker, H. W., Lambert, H., and Pascale, K. (1983). Analysis of the passive mechanical properties of rat carotid arteries. *Journal of Biomechanics*, 16(9), 703–715.

87. Sommer, G., Regitnig, P., Költringer, L., and Holzapfel, G. A. (2010). Biaxial mechanical properties of intact and layer-dissected human carotid arteries at physiological and supraphysiological loadings. *American Journal of Physiology-Heart and Circulatory Physiology*, 298(3), H898–H912.

88. Avril, S., Badel, P., and Duprey, A. (2010). Anisotropic and hyperelastic identification of in-vitro human arteries from full-field measurements. *Journal of Biomechanics*, 43(15), 2978–2985.

89. Kim, J., and Baek, S. (2011). Circumferential variations of mechanical behavior of the porcine thoracic aorta during the inflation test. *Journal of Biomechanics*, 44(10), 1941–1947.

90. Kim, J. H., Avril, S., Duprey, A., and Favre, J. P. (2012). Experimental characterization of rupture in human aortic aneurysms using a full-field measurement technique. *Biomechanics and Modeling in Mechanobiology*, 11(6), 841–854.

91. Romo, A., Avril, S., Badel, P., Molimard, J., Duprey, A., and Favre, J. P. (2012). Mechanical characterization of the thoracic ascending aorta. *IRCOBI Conference 2012*, IRC-12-72. http://www.ircobi.org/downloads/irc12/pdf_files/72.pdf.

92. Genovese, K., Lee, Y. U., Lee, A. Y., and Humphrey, J. D. (2013). An improved panoramic digital image correlation method for vascular strain analysis and material characterization. *Journal of the Mechanical Behavior of Biomedical Materials*, 27, 132–142.

93. Sutton, M. A., Ke, X., Lessner, S. M., Goldbach, M., Yost, M., Zhao, F., and Schreier, H. W. (2008). Strain field measurements on mouse carotid arteries using microscopic three-dimensional digital image correlation. *Journal of Biomedical Materials Research Part A*, 84(1), 178–190.

94. Bersi, M. R., Bellini, C., Di Achille, P., Humphrey, J. D., Genovese, K., and Avril, S. (2016). Novel methodology for characterizing regional variations in the material properties of murine aortas. *Journal of Biomechanical Engineering*, 138(7), 071005.

95. Davis, F. M., Luo, Y., Avril, S., Duprey, A., and Lu, J. (2015). Pointwise characterization of the elastic properties of planar soft tissues: Application to ascending thoracic aneurysms. *Biomechanics and Modeling in Mechanobiology*, 14(5), 967–978.

96. Nederveen, A. J., Avril, S., and Speelman, L. (2014). MRI strain imaging of the carotid artery: Present limitations and future challenges. *Journal of Biomechanics*, 47(4), 824–833.

97. Humphrey, J. D. (2009). Vascular mechanics, mechanobiology, and remodeling. *Journal of Mechanics in Medicine and Biology*, 9(2), 243–257.

98. Collins, R. and Hu, W. C. L. (1972). Dynamic deformation experiments on aortic tissue. *Journal of Biomechanics*, 5(4), 333–337.

99. Pham, T., Martin, C., Elefteriades, J., and Sun, W. (2013). Biomechanical characterization of ascending aortic aneurysm with concomitant bicuspid aortic valve and bovine aortic arch. *Acta Biomaterialia*, 9(8), 7927–7936.

100. Zemánek, M., Burša, J., and Děták, M. (2009). Biaxial tension tests with soft tissues of arterial wall. *Engineering Mechanics*, 16(1), 3–11.

101. Adham, M., Gournier, J. P., Favre, J. P., De La Roche, E., Ducerf, C., Baulieux, J., Barral, X., and Pouyet, M. (1996). Mechanical characteristics of fresh and frozen human descending thoracic aorta. *Journal of Surgical Research*, 64(1), 32–34.

102. Armentano, R. L., Santana, D. B., Cabrera Fischer, E. I., Graf, S., Campos, H. P., Germán, Y. Z., Saldías, M. D., and Alvarez, I. (2006). An in-vitro study of cryopreserved and fresh human arteries: A comparison with ePTFE prostheses and human arteries studied non-invasively in-vivo. *Cryobiology*, 52(1), 17–26.

103. Venkatasubramanian, R. T., Grassl, E. D., Barocas, V. H., Lafontaine, D., and Bischof, J. C. (2006). Effects of freezing and cryopreservation on the mechanical properties of arteries. *Annals of Biomedical Engineering*, 34(5), 823–832.

104. Chow, M.-J. and Zhang, Y. (2011). Changes in the mechanical and biochemical properties of aortic tissue due to cold storage. *Journal of Surgical Research*, 171(2), 434–442.

105. Stemper, B. D., Yoganandan, N., Stineman, M. R., Gennarelli, T. A., Baisden, J. L., and Pintar, F. A. (2007). Mechanics of fresh, refrigerated, and frozen arterial tissue. *Journal of Surgical Research*, 139(2), 236–242.

106. Sato, M., Hayashi, K., Niimi, H., Moritake, K., Okumura, A., and Handa, H. (1979). Axial mechanical properties of arterial walls and their anisotropy. *Medical & Biological Engineering & Computing*, 17(2), 170–176.

107. Tanaka, T. T., and Fung, Y.-C. (1974). Elastic and inelastic properties of the canine aorta and their variation along the aortic tree. *Journal of Biomechanics*, 7(4), 357–370.

108. Holzapfel, G. A. et al., 2005. Determination of layer-specific mechanical properties of human coronary arteries with nonatherosclerotic intimal thickening and related constitutive modeling. *American Journal of Physiology. Heart and Circulatory Physiology*, 289(5), H2048–H2058.

109. Weisbecker, H., Viertler, C., Pierce, D. M., and Holzapfel, G. A. (2013). The role of elastin and collagen in the softening behavior of the human thoracic aortic media. *Journal of Biomechanics*, 46(11), 1859–1865.

110. Farand, P., Garon, A., and Plante, G. E. (2007). Structure of large arteries: Orientation of elastin in rabbit aortic internal elastic lamina and in the elastic lamellae of aortic media. *Microvascular Research*, 73(2), 95–99.

111. Fung, Y. C. (1993). *Biomechanics. Mechanical Properties of Living Tissues*. New York: Springer.

112. Humphrey, J. D. (1995). Mechanics of the arterial wall: Review and directions. *Critical Reviews in Biomedical Engineering*, 23, 1–162.

113. Hill, M. R., Duan, X., Gibson, G. A., Watkins, S., and Robertson, A. M. (2012). A theoretical and non-destructive experimental approach for direct inclusion of measured collagen orientation and recruitment into mechanical models of the artery wall. *Journal of Biomechanics*, 45, 762–771.

114. Trabelsi, O., Duprey, A., Favre, J. P., and Avril, S. (2016). Predictive models with patient specific material properties for the biomechanical behavior of ascending thoracic aneurysms. *Annals of Biomedical Engineering*, 44(1), 84–98.

115. Franquet, A., Avril, S., Le Riche, R., Badel, P., Schneider, F. C., Li, Z. Y., Boissier, C., and Favre, J. P. (2013). A new method for the in-vivo identification of mechanical properties in arteries from cine MRI images: Theoretical framework and validation. *IEEE Transactions on Medical Imaging*, 32(8), 1448–1461.

116. Franquet, A., Avril, S., Le Riche, R., Badel, P., Schneider, F. C., Boissier, C., and Favre, J. P. (2013). Identification of the in-vivo elastic properties of common carotid arteries from MRI: A study on subjects with and without atherosclerosis. *Journal of the Mechanical Behavior of Biomedical Materials*, 27, 184–203.

117. Hayashi, K., Sato, M., Handa, H., and Moritake, K. (1974). Biomechanical study of the constitutive laws of vascular walls. *Experimental Mechanics*, 14(11), 440–444.

118. Haskett, D., Johnson, G., Zhou, A., Utzinger, U., and van de Geest, J. (2010). Microstructural and biomechanical alterations of the human aorta as a function of age and location. *Biomechanics and Modeling in Mechanobiology*, 9, 725–736.

119. Zeinali-Davarani, S., Wang, Y., Chow, M. J., Turcotte, R., and Zhang, Y. (2015). Contribution of collagen fiber undulation to regional biomechanical properties along porcine thoracic aorta. *Journal of Biomechanical Engineering*, 137(5), 51001.

120. Sokolis, D. P., Boudoulas, H., and Karayannacos, P. E. (2002). Assessment of the aortic stress–strain relation in uniaxial tension. *Journal of Biomechanics*, 35(9), 1213–1223.

121. Roy, C. S. (1881). The elastic properties of the arterial wall. *The Journal of Physiology*, 3(2), 125–159.

122. Chow, M.-J., Turcotte, R., Lin, C. P., and Zhang, Y. (2014). Arterial extracellular matrix: A mechanobiological study of the contributions and interactions of elastin and collagen. *Biophysical Journal*, 106(12), 2684–2692.

123. Ferruzzi, J., Collins, M. J., Yeh, A. T., and Humphrey, J. D. (2011). Mechanical assessment of elastin integrity in fibrillin-1-deficient carotid arteries: Implications for Marfan syndrome. *Cardiovascular Research*, 92(2), 287–295.

124. Fonck, E., Prod'hom, G., Roy, S., Augsburger, L., Rüfenacht, D. A., and Stergiopulos, N. (2007). Effect of elastin degradation on carotid wall mechanics as assessed by a constituent-based biomechanical model. *American Journal of Physiology. Heart and Circulatory Physiology*, 292(6), H2754–H2763.

125. Rezakhaniha, R., Fonck, E., Genoud, C., and Stergiopulos, N. (2011). Role of elastin anisotropy in structural strain energy functions of arterial tissue. *Biomechanics and Modeling in Mechanobiology*, 10(4), 599–611.

126. Ní Annaidh, A., Destrade, M., Gilchrist, M. D., and Murphy, J. G. (2013). Deficiencies in numerical models of anisotropic nonlinearly elastic materials. *Biomechanics and Modeling in Mechanobiology*, 12, 781–791.

127. Vergori, L., Destrade, M., McGarry, P., and Ogden, R. W. (2013). On anisotropic elasticity and questions concerning its finite element implementation. *Computational Mechanics*, 52(5), 1185–1197.

128. McGrath, J. C., Deighan, C., Briones, A. M., Shafaroudi, M. M., McBride, M., Adler, J., Arribas, S. M., Vila, E., and Daly, C. J. (2005). New aspects of vascular remodelling: The involvement of all vascular cell types. *Experimental Physiology*, 90(4), 469–475.

129. Bellini, C., Ferruzzi, J., Roccabianca, S., Di Martino, E. S., and Humphrey, J. D. (2014). A microstructurally motivated model of arterial wall mechanics with mechanobiological implications. *Annals of Biomedical Engineering*, 42(3), 488–502.

130. Mousavi, J., and Avril, S. (2017). Patient-specific stress analyses in the ascending thoracic aorta using a finite-element implementation of the constrained-mixture theory. *Biomechanics and Modeling in Mechanobiology*, 16(5), 1765–1777.

131. Hollander, Y., Durban, D., Lu, X., Kassab, G. S., and Lanir, Y. (2011). Experimentally validated microstructural 3D constitutive model of coronary arterial media. *Journal of Biomechanical Engineering*, 133(3), 031007.

132. Braeu, F. A., Seitz, A., Aydin, R. C., and Cyron, C. J. (2016). Homogenized constrained mixture models for anisotropic volumetric growth and remodeling. *Biomechanics and Modeling in Mechanobiology*, 16, 889–906.

133. Masson, I., Boutouyrie, P., Laurent, S., Humphrey, J. D., and Zidi, M. (2008). Characterization of arterial wall mechanical behavior and stresses from human clinical data. *Journal of Biomechanics*, 41(12), 2618–2627.

134. Stålhand, J., Klarbring, A., and Karlsson, M. (2004). Towards in-vivo aorta material identification and stress estimation. *Biomechanics and Modeling in Mechanobiology*, 2(3), 169–186.

135. Avril, S. (2017). Hyperelasticity of soft tissues and related inverse problems. In S. Avril and S. Evans (Eds.), *Material Parameter Identification and Inverse Problems in Soft Tissue Biomechanics* (pp. 37–66). Cham, Switzerland: Springer International Publishing.

136. Wittek, A., Karatolios, K., Fritzen, C. P., Bereiter-Hahn, J., Schieffer, B., Moosdorf, R., Vogt, S., and Blase, C. (2016). Cyclic three-dimensional wall motion of the human ascending and abdominal aorta characterized by time-resolved three-dimensional ultrasound speckle tracking. *Biomechanics and Modeling in Mechanobiology*, 15(5), 1375–1388.

137. Doyle, B. J., and Norman, P. E. (2016). Computational biomechanics in thoracic aortic dissection: Today's approaches and tomorrow's opportunities. *Annals of Biomedical Engineering*, 44(1), 71–83.

138. Okamoto, R. J., Wagenseil, J. E., DeLong, W. R., Peterson, S. J., Kouchoukos, N. T., and Sundt 3rd, T. M. (2002). Mechanical properties of dilated human ascending aorta. *Annals of Biomedical Engineering*, 30(5), 624–635.

139. Vorp, D. A., Schiro, B. J., Ehrlich, M. P., Juvonen, T. S., Ergin, M. A., and Griffith, B. P. (2003). Effect of aneurysm on the tensile strength and biomechanical behaviour of the ascending thoracic aorta. *Annals of Thoracic Surgery*, 75(4), 1210–1214.

140. Peterson, S. J., Sundt III, T. M., Kouchoukos, N. T., Yin, F. C. P., and Okamoto, R. J. (Eds.). (1999). Biaxial mechanical properties of dilated human ascending aortic tissue. BMES/EMBS Conference. *Proceedings of the First Joint*, October 13–16, Atlanta, GA.

141. Koullias, G., Modak, R., Tranquilli, M., Korkolis, D. P., Barash, P., and Elefteriades, J. A. (2005). Mechanical deterioration underlies malignant behavior of aneurysmal human ascending aorta. *Journal of Thoracic and Cardiovascular Surgery*, 130, 677–683.

142. Choudhury, N., Bouchot, O., Rouleau, L., Tremblay, D., Cartier, R., Butany, J., Mongrain, R., and Leask, R. L. (2008). Local mechanical and structural properties of healthy and diseased human ascending aorta tissue. *Cardiovascular Pathology*, 18(2), 83–91.

143. Khanafer, K., Duprey, A., Zainal, M., Schlicht, M., Williams, D., and Berguer, R. (2011). Determination of the elastic modulus of ascending thoracic aortic aneurysm at different ranges of pressure using uniaxial tensile testing. *Journal of Thoracic and Cardiovascular Surgery*, 142(3), 682–686.

144. Iliopoulos, D. C., Kritharis, E. P., Giagini, A. T., Papadodima, S. A., and Sokolis, D. P. (2008). Ascending thoracic aortic aneurysms are associated with compositional remodeling and vessel stiffening but not weakening in age-matched subjects. *Journal of Thoracic and Cardiovascular Surgery*, 137(1), 101–109.

145. Mohan, D., and Melvin, J. W. (1982). Failure properties of passive human aortic tissue. I—Uniaxial. Tension tests. *Journal of Biomechanics*, 15(11), 887–902.

146. McLean, N. F., Dudek, N. L., and Roach, M. R. (1999). The role of radial elastic properties in the development of aortic dissections. *Journal of Vascular Surgery*, 29, 703–710.

147. Sommer, G., Gasser, T. C., Regitnig, P., Auer, M., and Holzapfel, G. A. (2008). Dissection properties of the human aortic media: An experimental study. *ASME Journal of Biomechanical Engineering*, 130, 021007.

148. Mohan, D., and Melvin, J. W. (1982). Failure properties of passive human aortic tissue. II—Biaxial. Tension tests. *Journal of Biomechanics*, 16(1), 31–44.

149. Groenink, M., Langerak, S. E., Vanbavel, E., van der Wall, E. E., Mulder, B. J., van der Wal, A. C., and Spaan, J. A. (1999). Dependence of wall stress in the human thoracic aorta on age and pressure. *Cardiovascular Research*, 43, 471–480.

150. Sherebrin, M., Hegney, J. E., and Roach, M. R. (1989). Effects of age on the anisotropy of the descending human thoracic aorta determined by uniaxial tensile testing and digestion by NaOH under load. *Canadian Journal of Physiology and Pharmacology*, 67, 871–878.

151. Pasta, S., Phillippi, J. A., Gleason, T. G., and Vorp, D. A. (2012). Effect of aneurysm on the mechanical dissection properties of the human ascending thoracic aorta. *Journal of Thoracic and Cardiovascular Surgery*, 143(2), 460–467.

152. Pasta, S., Phillippi, J. A., Tsamis, A., D'Amore, A., Raffa, G. M., Pilato, M., Scardulla, C. et al. (2016). Constitutive modeling of ascending thoracic aortic aneurysms using microstructural parameters. *Medical Engineering & Physics*, 38(2), 121–130.

153. Martufi, G., Forneris, A., Appoo, J. J., and Di Martino, E. S. (2016). Is there a role for biomechanical engineering in helping to elucidate the risk profile of the thoracic aorta? *The Annals of Thoracic Surgery*, 101(1), 390–398.

154. de Virgilio, C., Nelson, R. J., Milliken, J., Snyder, R., Chiang, F., MacDonald, W. D., and Robertson, J. M. (1990). Ascending aortic dissection in weight lifters with cystic medial degeneration. *The Annals of Thoracic Surgery*, 49(4), 638–642.

155. Weisbecker, H., Pierce, D. M., Regitnig, P., and Holzapfel, G. A. (2012). Layer-specific damage experiments and modeling of human thoracic and abdominal aortas with non-atherosclerotic intimal thickening. *Journal of Mechanical Behavior of Biomedical Materials*, 12, 93–106.

156. Barker, A. J., Markl, M., Bürk, J., Lorenz, R., Bock, J., Bauer, S., Schulz-Menger, J., and von Knobelsdorff-Brenkenhoff, F. (2012). Bicuspid aortic valve is associated with altered wall shear stress in the ascending aorta. *Circulation: Cardiovascular Imaging*, 5, 457–466.

157. Hope, M. D., Sigovan, M., Wrenn, S. J., Saloner, D., and Dyverfeldt, P. (2014). Magnetic resonance imaging hemodynamic markers of progressive bicuspid aortic valve related aortic disease. *Journal of Magnetic Resonance Imaging*, 40, 140–145.

158. Pasta, S., Rinaudo, A., Luca, A., Pilato, M., Scardulla, C., Gleason, T. G., and Vorp, D. A. (2013). Difference in hemodynamic and wall stress of ascending thoracic aortic aneurysms with bicuspid and tricuspid aortic valve. *Journal of Biomechanics*, 46, 1729–1738.

159. Al-Atassi, T., Hynes, M., Sohmer, B., Lam, B.-K., Mesana, T., and Boodhwani, M. (2015). Aortic root geometry in bicuspid aortic insufficiency versus stenosis: Implications for valve repair. *European Journal of Cardiothoracic Surgery*, 47, e151–e154.

160. Condemi, F., Campisi, S., Viallon, M., Troalen, T., Xuexin, G., Barker, A. J., Markl, M. et al. (2017). Fluid- and biomechanical analysis of ascending thoracic aorta aneurysm with concomitant aortic insufficiency. *Annals of Biomedical Engineering*, 45(12), 2921–2932.

161. Youssefi, P., Gomez, A., He, T., Anderson, L., Bunce, N., Sharma, R., Figueroa, C. A., and Jahangiri, M. (2017). Patient-specific computational fluid dynamics—assessment of aortic hemodynamics in a spectrum of aortic valve pathologies. *The Journal of Thoracic and Cardiovascular Surgery*, 153(1), 8–20.

162. Thubrikar, M. J., Agali, P., and Robicsek, F. (1999). Wall stress as a possible mechanism for the development of transverse intimal tears in aortic dissections. *Journal of Medical Engineering & Technology*, 23, 127–134.

163. Tam, A. S. M., Sapp, M. C., and Roach, M. R. (1998). The effect of tear depth on the propagation of aortic dissections in isolated porcine thoracic aorta. *Journal of Biomechanics*, 31, 673–676.

164. Tiessen, I. M., and Roach, M. R. (1993). Factors in the initiation and propagation of aortic dissections in human autopsy aortas. *Journal of Biomechanical Engineering*, 115(1), 123–125.

165. Nathan, D. P., Xu, C., Gorman, J. H., Fairman, R. M., Bavaria, J. E., Gorman, R. C., Chandran, K. B., and Jackson, B. M. (2011). Pathogenesis of acute aortic dissection: A finite element stress analysis. *The Annals of Thoracic Surgery*, 91(2), 458–463.

166. Beller, C. J., Labrosse, M. R., Thubrikar, M. J., and Robicsek, F. (2004). Role of aortic root motion in the pathogenesis of aortic dissection. *Circulation*, 109(6), 763–769.

167. Mercer, J. L. (1969). Movement of the aortic annulus. *The British Journal of Radiology*, 42(500), 623–626.

168. Kozerke, S., Scheidegger, M. B., Pedersen, E. M., and Boesiger, P. (1999). Heart motion adapted cine phase-contrast flow measurements through the aortic valve. *Magnetic Resonance in Medicine*, 42(5), 970–978.

169. Stuber, M., Scheidegger, M. B., Fischer, S. E., Nagel, E., Steinemann, F., Hess, O. M., and Boesiger, P. (1999). Alterations in the local myocardial motion pattern in patients suffering from pressure overload due to aortic stenosis. *Circulation*, 100(4), 361–368.

170. Muhs, B. E., Vincken, K. L., van Prehn, J., Stone, M. K. C., Bartels, L. W., Prokop, M., Moll, F. L., and Verhagen, H. J. M. (2006). Dynamic cine-CT angiography for the evaluation of the thoracic aorta; insight in dynamic changes with implications for thoracic endograft treatment. *European Journal of Vascular Endovascular Surgery*, 32, 532–536.

171. Lu, T. L. C., Huber, C. H., Rizzo, E., Dehmeshki, J., von Segesser, L. K., and Qanadli, S. D. (2009). Ascending aorta measurements as assessed by ECG-gated multi-detector computed tomography: A pilot study to establish normative values for transcatheter therapies. *European Radiology*, 19, 664–669.

172. Fukui, T., Matsumoto, T., Tanaka, T., Ohashi, T., Kumagai, K., Akimoto, H., Tabayashi, K., and Sato, M. (2005). In-vivo mechanical properties of thoracic aneurysmal wall estimated from in-vitro biaxial tensile test. *Biomedical Materials and Engineering*, 15, 295–305.

173. García-Herrera, C. M. and Celentano, D. J. (2013). Modelling and numerical simulation of the human aortic arch under in-vivo conditions. *Biomechanics and Modeling in Mechanobiology*, 12(6), 1143–1154.

174. Trabelsi, O., Davis, F. M., Rodriguez-Matas, J. F., Duprey, A., and Avril, S. (2015). Patient specific stress and rupture analysis of ascending thoracic aneurysms. *Journal of Biomechanics*, 48(10), 1836–1843.

175. Duprey, A., Trabelsi, O., Vola, M., Favre, J. P., and Avril, S. (2016). Biaxial rupture properties of ascending thoracic aortic aneurysms. *Acta Biomaterialia*, 42, 273–285.

176. Martin, C., Sun, W., Pham, T., and Elefteriades, J. (2013). Predictive biomechanical analysis of ascending aortic aneurysm rupture potential. *Acta Biomaterialia*, 9(12), 9392–9400.

7

Atherosclerosis and Mechanical Forces

M. Kozakova and C. Palombo

Contents

7.1 Atherosclerosis

Atherosclerosis is a degenerative process of the arterial wall, leading to arterial diameter narrowing and lumen occlusion, which result in an inadequate oxygen supply to organs perfused by the affected arteries. Atherosclerotic lesions occur in both elastic and muscular arteries; the aorta is the first artery to be involved, followed by the carotid arteries, the coronary arteries, and the ileofemoral arteries. Major clinical manifestations of the atherosclerotic process include ischemic heart disease, ischemic stroke, and peripheral arterial disease.

Atherosclerosis is a slow process that starts in childhood and progresses with age. Although its exact etiology is unknown, many factors accelerating its progression have been identified over the years. These include nonmodifiable factors, such as sex, age, and genetic predisposition, and modifiable factors, such as high blood pressure, smoking, blood lipids, obesity, diabetes mellitus, and chronic inflammation. The significant role played by modifiable risk factors in the atherosclerotic process has been confirmed by a decline in cardiovascular mortality rates with a widespread use of prevention/treatment for these risk factors (Doll 2005; Turnbull 2009; Baigent 2010; Ninomiya 2013; Herrington et al. 2016). Although the mortality rate of atherosclerosis-related vascular diseases has decreased, such diseases are still a leading cause of death worldwide, and their incidence continues to rise as a result of population aging and the worldwide epidemic of obesity and type 2 diabetes mellitus (Barquera 2015). The World Health Organization estimates that 17.5 million people died from cardiovascular diseases in

2015 (31% of all deaths), and of these deaths, 7.4 million were due to ischemic heart disease and 6.7 million were due to stroke. Therefore, developing an understanding of the atherosclerotic process activation and progression is still an important medical task.

7.2 Arterial Wall and Classification and Development of Atherosclerotic Lesions

The atherosclerotic process develops within the arterial wall, with the participation of all its components. The arterial wall is composed of three layers: the tunica intima, the tunica media, and the tunica adventitia. The tunica intima is the innermost layer formed by a single stratum of endothelial cells (ECs) supported by an internal elastic lamina. Endothelial cells are in direct contact with the blood flow; in response to hemodynamic stimuli, ECs release a wide range of factors acting in an autocrine and paracrine manner to maintain vascular homeostasis (Deanfield 2007). A loss of normal endothelial function is believed to be a key event in the initiation of the atherosclerotic process (Bonetti 2003). The tunica media consists of layers of smooth muscle cells (SMCs) that are organized in groups of cells oriented perpendicularly to the longitudinal axis of the artery and reinforced by a network of type III collagen fibers to prevent excessive wall stretching. Each cellular group is embedded into a system of similarly oriented elastic fibers that endow the artery with compliance and recoil during the cardiac cycle (Clark 1985 and 1979). The tunica adventitia, or the outermost layer, is made up of connective tissue containing a network of vasa vasorum and nerves mediating the vascular tone.

Changes in the arterial wall may occur both as a normal adaptive response to altered hemodynamic and mechanical conditions and as a pathological process. Although the distinction between adaptive response and early atherosclerotic changes is not always clear, the accretion of lipids and the formation of necrotic core and fibrous cap are understood to characterize the atherosclerotic process (Virmani 2000; Chen 2010). A modified American Heart Association (AHA) classification distinguishes seven categories of vascular lesions that include intimal thickening, intimal xanthoma ("fatty streak"), pathological intimal thickening, fibrous cap atheroma, thin fibrous cap atheroma, calcified nodule, and fibrocalcific plaque (Figure 7.1a–b) (Virmani 2000). Intimal xanthoma and intimal thickening may exist, without progressing to more advanced lesions.

Intimal xanthomas are focal accumulations of foam cells without necrotic core and fibrous cap. They are already present in some fetal aortas and in infants in the first 6 months of life (Stary 2000; Milei 2008). Xanthomas reflect the mother's risk factors (Napoli 1997), and their number decreases in subsequent years (Stary 2000). Adaptive intimal thickening represents an accumulation of SMCs within the intima in the absence of lipids and foam cells. It develops spontaneously after birth at predilection sites, that is, sites with low or oscillatory shear stress, such as branching points and inner curvature of the vessels (Wentzel 2012). The predilection sites are characterized by changes in endothelial turnover and gene expression (Wentzel 2012) and may provide a locus for initial lesion development (Schwartz 1995). However, the transition of nonatherosclerotic intimal

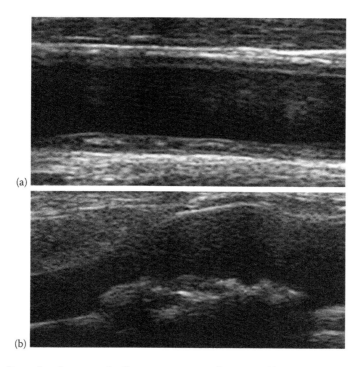

(a)

(b)

Figure 7.1   B-mode ultrasound of common carotid artery. (a) Transition of pathological intimal thickening to atheroma, and (b) large irregular fibrocalcific plaque.

thickening to pathological thickening is not well understood. The role of enzymes capable of atherogenic lipoproteins retention and aggregation has been proposed (Guyton 1993; Tabas 1993). Pathological intimal thickening comprises, in addition to SMCs and proteoglycan-rich matrix, areas of extracellular lipid accumulation (Figure 7.1a) (Virmani 2000).

Fibrous cap atheroma is the first of advanced atherosclerotic lesions and is composed of a lipid-rich necrotic core encapsulated by fibrous tissue (Figure 7.2). The necrotic core contains necrotic debris and lipid pools infiltrated by macrophages; it is thought to be caused by apoptosis and secondary necrosis of foam cells and SMCs (Clarke 2009; Moore 2011). The fibrous cap consists of collagen, elastin, and proteoglycans produced by synthetic phenotype of SMCs (Kragel 1989; Stary 1995). An expansion of the necrotic core and thinning and weakening of the fibrous cap are strong predictors of plaque vulnerability. Thin fibrous cap atheroma is defined by a cap thickness lower than 65 μm, rare SMCs, and increased infiltration by inflammatory cells (macrophages and lymphocytes) (Fishbein 1996; Burke 1997). Lesions with this type of cap are the most likely to rupture (Burke 1997). Thinning of the fibrous cap involves two possible mechanisms that occur concurrently. The first mechanism is a gradual loss of SMCs (van der Wal 1994), and the second one is the degradation of collagen by proteolytic enzymes (plasminogen activators, cathepsin, and matrix metalloproteinases [MMPs]) produced by infiltrating macrophages (Moreno 1994; Shah 2001; Hansson 2015). Sudden changes in endothelial shear stress and tensile or

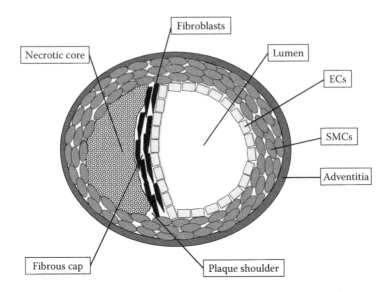

Figure 7.2   Schematic of a blood vessel with fibrous cap atheroma.

pulsatile stress, induced by physical or psychological triggers, may elicit plaque rupture (Li 2009; Mittleman 2011).

On rupture, the lipid-rich plaques expose the highly thrombogenic necrotic core to circulating blood, which causes the activation of tissue factors that start the coagulation cascade, leading to platelet activation and aggregation, with the subsequent formation of a superimposed thrombus (i.e., atherothrombosis) (Badimon 2014). The magnitude of thrombotic response is variable and is supposed to be determined by the classic Virchow's triad: thrombogenicity of the exposed plaque material, local flow disturbances, and systemic thrombotic propensity. The superimposed thrombus may compromise the arterial lumen, leading to manifestations of acute ischemic syndromes (acute coronary syndrome or ischemic stroke).

Although plaque rupture is the most common cause of acute ischemic events, these may also occur as a consequence of plaque erosion or, rarely, calcified nodules. Plaque erosion reflects the loss of the antithrombotic properties of the plaque's surface, which is caused by damage to the intima and the exposition of medial SMCs and proteoglycans to the circulating blood (Burke 1997). Calcified nodules are characterized by nodular calcifications protruding into the lumen through a fibrous cap (Burke 1997; Virmani 2000).

Finally, fibrocalcific lesion describes a collagen-rich plaque containing large areas of calcification (Figure 7.1b). The necrotic core is often present at the site of calcification or in the upstream or downstream vicinity, suggesting that these lesions represent a healed plaque rupture (Burke 2001) and that plaque healing plays an important role in the development and progression of chronic stenotic atherosclerotic lesions.

Identification and quantification of atherosclerotic lesions in the aorta, the coronary arteries, or the carotid artery are now used to refine the stratification of cardiovascular risk and to guide preventive/therapeutic strategies. The presence of calcified aortic plaques in the thoracic aorta, as detected by X-ray, is associated with a two-fold increase in the risk of cardiovascular death in both men and women (Witteman 1990). The amount of coronary calcification, as assessed by electron beam tomography, is associated with coronary heart events (Kondos 2003; Vliegenthart 2005). The measurement of the carotid wall thickness and/or the detection of carotid plaque by ultrasonography (US) improve the cardiovascular risk estimation over traditional risk factors (Nambi 2010; Vlachopoulos 2015). Characterization of the carotid plaque composition by means of magnetic resonance imaging (MRI) or US allows for the identification of vulnerable plaques with large lipid-rich necrotic zones and thin fibrous caps (DeMaria 2006; Yuan 2008).

7.3 Pathophysiological Mechanisms of Atherosclerosis

The atherosclerotic process derives from the interplay between disturbed blood flow, endothelial dysfunction, subendothelial retention of lipoproteins, and inflammatory response (Mannarino 2008; Tabas 2015). Endothelial dysfunction represents a switch from nitric oxide (NO)-mediated atheroprotective signaling toward redox signaling (Deanfield 2007; Rajendran 2013). The major reactive oxygen species (ROS) in ECs are superoxide anions ($O_2^{\bullet-}$), hydrogen peroxide (H_2O_2), and hydroxyl radicals ($^{\bullet}OH$). $O_2^{\bullet-}$ is extremely unstable and, in the presence of superoxide dismutase, generates H_2O_2, which is stable, is freely diffusible across the biological membrane, and reacts with cysteine groups in proteins to alter their activity and function (Rhee 2006). Among proteins susceptible to be modified by H_2O_2 are phosphatases, transcription factors, ion channels, antioxidants, metabolic enzymes, structural proteins, and protein kinases (Thomas 2008). In ECs, H_2O_2 modulates cell growth, proliferation and survival, cytoskeletal reorganization, vasodilating, and inflammatory responses (Bretón-Romero and Lamas 2014).

The atherosclerotic process is initiated in predilection lesion-prone areas that display a unique endothelial dysfunctional phenotype (proinflammatory and prothrombotic), which is supposed to be activated by biomechanical forces present in these areas (a low average shear stress and a high oscillatory shear index) (Tabas 2015). Lesion-prone areas are also characterized by their predisposition to subendothelial retention of apolipoprotein B (apoB)-containing lipoproteins, which further exacerbate endothelial dysfunction (Tabas 2007). The combination of endothelial dysfunction and apoB retention triggers a low-grade inflammatory response (Yuan 2008). This response leads to the proliferation and migration of vascular SMCs, the recruitment of monocytes, and their differentiation into lipid-loaded macrophages (foam cells); in turn, this leads to matrix degradation and accumulation of cellular, extracellular, and lipid material in the subendothelial space. In addition to macrophages and synthetic phenotype of SMCs, the cellular components of atherosclerotic lesions comprise T cells, B cells, dendritic cells, and mast cells, which synthesize a number of cytokines, such as the tumor necrosis factor and interleukin-1 (Kuiper 2007). Atherosclerotic lesions frequently undergo a partial resolution process, resulting in the formation of a necrotic core and an overlying fibrous cap (fibroatheroma) (Figure 7.2).

Although the pathophysiological mechanism of the atherosclerotic process is universal, the presence of individual risk factors may modify the disease presentation in each individual patient.

It is evident that atherosclerosis is a multifaceted process that reflects an interaction between biological and mechanical factors. Blood vessels are permanently exposed to mechanical forces; the two main forces acting on vessel wall are shear stress, caused by the movement of blood, and circumferential stress, generated by intraluminal pressure. These forces are intimately related through the material properties of the vessel wall, and both the forces participate in the initiation and progression of the atherosclerotic process. Indeed, the first atherosclerotic changes develop in regions with composite blood flow, and mechanical loads have an impact on the composition and vulnerability of advanced atherosclerotic lesions. Shear stress mainly modulates the function of ECs, but it also has an impact on vascular SMCs. On the contrary, cyclic stretching, as induced by pulsating circumferential stress, activates biochemical signaling–primarily in vascular SMCs, and also provides mechanical stimulation to ECs. However, the complexity of the vascular environment and the crosstalk between different components of the vessel wall make it difficult to pinpoint the exact impact of mechanical forces on different types of cells (Jufri 2015).

7.4 Shear Stress and Atherosclerosis

Shear stress is the tangential stress created by friction of the flowing blood on the endothelial surface of the arterial wall. Stress induces mechanotransduction, that is, the conversion of mechanical stresses into biochemical responses (Gimbrone 2000; Davies 2009). Specifically, endothelial shear stress stimulates mechanoreceptors on the surface of ECs, which, in turn, release factors regulating vascular homeostasis through vascular tone, permeability, anticoagulant activity, and responses to inflammation and injury (Traub 1998; Li 2005). Shear stress mechanotransduction in the endothelium requires several sequential steps (Davies 2009): physical deformation of the cell surface and intracellular transmission of stress (mechanotransmission) and conversion of mechanical force to chemical activity ("true" mechanotransduction), leading to a downstream biochemical signaling response with feedback (Figure 7.3). A number of membrane-associated molecules and membrane microdomains have been proposed as potential shear stress sensors, including ion channels, tyrosine kinases receptors, adhesion molecules, the glycocalyx, primary cilia, and caveolae (Wang 1993; Tzima 2005; Kwak 2014). Cytoskeletal filaments, distributed throughout the body of ECs, transmit the stress to multiple subcellular sites, where the coupling of mechanical forces to chemical activity occurs (Davies 1995; Malek 1996). Downstream signaling responses include the activation of secondary signaling pathways and of transcription factors regulating endothelial gene expression (proatherogenic genes vs. atheroprotective genes) (Chien 1998; Nagel 1999; Hay 2003). As a result, multiple biological responses are triggered, and, in the case of sustained blood flow alteration, the endothelium develops different adaptive phenotypes that

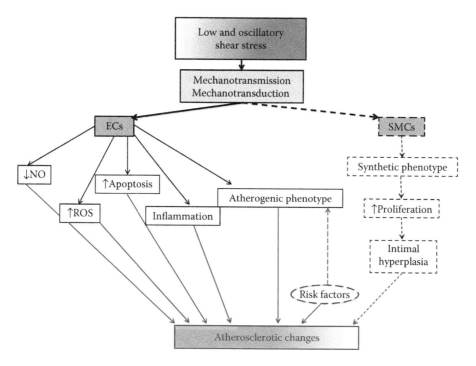

Figure 7.3 Schematic representing the mechanisms through which low and oscillatory shear stresses may participate in the initiation and progression of the atherosclerotic process.

may react differently with coexisting risk factors, such as high cholesterol, hypertension, obesity, diabetes, and smoking (Dai 2004; Passerini 2004).

Between the various shear-induced signaling molecules, NO and ROS have been shown to play a central role in vascular homeostasis and diseases (Hsieh 2014; Stocker 2004) (Figure 7.3). Nitric oxide exerts atheroprotective effects by preventing the expression of cell adhesion molecules, reducing platelet aggregation, inhibiting SMCs proliferation and ECs apoptosis, and regulating vascular permeability. Excessive ROS production causes a decrease in endothelial NO synthase (eNOS) expression and NO bioavailability, thus reducing its atheroprotective effect (Hsieh 2014). Furthermore, the imbalance between $O_2^{\bullet-}$ and NO results in the formation of peroxynitrite, a potent mediator of low-density lipoprotein (LDL) oxidation (White 1994; Hsiai 2007). Oxidized LDL is thought to promote atherosclerosis through complex inflammatory and immunological mechanisms that lead to lipid dysregulation and foam cell formation (Kita 2001).

Shear stress also regulates the vascular function of SMCs by changing their phenotypic behaviors, such as cell differentiation and proliferation (Figure 7.3). In regions of high shear stress, the alignment of SMCs is parallel to the shear stress direction; their proliferation is inhibited and depends on the cell-cycle arrest. By contrast, in regions of low shear stress, the alignment of SMCs is perpendicular to the shear stress direction, and their proliferation is accelerated (Sterpetti 1992 and 1993; Qiu 2013). Oscillatory shear stress also shifts the phenotypic transformation of SMCs toward the synthetic phenotype and induces their proliferation (Asada 2005).

7.4.1 Flow Pattern and Shear Stress

In a straight segment of artery, the hemodynamic flow pattern is typically laminar (Figure 7.4a) (Tortoli 2006 and 2011) and generates pulsatile, unidirectional shear stress whose magnitude varies between 1.5 and 3 Pa over the cardiac cycle. This unidirectional laminar shear stress enhances the production of NO via two mechanisms. Immediately after the onset of shear, there is an acute activation of the endothelial eNOS, leading to NO release within a few seconds. Over a period of several hours, shear stress stimulates eNOS mRNA expression (Nishida 1992; Fleming 1999; Davis 2004). Prolonged laminar shear stress also reduces $O_2^{\bullet-}$ formation (Boo 2003).

However, the vascular tree is not simply straight; it comprises curved, branched, and stenotic segments with complex hemodynamic features (Figure 7.4b), generating low, oscillatory (bidirectional), or high shear stress. In particular, in the area of inner curvature, a low (<1.0–1.5 Pa) unidirectional shear stress is present; at the lateral walls in a bifurcation, at the ostia of branches, and downstream of a stenosis, low oscillatory shear stress occurs; upstream and at the most stenotic site of plaque, high (>3.0 Pa) shear stress occurs (Thim 2012; Wentzel 2012). In vitro and in vivo animal studies have demonstrated that low shear stress and oscillatory shear stress increase $O_2^{\bullet-}$ and endothelin-1 production (Ziegler 1998; McNally 2003; Lu 2004; Ding 2015); provoke apoptosis of ECs (Tricot 2000); upregulate the expression of adhesion molecules and proinflammatory cytokines (Nagel 1994; Chappell 1998); induce oxidative transformation of LDL cholesterol and its subendothelial accumulation (White 1994; Asada 2005; Liu 2002); and promote SMCs differentiation, proliferation, and migration (Haga 2003; Goldman 2007) as well as extracellular matrix (ECM) degradation in the vascular wall and in the fibrous cap (Magid 2003; Chatzizisis 2011).

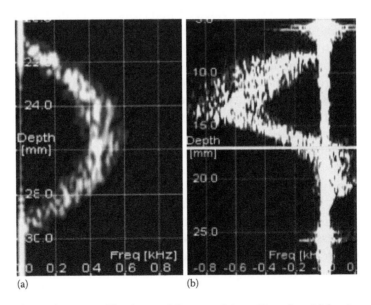

Figure 7.4 Flow velocity profile obtained from multigate Doppler: (a) laminar symmetric flow, and (b) flow in stenotic carotid artery.

Shear stress not only influences the initiation of the atherosclerotic process but also modifies plaque configuration, as the relationship between shear stress and atherosclerosis is reciprocal. As plaque develops, the flow, and, consequently, the shear stress around the plaque, adjusts (Figure 7.3b), which further shapes the plaque's growth and composition. In a setting of low shear stress and enhanced inflammation, the balance between ECM synthesis and degradation is shifted toward degradation (Magid 2003; Chatzizisis 2007 and 2011). Therefore, plaques in regions of low shear stress contain low amounts of SMCs and collagen, high quantities of macrophages, and large lipid cores. Inflammation and ECM degradation also involve the vascular media, promoting an excessive expansive remodeling that further exacerbates the low local shear stress (Chatzizisis 2007 and 2011; Koskinas 2010). Low shear stress fosters additional lipid accumulation and matrix degradation, thus increasing the vulnerability of the plaque. When expansive remodeling is exhausted, enduring plaque growth narrows the vascular lumen and, in so doing, alters the flow pattern and shear stress distribution around the plaque. The downstream segment of plaque is subjected to low shear stress, which could lead to apoptosis of ECs and inflammation and accumulation of macrophages. These processes reduce the tissue strength, yet they might be opposed by SMC proliferation and ECM synthesis, stimulated by augmented cyclic strain. Therefore, the atherosclerotic lesion may progress in the downstream region, but its risk of rupture is relatively low because of the stimuli activating SMCs (Williams 1998; Slager 2005). The upstream segment up to the point of maximal stenosis is exposed to high shear stress and shows enhanced accumulation of macrophages, intraplaque hemorrhage, thin fibrous cap, and a greater incidence of plaque rupture (Slager 2005; Cicha 2011; Morbiducci 2016). Several mechanisms have been suggested to explain cap destabilization induced by a high shear stress. High shear stress increases NO and plasmin production by the endothelium. Nitric oxide has been shown to suppress SMC proliferation and upregulate MMP expression by human macrophages, whereas plasmin has been shown to activate specific MMPs (MMP-1, -3, -9, -10, and -13) (Lijnen 2001; Death 2002; Kenagy 2002).

As can be seen, low, oscillatory, or high shear stresses are important determinants of the atherosclerotic process initiation and progression, as well as of plaque vulnerability. However, the endothelial response to shear stress is also modulated by the presence of risk factors such as hyperlipidemia, hypertension, and smoking (Edirisinghe 2010; Singh 2010; Koskinas 2013).

The evaluation of shear stress in clinical practice has become possible, thanks to the integration of different imaging techniques, such as computed tomography, intravascular Doppler US, and MRI, with computational flow dynamics (Yim 2005; Sui 2008; Chaichana 2013; Sun 2014). In addition, MRI and multigate Doppler (Figure 7.4a–b) can directly image flow profile patterns in arteries, together with the distribution and magnitude of wall shear stress (Tortoli 2006 and 2011; Sui 2008). Using these methods, the role of shear stress in atherosclerosis development and plaque vulnerability has been demonstrated in vivo. In patients with unilateral carotid plaques, wall shear stress in the common carotid artery with plaque was lower than that in the contralateral artery free of plaque (Gnasso 1997). In coronary arteries, regions of low shear stress developed progressive atherosclerosis and outward remodeling, areas of physiological shear stress remained quiescent, and areas of increased shear stress exhibited outward remodeling (Stone 2003). In coronary stents, the neointimal thickness was inversely correlated to shear stress (Wentzel 2001). Plaque ulceration in areas of high shear stress was demonstrated in the coronary and carotid arteries by intravascular US and MRI, respectively (Groen 2007; Fukumoto 2008; Tang 2009).

7.5 Arterial Wall Stretch/Stress and Atherosclerosis

The pulsatile nature of blood flow exposes the vessel to cyclic mechanical stretch or strain. Stretch describes the change in dimension of the vessel, and strain expresses the ratio of this change in dimension to its original dimension. The force per unit area that produces the deformation is called stress (Nichols et al. 2011). During systole, blood vessels experience both longitudinal and circumferential stretches that are counteracted by the vessels' elasticity. Under physiological conditions, a large elastic artery such as the aorta undergoes about 10% circumferential strain between diastole and systole (Bell 2014).

Cyclic stretch is the predominant mechanical factor that influences the structural organization and signaling of vascular SMCs (Figure 7.5). Similarly to ECs, SMCs are able to propagate mechanical signals from outside to inside the cell and convert mechanical stimuli into biochemical cues that ultimately lead to functional changes in vascular SMCs (mechanotransduction) (Ye 2014). Mechanosensitive proteins that capture and propagate mechanical signals within and between SMCs are integrin,

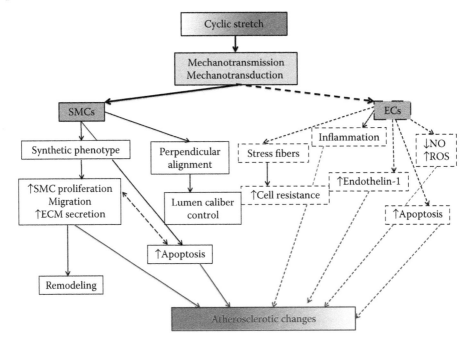

Figure 7.5 Schematic representing the mechanisms through which cyclic wall stretch may participate in the initiation and progression of the atherosclerotic process.

cadherin junctions, actin, intermediate filaments, and microtubules. Integrin proteins connect ECM to actin filaments within the cell, allowing forces to be transmitted from outside to inside the cells (Wiesner 2005). Cadherin junctions couple adjacent vascular SMCs together and propagate mechanical signals from one cell to the next (Ye 2014). Actin, intermediate filaments, and microtubules propagate mechanical signals throughout the cytoplasm of SMCs (Gimbrone 1975; Philippova 1998; Kim 2008). On sensing mechanical stimuli, the cell activates signaling pathways that mediate changes in SMC proliferation, migration, contraction, and gene expression.

Vascular SMCs in healthy adult vessels display a contractile phenotype, characterized by a slow proliferation rate and the expression of contractile markers. The contractile nature of SMCs allows them to regulate the myogenic vascular tone, blood pressure, and intravascular blood flow. In disease, SMCs switch from contractile to synthetic phenotype, which is characterized by decreased expression of contractile markers and increased rate of proliferation, migration, and secretion of ECM components.

Experimental data regarding the impact of stretch on SMC phenotype are contradicting, depending on the model used. In vitro studies on cultured cells have demonstrated that in response to cyclic stretch, vascular SMCs undergo phenotypic switching from contractile to synthetic phenotype (Hu 2014; Rodríguez 2015). By contrast, in ex vivo model, where the stretch was applied to a segment of portal vein, SMCs adopted a contractile pattern (Turczynska 2012). The discrepancy between both models may be explained by the fact that, in the wall of a real vessel, an interaction occurs between SMCs and ECs (Mantella 2015). Vascular SMCs cocultured with ECs display different gene expressions as compared with monocultured SMCs (Heydarkhan-Hagvall 2003).

As vascular SMCs adopt their synthetic phenotype, the rates of proliferation and migration increase. Indeed, in vitro studies have shown that cyclic stretch increases both proliferation and migration of SMCs through the activation of various mechanisms and pathways (Li 2003; Mata-Greenwood 2005; Chiu 2013; Scherer 2014; Song 2013). Stretch exposure also promotes apoptosis of vascular SMCs (Wernig 2003; Cheng 2012), and the fact that both proliferation and apoptosis are upregulated by stretch suggests the existence of a compensatory mechanism counteracting the increase or decrease in cell survival (Mantella 2015). Finally, stretch affects the alignment of vascular SMCs, and the alignment response to stretch seems to depend on its frequency and degree (Liu 2008). Graded stretch of cultured aortic SMCs caused a graded alignment of SMCs, from a minimum of completely random orientation to a maximum of approximately 80°–85° (nearly perpendicular) to the stretch vector (Standley 2002; Chen 2003). Anatomical alignment of vascular SMCs relative to the biophysical stretching exerted by pulsatile blood flow is important for the control of the vascular lumen caliber (Standley 2002).

Increased proliferation and migration of SMCs, together with increased ECM secretion, result in inward vascular remodeling, characterized by decreased vascular lumen, increased wall thickness, and increased vascular resistance. Such a remodeling allows the vessel to maintain an almost-normal wall stress in conditions of persistently increased blood pressure, as, according to the Laplace's law, the wall stress is directly proportional to intraluminal pressure and diameter and inversely proportional to wall thickness (Mayet 2003).

Mechanical stretch primarily affects the tunica media, that is, vascular SMCs; however, it also triggers biochemical signaling in ECs (Figure 7.5). Mechanoreceptor proteins that participate in stretch signal mechanotransduction in ECs are stretch-activated channels, integrin and focal adhesion kinase (Naruse 1998; Katsumi 2005; Zebda 2012). Within the cell, the stretch stimulates the occurrence of stress fibers, that is, actin filaments, which increase the resistance of the cell against the applied stress (Tojkander 2012). To minimize the alteration in intracellular strain, the stress fibers reorient perpendicularly to the direction of stretch (Wang 2001).

Similarly to shear stress, pathological stretch in ECs may alter the balance between NO and ROS in favor of ROS, stimulate the expression of proteins associated with the recruitment of inflammatory cells (interleukin-6, vascular cell adhesion molecule 1, and intercellular adhesion molecule), promote apoptosis of ECs, and increase MMP-2 and MMP-14 activity in the ECM (Kobayashi 2003; Wang 2003; Ali 2004; Kou 2009). Stretch was also found to increase endothelin-1 levels in human umbilical vein ECs (Cheng 2001). All these mechanisms may impair vascular homeostasis and initiate a cascade of alterations leading to atherosclerosis.

Estimation of the vascular mechanical load in vivo is usually performed by calculation of circumferential tensile wall stress (the cause) by using Laplace's equation (tensile stress = blood pressure × luminal diameter/wall thickness [Pa]) or the circumferential strain (the effect, defined as systolic luminal diameter − diastolic luminal diameter/diastolic luminal diameter [%]). Clinical studies using these approximations demonstrated that the arterial wall thickness increases with increasing tensile wall stress and that such an increase can be considered an adaptive intimal medial thickening and not an atherosclerotic process (Bots 1997; Chironi 2009; Kozakova 2008 and 2015; Palombo 2015).

7.6 Arterial Stiffness and Atherosclerosis

Numerous clinical studies have demonstrated the association between arterial stiffness and atherosclerotic burden (van Popele 2001; Oberoi 2013; Tsao 2014; Palombo 2016). Arterial stiffening reflects the degenerative changes in the ECM in the medial layer and is characterized by elastin fatigue fracture and collagen deposition and crosslinking. From the pathological point of view, arterial stiffening is distinct from atherosclerosis, which typically involves the intimal layer and is characterized by lipid accumulation, inflammatory cell and SMC migration, and foam cell formation. Yet, several factors have been suggested to link atherosclerosis to arterial stiffness, including the mechanical forces at the blood–wall interface. In fact, arterial stiffening alters the mechanical properties of the vascular wall and increases intraluminal blood pressure and thus the mechanical forces to which ECs and SMCs are exposed.

Arterial stiffening decreases wall compliance, and this, in turn, reduces cyclic stretch. Reduction in cyclic stretch has been shown to decrease eNOS activity

(Thacher 2010). In ECs cultured in distensible Silastic® tubes and exposed to realistic pulsatile perfusion, the combined phasic shear and stretch enhanced eNOS activity, whereas the eNOS activity was not stimulated in cells cultured in stiff tubes and exposed to identical pulsatile perfusion (Peng 2003). These observations suggest that the ability of the vessel wall to stretch affects endothelial mechanotransduction far more than a pulsatile flow stimulus. The decrease in cyclic stretch has also been shown to induce changes to SMCs phenotype and to increase MMP-2 expression (Gambillara 2008).

Within stiffer arteries, the speed of propagation of the arterial pulse through aorta is increased, and the increased speed of the forward traveling wave implies an earlier reflection of the backward wave from the periphery. The backward wave arrives at the ascending aorta in systole, instead of arriving in diastole, and this shift in timing leads to an augmentation of the aortic systolic pressure and to the generation of slow oscillating shear stress at the intima–lumen interface (Beraia 2014). As mentioned earlier, prolonged slow oscillating shear stress stimulates mitochondrial production of ROS, downregulates eNOS expression, and induces the expression of adhesion molecules and endothelin-1 (Chappell 1998; Ziegler 1998; Takabe 2011).

7.7 Role of Plaque Composition and Mechanical Forces in Plaque Vulnerability and Rupture

A plaque ruptures if the local stress exceeds the strength of the fibrous cap. The balance between local stress and fibrous cap strength is determined by the intrinsic properties of individual plaque (vulnerability) and by the extrinsic forces on the plaque (trigger force). Plaque geometry plays an important role in this relationship, as it determines the distribution and magnitude of hemodynamic forces, as well as the distribution of internal stresses (Kwak 2014; Lee 2017).

An ex vivo study of coronary plaque demonstrated that plaque containing eccentric lipid pools is fissured at the junction of the plaque cap with the more normal intima, and the computer modeling of different forms of plaque confirmed that, in systole, eccentric pools of lipid concentrate stress on the plaque cap near the edge of the plaque (Kumar 2005). The increased vulnerability of this shoulder region (Figure 7.2) also depends on shape of the lumen and geometry of remodeled vessel (Richardson 1989). Therefore, the entire vascular segment containing atherosclerotic plaque should be considered when studying the factors triggering plaque rupture. The concentration of mechanical stress in the fibrous cap is supposed to reflect the inability of the soft lipid core to bear the large mechanical stresses that develop during a sudden elevation of blood pressure. The softer the lipid core, the lesser the stress it can bear and, correspondingly, the more the stress redistributed to the adjacent fibrous cap (Falk 1995). Repetitive cyclic stretching, compression, bending, flexion, shear, and pressure fluctuations may fatigue and weaken the fibrous cap, which may ultimately rupture spontaneously, that is, without being triggered by a sudden increase in blood pressure. Yet, the rupture is not always located in the area of greatest stress. Histological findings have shown that the site of tearing is also influenced by the variation in the mechanical strength of the cap tissue due to the focal accumulation of macrophages and foam cells that represent weak points in the fibrous cap (Richardson 1989; Lendon 1991).

The role of plaque composition in plaque vulnerability has been clearly established (Shah 2003; Gupta 2013), and the capability of different imaging techniques to determine the structure of atherosclerotic plaque has been tested (Goel 2015). Magnetic resonance imaging is able to provide information on the thickness of the fibrous cap and possible irregularities and discontinuities at its surface, as well as on the volume of the lipid-rich necrotic core, intraplaque hemorrhage, neovascularization, and signs of vascular wall inflammation (Fayad 2001; Saloner 2007; Goel 2015). Ultrasonography can provide useful data on intraplaque hemorrhage, inflammation, lipid core, vasa vasorum, and neovascularization (Puato 2003; Claessen 2012; Goel 2015). Optical coherence tomography (OCT) can supply detailed information on plaque composition, macrophage infiltration, and fibrous cap thickness (van Soest G 2009), whereas positron emission tomography (PET) seems to be a promising tool for the detection of inflammation (Rudd 2007). Both MRI and US may also depict plaque geometry and surface, as well as the geometry of the surrounding remodeled vessel (Yao 1998; Fenster 2006; Saloner 2007).

The appraisal of the interplay between mechanical forces and atherosclerotic plaque is challenging, as vascular structures and plaques are composed of various materials with different mechanical properties (Arroyo 1999). Furthermore, it is difficult to replicate the mechanical behavior of diseased tissue in vivo, and access to human tissue for in vitro mechanical testing is limited. Therefore, computational analyses mimicking the vivo environment have been introduced. Finite element (FE) analysis, allowing for the evaluation of complex structures by breaking them down into smaller simpler sections, has been used to assess the three-dimensional stress distribution within plaque of certain geometrical and structural characteristics under certain loading and boundary conditions (Li 2008; Holzapfel 2014). The stress distributions in plaque have been shown to be a function of both the geometry and mechanical properties of the tissue (Vito 2003).

In computational analyses, the arterial tissue is considered nonlinearly elastic and anisotropic. It is treated as a fiber-reinforced material, with fibers corresponding to the collagenous component of the material, and is modeled by an anisotropic strain-energy function (Holzapfel 2014). Important determinants of plaque rupture used in FE models are the level and location of the peak circumferential stress, which has been suggested to govern plaque failure (Mohan 1983; Cheng 1993). An experimental study comparing coronary artery lesions causing lethal myocardial infarction with stable coronary lesions demonstrated that, at a mean intraluminal pressure of 110 mmHg, plaque rupture occurred in a region where computed stress was higher than 300 kPa (Cheng 1993). Currently, this value is used in the majority of FE studies as a threshold stress value that induces rupture. However, in vivo plaque rupture, as previously mentioned, does not always occur in the region of highest stress, and, on the other hand, not every plaque ruptures at a stress level of 300 kPa. Cap inclusions located in the area of high stress, such as calcified macrophages and SMCs that have undergone apoptosis, can increase the stress to nearly 600 kPa when the cap thickness is less than 65 μm (Vengrenyuk 2006). Another possible hemodynamic mechanism of plaque rupture may exist through the axial tensile stress induced by the blood pressure drop over a severely stenotic lesion in conditions of high blood flow. Computational fluid dynamic analyses have shown that a pressure drop of 20 mmHg could induce more than 10 kPa of axial tensile stress in a 75-μm-thick cap (Doriot 2003; Slager 2005).

However, it should be considered that the arterial geometry extracted from in vivo imaging (MRI, US, CT, and PET) is not in a stress-free state, as the arterial tissue is submitted to different loading forces, such as pulsatile pressure and longitudinal tension. Ignoring these initial stresses in computational models may affect the resulting peak cap stress in different plaque geometries (Speelman 2011). Finally, most of the biological tissues, including the arterial wall, are not free of stress, even when all external loads are removed. The stresses and strains that remain in a vessel free of external load (at zero blood pressure) are termed "residual" and have proved to be important in determining the wall stress distribution under physiological pressure (Greenwald 1997; Ohayon 2007). An ex vivo study of human vulnerable plaque has demonstrated that residual stress/strain present in vulnerable plaque dramatically influences the spatial stress distribution and highlights new sites of stress concentration (Wang 2017). Some FE studies have reported that the inclusion of residual stresses/strains in the arterial model allows for a more accurate evaluation of stress distribution within atherosclerotic plaque (Ohayon 2007; Wang 2017).

Finite element studies of diseased arteries confirmed that the lipid pool size and the thickness of fibrous cap are key structural features defining the risk of plaque rupture (Versluis 2006; Holzapfel 2007; Akyildiz 2011). They also indicated that the most common rupture point is at the shoulder of the cap (Cheng 1993; Imoto 2005) (Figure 7.2). The limitations of these studies stem from the generalized assumptions made about the material properties, residual stresses, and rupture threshold values included in the mathematical models.

7.8 Conclusion

Mechanical forces play an important role in the initiation and progression of atherosclerotic process, as well as in the destabilization of advanced atherosclerotic lesions. The interactions between mechanical forces and biological factors, as well as the relationships between flow, pressure, and material properties of the vessel wall, are extremely complex and vary from one individual to another. Thus, an accurate assessment of the impact of mechanical factors on the vessel wall in each individual patient is not currently possible. Yet, using different imaging techniques, useful information can be obtained regarding blood flow velocity, volume, and profile; geometry and stiffness of atherosclerotic lesions and the surrounding vessel; and plaque volume, composition, and inflammation. Correct interpretation of these data, together with the knowledge of vascular biology and the use of computational analysis, may help in clinical decision-making and/or cardiovascular risk prevention. Some progress has already been made in the field of plaque stabilization, toward altering the structure, content, or function of the plaque and/or its overlying endothelium, to either prevent or reduce the severity of plaque rupture.

References

Akyildiz AC, Speelman L, van Brummelen H et al. 2011. Effects of intima stiffness and plaque morphology on peak cap stress. *Biomed Eng Online* 10:25.

Ali MH, Pearlstein DP, Mathieu CE, Schumacker PT. 2004. Mitochondrial requirement for endothelial responses to cyclic strain: Implications for mechanotransduction. *Am J Physiol Lung Cell Mol Physiol* 287:L486–L496.

Arroyo LH, Lee RT. 1999. Mechanisms of plaque rupture: Mechanical and biologic interactions. *Cardiovasc Res* 41:369–375.

Asada H, Paszkowiak J, Teso D et al. 2005. Sustained orbital shear stress stimulates smooth muscle cell proliferation via the extracellular signal-regulated protein kinase 1/2 pathway. *J Vasc Surg* 44:772–780.

Badimon L, Vilahur G. 2014. Thrombosis formation on atherosclerotic lesions and plaque rupture. *J Intern Med* 276:618–632.

Baigent C, Blackwell L, Emberson J et al.; Cholesterol Treatment Trialists' (CTT) Collaboration. 2010. Efficacy and safety of more intensive lowering of LDL cholesterol: A meta-analysis of data from 170,000 participants in 26 randomised trials. *Lancet* 376:1670–1681.

Barquera S, Pedroza-Tobías A, Medina C et al. 2015. Global overview of the epidemiology of atherosclerotic cardiovascular disease. *Arch Med Res* 46:328–338.

Bell V, Mitchell WA, Sigurðsson S et al. 2014. Longitudinal and circumferential strain of the proximal aorta. *J Am Heart Assoc* 3:e001536.

Beraia G, Beraia M. 2014. Wave reflection at the boundary layers and initial factors of atherosclerosis. *Int J Med Phys Clin Eng Rad Oncol* 3:71–81.

Bonetti PO, Lerman LO, Lerman A. 2003. Endothelial dysfunction: A marker of atherosclerosis risk. *Atheroscler Thromb Vasc Biol* 23:168–175.

Boo YC, Jo H. 2003. Flow-dependent regulation of endothelial nitric oxide synthase: Role of protein kinases. *Am J Physiol Cell Physiol* 285:C499–C508.

Bots ML, Hofman A, Grobbee DE. 1997. Increased common carotid artery intima-media thickness. Adaptive response or a reflection of atherosclerosis? Finding from the Rotterdam study. *Stroke* 28:2442–2447.

Bretón-Romero R, Lamas S. 2014. Hydrogen peroxide signaling in vascular endothelial cells. *Redox Biol* 2:529–534.

Burke AP, Farb A, Malcom GT, Liang YH, Smialek J, Virmani R. 1997. Coronary risk factors and plaque morphology in men with coronary disease who died suddenly. *N Engl J Med* 336:1276–1282.

Burke AP, Kolodgie FD, Farb A et al. 2001. Healed plaque ruptures and sudden coronary death: Evidence that subclinical rupture has a role in plaque progression. *Circulation* 103:934–940.

Chaichana T, Sun Z, Jewkes J. 2013. Haemodynamic analysis of the effect of different types of plaques in the left coronary artery. *Comput Med Imaging Graph* 37:197–206.

Chappell DC, Varner SE, Nerem RM, Medford RM, Alexander RW. 1998. Oscillatory shear stress stimulates adhesion molecule expression in cultured human endothelium. *Circ Res* 82:532–539.

Chatzizisis YS, Baker AB, Sukhova GK et al. 2011. Augmented expression and activity of extracellular matrix-degrading enzymes in regions of low endothelial shear stress colocalize with coronary atheromata with thin fibrous caps in pigs. *Circulation* 123:621–630.

Chatzizisis YS, Coskun AU, Jonas M, Edelman ER, Feldman CL, Stone PH. 2007. Role of endothelial shear stress in the natural history of coronary atherosclerosis and vascular remodeling: Molecular, cellular, and vascular behavior. *J Am Coll Cardiol* 49:2379–2393.

Chen Q, Li W, Quan Z, Sumpio BE. 2003. Modulation of vascular smooth muscle cell alignment by cyclic strain is dependent on reactive oxygen species and P38 mitogen-activated protein kinase. *J Vasc Surg* 37:660–668.

Chen Z, Ichetovkin M, Kurtz M et al. 2010. Cholesterol in human atherosclerotic plaque is a marker for underlying disease state and plaque vulnerability. *Lipids Health Dis* 9:61.

Cheng GC, Loree HM, Kamm RD, Fishbein MC, Lee RT. 1993. Distribution of circumferential stress in ruptured and stable atherosclerotic lesions. A structural analysis with histopathological correlation. *Circulation* 87:1179–1187.

Cheng TH, Shih NL, Chen SY et al. 2001. Reactive oxygen species mediate cyclic strain-induced endothelin-1 gene expression via ras/raf/extracellular signal-regulated kinase pathway in endothelial cells. *J Mol Cell Cardiol* 33:1805–1814.

Cheng WP, Wang BW, Chen SC, Chang H, Shyu KG. 2012. Mechanical stretch induces the apoptosis regulator PUMA in vascular smooth muscle cells. *Cardiovasc Res* 93:181–189.

Chien S, Li S, Shyy YJ. 1998. Effects of mechanical forces on signal transduction and gene expression in endothelial cells. *Hypertension* 31:162–169.

Chironi GN, Simon A, Bokov P, Levenson J. 2009. Correction of carotid intima-media thickness for adaptive dependence on tensile stress: Implication for cardiovascular risk assessment. *J Clin Ultrasound* 37:270–275.

Chiu CZ, Wang BW, Shyu KG. 2013. Effects of cyclic stretch on the molecular regulation of myocardin in rat aortic vascular smooth muscle cells. *J Biomed Sci* 20:50.

Cicha I, Wörner A, Urschel K et al. 2011. Carotid plaque vulnerability: A positive feedback between hemodynamic and biochemical mechanisms. *Stroke* 42:3502–3510.

Claessen BE, Maehara A, Fahy M, Xu K, Stone GW, Mintz GS. 2012. Plaque composition by intravascular ultrasound and distal embolization after percutaneous coronary intervention. *JACC Cardiovasc Imaging* 5:S111–S118.

Clark JM, Glagov S. 1979. Structural changes of arterial wall. I: Relationships and attachment of medial smooth muscle cells in normally distended and hyperdistended aortas. *Lab Invest* 40:587–602.

Clark JM, Glagov S. 1985. Transmural organization of the arterial wall: The lamellar unit revisited. *Atherosclerosis* 5:19–34.

Clarke MC, Bennett MR. 2009. Cause or consequence: What does macrophage apoptosis do in atherosclerosis? *Arterioscler Thromb Vasc Biol* 29:153–155.

Dai G, Kaazempur-Mofrad MR, Natarajan S et al. 2004. Distinct endothelial phenotypes evoked by arterial waveforms derived from atherosclerosis-susceptible and -resistant regions of human vasculature. *Proc Natl Acad Sci U S A* 101:14871–14876.

Davis ME, Grumbach IM, Fukai T, Cutchins A, Harrison DG. 2004. Shear stress regulates endothelial nitric-oxide synthase promoter activity through nuclear factor κB binding. *J Biol Chem* 279:163–168.

Davies PF. 1995. Flow-mediated endothelial mechanotransduction. *Physiol Rev* 75:519–560.

Davies PF. 2009. Hemodynamic shear stress and the endothelium in cardiovascular pathophysiology. *Nat Clin Pract Cardiovasc Med* 6:16–26.

Deanfield JE, Halcox JP, Rabelink TJ. 2007. Endothelial function and dysfunction: Testing and clinical relevance. *Circulation* 115:1285–1295.

Death AK, Nakhla S, McGrath KC et al. 2002. Nitroglycerin upregulates matrix metalloproteinase expression by human macrophages. *J Am Coll Cardiol* 39:1943–1950.

DeMaria AN, Narula J, Mahmud E, Tsimikas S. 2006. Imaging vulnerable plaque by ultrasound. *J Am Coll Cardiol* 47:C32–C39.

Ding Z, Liu S, Wang X et al. 2015. Hemodynamic shear stress via ROS modulates PCSK9 expression in human vascular endothelial and smooth muscle cells and along the mouse aorta. *Antioxid Redox Signal* 22:760–771.

Doll R, Peto R, Boreham J, Sutherland I. 2005. Mortality in relation to smoking: 50 years' observations on male British doctors. *Br J Cancer* 92:426–429.

Doriot PA. 2003. Estimation of the supplementary axial wall stress generated at peak flow by an arterial stenosis. *Phys Med Biol* 48:127–138.

Edirisinghe I, Rahman I. 2010. Cigarette smoke-mediated oxidative stress, shear stress, and endothelial dysfunction: Role of VEGFR2. *Ann N Y Acad Sci* 1203:66–72.

Falk E, Shah PK, Fuster V. 1995. Coronary plaque disruption. *Circulation* 92:657–671.

Fayad ZA. 2001. The assessment of the vulnerable atherosclerotic plaque using MR imaging: A brief review. *Int J Cardiovasc Imaging* 17:165–177.

Fenster A, Blake C, Gyacskov I, Landry A, Spence JD. 2006. 3D ultrasound analysis of carotid plaque volume and surface morphology. *Ultrasonics* 44:e153–e157.

Fishbein MC, Siegel RJ. 1996. How big are coronary atherosclerotic plaques that rupture? *Circulation* 94:2662–2666.

Fleming I, Busse R. 1999. Signal transduction of eNOS activation. *Cardiovasc Res* 43:532–541.

Fukumoto Y, Hiro T, Fujii T et al. 2008. Localized elevation of shear stress is related to coronary plaque rupture: A 3-dimensional intravascular ultrasound study with *in-vivo* color mapping of shear stress distribution. *J Am Coll Cardiol* 51:645–650.

Gambillara V, Thatcher T, Silacci P, Stergiopulos N. 2008. Effects of reduced cyclic stretch on vascular smooth muscle cell function of pig carotids perfused *ex vivo*. *Am J Hypertens* 21:425–431.

Gimbrone MA Jr, Cotran RS. 1975. Human vascular smooth muscle in culture. Growth and ultrastructure. *Lab Invest* 33:16–27.

Gimbrone MA Jr, Topper JN, Nagel T, Anderson KR, Garcia-Cardeña G. 2000. Endothelial dysfunction, hemodynamic forces, and atherogenesis. *Ann N Y Acad Sci* 902:230–239.

Gnasso A, Irace C, Carallo C et al. 1997. *In vivo* association between low wall shear stress and plaque in subjects with asymmetrical carotid atherosclerosis. *Stroke* 28:993–998.

Goel S, Miller A, Agarwal C et al. 2015. Imaging modalities to identity inflammation in an atherosclerotic plaque. *Radiol Res Pract* 2015:410967.

Goldman J, Zhong L, Liu SQ. 2007. Negative regulation of vascular smooth muscle cell migration by blood shear stress. *Am J Physiol Heart Circ Physiol* 292:H928–H938.

Greenwald SE, Moore JE Jr, Rachev A, Kane TP, Meister JJ. 1997. Experimental investigation of the distribution of residual strains in the artery wall. *J Biomech Eng* 119:438–444.

Groen H, Gijsen F, van der Lugt A et al. 2007. Plaque rupture in the carotid artery is localized at the high shear stress region: A case report. *Stroke* 38:2379–2381.

Gupta A, Baradaran H, Schweitzer AD et al. 2013. Carotid plaque MRI and stroke risk: A systematic review and meta-analysis. *Stroke* 44:3071–3077.

Guyton JR, Klemp KF. 1993. Transitional features in human atherosclerosis. Intimal thickening, cholesterol clefts, and cell loss in human aortic fatty streaks. *Am J Pathol* 143:1444–1457.

Haga M, Yamashita A, Paszkowiak J, Sumpio BE, Dardik A. 2003. Oscillatory shear stress increases smooth muscle cell proliferation and Akt phosphorylation. *J Vasc Surg* 37:1277–1284.

Hansson GK, Libby P, Tabas I. 2015. Inflammation and plaque vulnerability. *J Intern Med* 278:483–493.

Hay DC, Beers C, Cameron V, Thomson L, Flitney FW, Hay RT. 2003. Activation of NF-kappaB nuclear transcription factor by flow in human endothelial cells. *Biochim Biophys Acta* 1642:33–44.

Herrington W, Lacey B, Sherliker P, Armitage J, Lewington S. 2016. Epidemiology of atherosclerosis and the potential to reduce the global burden of atherothrombotic disease. *Circ Res* 118:535–546.

Heydarkhan-Hagvall S, Helenius G, Johansson BR, Li JY, Mattsson E, Risberg B. 2003. Co-culture of endothelial cells and smooth muscle cells affects gene expression of angiogenic factors. *J Cell Biochem* 89:1250–1259.

Holzapfel GA, Sommer G, Auer M, Regitnig P, Ogden RW. 2007. Layer-specific 3D residual deformations of human aortas with non-atherosclerotic intimal thickening. *Ann Biomed Eng* 35:530–545.

Holzapfel GA, Mulvihill JJ, Cunnane EM, Walsh MT. 2014. Computational approaches for analyzing the mechanics of atherosclerotic plaques: A review. *J Biomech* 47:859–869.

Hsiai TK, Hwang J, Barr ML et al. 2007. Hemodynamics influences vascular peroxynitrite formation: Implication for low-density lipoprotein apo-B-100 nitration. *Free Radical Bio Med* 42:519–529.

Hsieh HJ, Liu CA, Huang B, Tseng AH, Wang DL. 2014. Shear-induced endothelial mechanotransduction: The interplay between reactive oxygen species (ROS) and nitric oxide (NO) and the pathophysiological implications. *J Biomed Sci* 21:3.

Hu B, Song JT, Qu HY et al. 2014. Mechanical stretch suppresses microRNA-145 expression by activating extracellular signal-regulated kinase 1/2 and upregulating angiotensin-converting enzyme to alter vascular smooth muscle cell phenotype. *PLoS One* 9:e96338.

Imoto K, Hiro T, Fujii T et al. 2005. Longitudinal structural determinants of atherosclerotic plaque vulnerability: A computational analysis of stress distribution using vessel models and three-dimensional intravascular ultrasound imaging. *J Am Coll Cardiol* 46:1507–1515.

Jufri NF, Mohamedali A, Avolio A, Baker MS. 2015. Mechanical stretch: Physiological and pathological implications for human vascular endothelial cells. *Vasc Cell* 7:8.

Katsumi A, Naoe T, Matsushita T, Kaibuchi K, Schwartz MA. 2005. Integrin activation and matrix binding mediate cellular responses to mechanical stretch. *J Biol Chem* 280:16546–16549.

Kenagy RD, Fischer JW, Davies MG et al. 2002. Increased plasmin and serine proteinase activity during flow-induced intimal atrophy in baboon PTFE grafts. *Arterioscler Thromb Vasc Biol* 22:400–404.

Kim HR, Gallant C, Leavis PC, Gunst SJ, Morgan KG. 2008. Cytoskeletal remodeling in differentiated vascular smooth muscle is actin isoform dependent and stimulus dependent. *Am J Physiol Cell Physiol* 295:C768–C778.

Kita T, Kume N, Minami M et al. 2001. Role of oxidized LDL in atherosclerosis. *Ann N Y Acad Sci* 947:199–205.

Kobayashi S, Nagino M, Komatsu S et al. 2003. Stretch-induced IL-6 secretion from endothelial cells requires NF-kappaB activation. *Biochem Biophys Res Commun* 308:306–312.

Kondos GT, Hoff JA, Sevrukov A et al. 2003. Electron-beam tomography coronary artery calcium and cardiac events: A 37-month follow-up of 5635 initially asymptomatic low- to intermediate-risk adults. *Circulation* 107:2571–2576.

Koskinas KC, Chatzizisis YS, Papafaklis MI et al. 2013. Synergistic effect of local endothelial shear stress and systemic hypercholesterolemia on coronary atherosclerotic plaque progression and composition in pigs. *Int J Cardiol* 169:394–401.

Koskinas KC, Feldman CL, Chatzizisis YS et al. 2010. Natural history of experimental coronary atherosclerosis and vascular remodeling in relation to endothelial shear stress: A serial, in vivo intravascular ultrasound study. *Circulation* 121:2092–2101.

Kou B, Zhang J, Singer DR. 2009. Effects of cyclic strain on endothelial cell apoptosis and tubulogenesis are dependent on ROS production via NAD(P)H subunit p22phox. *Microvasc Res* 77:125–133.

Kozakova M, Palombo C, Morizzo C et al. 2015. Obesity and carotid artery remodeling. *Nutr Diabetes* 5:e177.

Kozakova M, Palombo C, Paterni M et al. 2008. Relationship between insulin sensitivity cardiovascular risk Investigators. Body composition and common carotid artery remodeling in a healthy population. *J Clin Endocrinol Metab* 93:3325–3332.

Kragel AH, Reddy SG, Wittes JT, Roberts WC. 1989. Morphometric analysis of the composition of atherosclerotic plaques in the four major epicardial coronary arteries in acute myocardial infarction and in sudden coronary death. *Circulation* 80:1747–1756.

Kuiper J, van Puijvelde GH, van Wanrooij EJ et al. 2007. Immunomodulation of the inflammatory response in atherosclerosis. *Curr Opin Lipidol* 18:521–526.

Kumar RK, Balakrishnan KR. 2005. Influence of lumen shape and vessel geometry on plaque stresses: Possible role in the increased vulnerability of a remodelled vessel and the "shoulder" of a plaque. *Heart* 91:1459–1465.

Kwak BR, Bäck M, Bochaton-Piallat ML et al. 2014. Biomechanical factors in atherosclerosis: Mechanisms and clinical implications. *Eur Heart J* 35:3013–3020.

Lee JM, Choi G, Hwang D et al. 2017. Impact of longitudinal lesion geometry on location of plaque rupture and clinical presentations. *JACC Cardiovasc Imaging* 10:677–688.

Lendon CL, Davies MJ, Born GVR, Richardson PD. 1991. Atherosclerotic plaque caps are locally weakened when macrophage density is increased. *Atherosclerosis* 87:87–90.

Li C, Wernig F, Leitges M, Hu Y, Xu Q. 2003. Mechanical stress-activated PKCdelta regulates smooth muscle cell migration. *FASEB J* 17:2106–2108.

Li YS, Haga JH, Chien S. 2005. Molecular basis of the effects of shear stress on vascular endothelial cells. *J Biomech* 38:1949–1971.

Li ZY, Tang T, U-King-Im J, Graves M, Sutcliffe M, Gillard JH. 2008. Assessment of carotid plaque vulnerability using structural and geometrical determinants. *Circ J* 72:1092–1099.

Li ZY, Taviani V, Tang T et al. 2009. The mechanical triggers of plaque rupture: Shear stress vs pressure gradient. *Br J Radiol* 82:S39–S45.

Lijnen HR. 2001. Plasmin and matrix metalloproteinases in vascular remodeling. *Thromb Haemost* 86:324–333.

Liu Y, Chen BP, Lu M et al. 2002. Shear stress activation of SREBP1 in endothelial cells is mediated by integrins. *Arterioscler Thromb Vasc Biol* 22:76–81.

Liu B, Qu MJ, Qin KR et al. 2008. Role of cyclic strain frequency in regulating the alignment of vascular smooth muscle cells in vitro. *Biophys J* 94:1497–1507.

Lu X, Kassab GS. 2004. Nitric oxide is significantly reduced in ex vivo porcine arteries during reverse flow because of increased superoxide production. *J Physiol Lond* 561:575–582.

Magid R, Murphy TJ, Galis ZS. 2003. Expression of matrix metalloproteinase-9 in endothelial cells is differentially regulated by shear stress. Role of c-Myc. *J Biol Chem* 278:32994–32999.

Malek AM, Izumo S. 1996. Mechanism of endothelial cell shape change and cytoskeletal remodeling in response to fluid shear stress. *J Cell Sci* 109:713–726.

Mannarino E, Pirro M. 2008. Molecular biology of atherosclerosis. *Clin Cases Miner Bone Metab* 5:57–62.

Mantella LE, Quan A, Verma S. 2015. Variability in vascular smooth muscle cell stretch-induced responses in 2D culture. *Vasc Cell* 7:7.

Mata-Greenwood E, Grobe A, Kumar S, Noskina Y, Black SM. 2005. Cyclic stretch increases VEGF expression in pulmonary arterial smooth muscle cells via TGF-beta1 and reactive oxygen species: A requirement for NAD(P)H oxidase. *Am J Physiol Lung Cell Mol Physiol* 289:L288–L289.

Mayet J, Hughes A. 2003. Cardiac and vascular pathophysiology in hypertension. *Heart* 89:1104–1109.

McNally JS, Davis ME, Giddens DP et al. 2003. Role of xanthine oxidoreductase and NAD(P)H oxidase in endothelial superoxide production in response to oscillatory shear stress. *Am J Physiol Heart Circ Physiol* 285:H2290–H2297.

Milei J, Ottaviani G, Lavezzi AM, Grana DR, Stella I, Matturri L. 2008. Perinatal and infant early atherosclerotic coronary lesions. *Can J Cardiol* 24:137–141.

Mittleman MA, Mostofsky E. 2011. Physical, psychological and chemical triggers of acute cardiovascular events: Preventive strategies. *Circulation* 124:346–354.

Mohan D, Melvin JW. 1983. Failure properties of passive human aortic tissue. II—Biaxial tension tests. *J Biomech* 16:31–44.

Moore KJ, Tabas I. 2011. Macrophages in the pathogenesis of atherosclerosis. *Cell* 145:341–355.

Morbiducci U, Kok AM, Kwak BR, Stone PH, Steinman DA, Wentzel JJ. 2016. Atherosclerosis at arterial bifurcations: Evidence for the role of haemodynamics and geometry. *Thromb Haemost* 115:484–492.

Moreno PR, Falk E, Palacios IF, Newell JB, Fuster V, Fallon JT. 1994. Macrophage infiltration in acute coronary syndromes. Implications for plaque rupture. *Circulation* 90:775–778.

Nagel T, Resnick N, Atkinson WJ, Dewey CF Jr, Gimbrone MA Jr. 1994. Shear stress selectively upregulates intercellular adhesion molecule-1 expression in cultured human vascular endothelial cells. *J Clin Invest* 94:885–891.

Nagel T, Resnick N, Dewey CF Jr, Gimbrone MA Jr. 1999. Vascular endothelial cells respond to spatial gradients in fluid shear stress by enhanced activation of transcription factors. *Arterioscler Thromb Vasc Biol* 19:1825–1832.

Nambi V, Chambless L, Folsom AR et al. 2010. Carotid intima-media thickness and presence or absence of plaque improves prediction of coronary heart disease risk: The ARIC (Atherosclerosis Risk In Communities) Study. *J Am Coll Cardiol* 55:1600–1607.

Napoli C, D'Armiento FP, Mancini FP et al. 1997. Fatty streak formation occurs in human fetal aortas and is greatly enhanced by maternal hypercholesterolemia. Intimal accumulation of low density lipoprotein and its oxidation precede monocyte recruitment into early atherosclerotic lesions. *J Clin Invest* 100:2680–2690.

Naruse K, Yamada T, Sokabe M. 1998. Involvement of SA channels in orienting response of cultured endothelial cells to cyclic stretch. *Am J Physiol* 274:H1532–H1538.

Nichols WW, O'Rourke MF, Vlachopoulos C. 2011. Properties of the arterial wall: Theory. In: *McDonald's Blood Flow in Arteries. Theoretical, Experimental and Clinical Principles*, Nichols WW, O'Rourke MF, Vlachopoulos C (Eds.), pp. 55–76. London, UK, Hooder Arnold.

Ninomiya T, Perkovic V, Turnbull F et al.; Blood Pressure Lowering Treatment Trialists' Collaboration. 2013. Blood pressure lowering and major cardiovascular events in people with and without chronic kidney disease: Meta-analysis of randomised controlled trials. *BMJ* 347:f5680.

Nishida K, Harrison DG, Navas JP et al. 1992. Molecular cloning and characterization of the constitutive bovine aortic endothelial cell nitric oxide synthase. *J Clin Invest* 90:2092–2096.

Oberoi S, Schoepf UJ, Meyer M et al. 2013. Progression of arterial stiffness and coronary atherosclerosis: Longitudinal evaluation by cardiac CT. *AJR Am J Roentgenol* 200:798–804.

Ohayon J, Dubreuil O, Tracqui P et al. 2007. Influence of residual stress/strain on the biomechanical stability of vulnerable coronary plaques: Potential impact for evaluating the
risk of plaque rupture. *Am J Physiol Heart Circ Physiol* 293:H1987–H1996.

Palombo C, Kozakova M. 2016. Arterial stiffness, atherosclerosis and cardiovascular risk:
Pathophysiologic mechanisms and emerging clinical indications. *Vascul Pharmacol* 77:1–7.

Palombo C, Morizzo C, Baluci M et al. 2015. Large artery remodeling and dynamics following simulated microgravity by prolonged head-down tilt bed rest in humans. *Biomed
Res Int* 2015:342565.

Passerini AG, Polacek DC, Shi G et al. 2004. Coexisting proinflammatory and antioxidative
endothelial transcription profiles in a disturbed flow region of the adult porcine aorta.
Proc Natl Acad Sci U S A 101:2482–2487.

Peng X, Haldar S, Deshpande S, Irani K, Kass DA. 2003. Wall stiffness suppresses Akt/eNOS
and cytoprotection in pulse-perfused endothelium. *Hypertension* 41:378–381.

Philippova MP, Bochkov VN, Stambolsky DV, Tkachuk VA, Resink TJ. 1998. T-cadherin
and signal-transducing molecules co-localize in caveolin-rich membrane domains of
vascular smooth muscle cells. *FEBS Lett* 429:207–210.

Puato M, Faggin E, Rattazzi M et al.; Study Group on Arterial Wall Structure. 2003. In vivo
noninvasive identification of cell composition of intimal lesions: A combined approach
with ultrasonography and immunocytochemistry. *J Vasc Surg* 38:1390–1395.

Qiu J, Zheng Y, Hu J et al. 2013. Biomechanical regulation of vascular smooth muscle cell
functions: From in vitro to in vivo understanding. *J R Soc Interface* 11:20130852.

Rajendran P, Rengarajan T, Thangavel J et al. 2013. The vascular endothelium and human
diseases. *Int J Biol Sci* 9:1057–1069.

Rhee SG. 2006. Cell signaling: H_2O_2, a necessary evil for cell signaling. Science 312:1882–1883.

Richardson PD, Davies MJ, Born GV. 1989. Influence of plaque configuration and stress distribution on fissuring of coronary atherosclerotic plaques. *Lancet* 2:941–944.

Rodríguez AI, Csányi G, Ranayhossaini DJ et al. 2015. MEF2B-Nox1 signaling is critical for
stretch-induced phenotypic modulation of vascular smooth muscle cells. *Arterioscler
Thromb Vasc Biol* 35:430–438.

Rudd JH, Myers KS, Bansilal S et al. 2007. (18)Fluorodeoxyglucose positron emission
tomography imaging of atherosclerotic plaque inflammation is highly reproducible:
Implications for atherosclerosis therapy trials. *J Am Coll Cardiol* 50:892–896.

Saloner D, Acevedo-Bolton G, Wintermark M, Rapp JH. 2007. MRI of geometric and compositional features of vulnerable carotid plaque. *Stroke* 38:637–641.

Scherer C, Pfisterer L, Wagner AH et al. 2014. Arterial wall stress controls NFAT5 activity in
vascular smooth muscle cells. *J Am Heart Assoc* 3:e000626.

Schwartz SM, deBlois D, O'Brien ER. 1995. The intima. Soil for atherosclerosis and restenosis.
Circ Res 77:445–465.

Shah K. 2003. Mechanisms of plaque vulnerability and rupture. *J Am Coll Cardiol* 41:S15–S22.

Shah PK, Galis ZS. 2001. Matrix metalloproteinase hypothesis of plaque rupture: Players
keep piling up but questions remain. *Circulation* 104:1878–1880.

Singh PK, Marzo A, Howard B et al. 2010. Effects of smoking and hypertension on wall shear
stress and oscillatory shear index at the site of intracranial aneurysm formation. *Clin
Neurol Neurosurg* 112:306–313.

Slager CJ, Wentzel JJ, Gijsen FJ et al. 2005. The role of shear stress in the generation of
rupture-prone vulnerable plaques. *Nat Clin Pract Cardiovasc Med* 2:401–407.

Song L, Yang J, Duan P et al. 2013. Downregulation of miR-223 and miR-153 mediates mechanical stretch-stimulated proliferation of venous smooth muscle cells via activation of the insulin-like growth factor-1 receptor. *Arch Biochem Biophys* 535:128–135.

Speelman L, Akyildiz AC, den Adel B et al. 2011. Initial stress in biomechanical models of atherosclerotic plaques. *J Biomech* 44:2376–2382.

Standley PR, Cammarata A, Nolan BP, Purgason CT, Stanley MA. 2002. Cyclic stretch induces vascular smooth muscle cell alignment via NO signaling. *Am J Physiol Heart Circ Physiol* 283:H1907–H1914.

Stary HC. 2000. Lipid and macrophage accumulations in arteries of children and the development of atherosclerosis. *Am J Clin Nutr* 72:1297S–1306S.

Stary HC, Chandler AB, Dinsmore RE et al. 1995. A definition of advanced types of atherosclerotic lesions and a histological classification of atherosclerosis. A report from the Committee on Vascular Lesions of the Council on Arteriosclerosis, American Heart Association. *Circulation* 92:1355–1374.

Sterpetti AV, Cucina A, D'Angelo LS, Cardillo B, Cavallaro A. 1992. Response of arterial smooth muscle cells to laminar flow. *J Cardiovasc Surg* 33:619–624.

Sterpetti AV, Cucina A, D'Angelo LS, Cardillo B, Cavallaro A. 1993. Shear stress modulates the proliferation rate, protein synthesis, and mitogenic activity of arterial smooth muscle cells. *Surgery* 113:691–699.

Stocker R, Keaney JF Jr. 2004. Role of oxidative modifications in atherosclerosis. *Physiol Rev* 84:1381–1478.

Stone PH, Coskun AU, Kinlay S et al. 2003. Effect of endothelial shear stress on the progression of coronary artery disease, vascular remodeling, and in-stent restenosis in humans: *In vivo* 6-month follow-up study. *Circulation* 108:43–44.

Sui B, Gao P, Lin Y, Gao B, Liu L, An J. 2008. Assessment of wall shear stress in the common carotid artery of healthy subjects using 3.0-tesla magnetic resonance. *Acta Radiol* 49:442–449.

Sun Z, Xu L. 2014. Computational fluid dynamics in coronary artery disease. *Comput Med Imaging Graph* 38:651–663.

Tabas I, Li Y, Brocia RW, Xu SW, Swenson TL, Williams KJ. 1993. Lipoprotein lipase and sphingomyelinase synergistically enhance the association of atherogenic lipoproteins with smooth muscle cells and extracellular matrix. A possible mechanism for low density lipoprotein and lipoprotein(a) retention and macrophage foam cell formation. *J Biol Chem* 268:20419–20432.

Tabas I, García-Cardeña G, Owens GK. 2015. Recent insights into the cellular biology of atherosclerosis. *J Cell Biol* 209:13–22.

Tabas I, Williams KJ, Borén J. 2007. Subendothelial lipoprotein retention as the initiating process in atherosclerosis: Update and therapeutic implications. *Circulation* 116:1832–1844.

Takabe W, Jen N, Ai L et al. 2011. Oscillatory shear stress induces mitochondrial superoxide production: Implication of NADPH oxidase and c-Jun NH2-terminal kinase signaling. *Antioxid Redox Signal* 15:1379–1388.

Tang D, Teng Z, Canton G et al. 2009. Sites of rupture in human atherosclerotic carotid plaques are associated with high structural stresses: An *in vivo* MRI-based 3D fluid–structure interaction study. *Stroke* 40:3258–3263.

Thacher T, Silacci P, Stergiopulos N, da Silva RF. 2010. Autonomous effects of shear stress and cyclic circumferential stretch regarding endothelial dysfunction and oxidative stress: An ex vivo arterial model. *J Vasc Res* 47:336–345.

Thim T, Hagensen MK, Hørlyck A et al. 2012. Wall shear stress and local plaque development in stenosed carotid arteries of hypercholesterolemic minipigs. *J Cardiovasc Dis Res* 3:76–83.

Thomas SR, Witting PK, Drummond GR. 2008. Redox control of endothelial function and dysfunction: Molecular mechanisms and therapeutic opportunities. *Antioxid Redox Signal* 10:1713–1765.

Tojkander S, Gateva G, Lappalainen P. 2012. Actin stress fibers-assembly, dynamics and biological roles. *J Cell Sci* 125:1855–1864.

Tortoli P, Morganti T, Bambi G, Palombo C, Ramnarine KV. 2006. Noninvasive simultaneous assessment of wall shear rate and wall distension in carotid arteries. *Ultrasound Med Biol* 32:1661–1670.

Tortoli P, Palombo C, Ghiadoni L, Bini G, Francalanci L. 2011. Simultaneous ultrasound assessment of brachial artery shear stimulus and flow-mediated dilation during reactive hyperemia. *Ultrasound Med Biol* 37:1561–1570.

Traub O, Berk BC. 1998. Laminar shear stress: Mechanisms by which endothelial cells transduce an atheroprotective force. *Arterioscler Thromb Vasc Biol* 18:677–685.

Tricot O, Mallat Z, Heymes C, Belmin J, Lesèche G, Tedgui A. 2000. Relation between endothelial cell apoptosis and blood flow direction in human atherosclerotic plaques. *Circulation* 101:2450–2453.

Tsao CW, Pencina KM, Massaro JM et al. 2014. Cross-sectional relations of arterial stiffness, pressure pulsatility, wave reflection, and arterial calcification. *Arterioscler Thromb Vasc Biol* 34:2495–2500.

Turczynska KM, Sadegh MK, Hellstrand P, Swärd K, Albinsson S. 2012. MicroRNAs are essential for stretch-induced vascular smooth muscle contractile differentiation via microRNA (miR)-145-dependent expression of L-type calcium channels. *J Biol Chem* 287:19199–19206.

Turnbull FM, Abraira C, Anderson RJ et al.; Control Group. 2009. Intensive glucose control and macrovascular outcomes in type 2 diabetes. *Diabetologia* 52:2288–2298.

Tzima E, Irani-Tehrani M, Kiosses WB et al. 2005. A mechanosensory complex that mediates the endothelial cell response to fluid shear stress. *Nature* 437:426–431.

van der Wal AC, Becker AE, van der Loos CM, Das PK. 1994. Site of intimal rupture or erosion of thrombosed coronary atherosclerotic plaques is characterized by an inflammatory process irrespective of the dominant plaque morphology. *Circulation* 89:36–44.

Van Popele NM, Grobbee DE, Bots ML et al. 2001. Association between arterial stiffness and atherosclerosis. The Rotterdam Study. *Stroke* 32:454–460.

van Soest G, Goderie TP, Gonzalo N et al. 2009. Imaging atherosclerotic plaque composition with intracoronary optical coherence tomography. *Neth Heart J* 17:448–450.

Vengrenyuk Y, Carlier S, Xanthos S et al. 2006. A hypothesis for vulnerable plaque rupture due to stress-induced debonding around cellular microcalcifications in thin fibrous caps. *Proc Natl Acad Sci U S A* 103:14678–14683.

Versluis A, Bank AJ, Douglas WH. 2006. Fatigue and plaque rupture in myocardial infarction. *J. Biomech* 39:339–347.

Virmani R, Kolodgie FD, Burke AP, Farb A, Schwartz SM. 2000. Lessons from sudden coronary death: A comprehensive morphological classification scheme for atherosclerotic lesions. *Arterioscler Thromb Vasc Biol* 20:1262–1275.

Vito RP, Dixon SA. 2003. Blood vessel constitutive models-1995–2002. *Annu Rev Biomed Eng* 5:413–439.

Vlachopoulos C, Xaplanteris P, Aboyans V et al. 2015. The role of vascular biomarkers for primary and secondary prevention. A position paper from the European Society of

Cardiology Working Group on Peripheral Circulation: Endorsed by the Association for Research into Arterial Structure and Physiology (ARTERY) Society. *Atherosclerosis* 241:507–532.

Vliegenthart R, Oudkerk M, Hofman A et al. 2005. Coronary calcification improves cardiovascular risk prediction in the elderly. *Circulation* 112:572–577.

Wang BW, Chang H, Lin S, Kuan P, Shyu KG. 2003. Induction of matrix metalloproteinases-14 and -2 by cyclical mechanical stretch is mediated by tumor necrosis factor-alpha in cultured human umbilical vein endothelial cells. *Cardiovasc Res* 59:460–469.

Wang JH, Goldschmidt-Clermont P, Wille J, Yin FC. 2001. Specificity of endothelial cell reorientation in response to cyclic mechanical stretching. *J Biomech* 34:1563–1572.

Wang L, Zhu J, Samady H et al. 2017. Effects of residual stress, axial stretch, and circumferential shrinkage on coronary plaque stress and strain calculations: A modeling study using ivus-based near-idealized geometries. *J Biomech Eng* 139(1):0145011–01450111.

Wang N, Butler JP, Ingber DE. 1993. Mechanotransduction across the cell-surface and through the cytoskeleton. *Science* 260:1124–1127.

Wernig F, Mayr M, Xu Q. 2003. Mechanical stretch-induced apoptosis in smooth muscle cells is mediated by beta1-integrin signaling pathways. *Hypertension* 41:903–911.

Wentzel JJ, Chatzizisis YS, Gijsen FJ, Giannoglou GD, Feldman CL, Stone PH. 2012. Endothelial shear stress in the evolution of coronary atherosclerotic plaque and vascular remodelling: Current understanding and remaining questions. *Cardiovasc Res* 96:234–243.

Wentzel JJ, Krams R, Schuurbiers JCH et al. 2001. Relationship between neointimal thickness and shear stress after Wallstent implantation in human coronary arteries. *Circulation* 103:1740–1745.

White CR, Brock TA, Chang LY et al. 1994. Superoxide and peroxynitrite in atherosclerosis. *Proc Natl Acad Sci U S A* 91:1044–1048.

Wiesner S, Legate KR, Fässler R. 2005. Integrin-actin interactions. *Cell Mol Life Sci* 62: 1081–1099.

Williams B. 1998. Mechanical influences on vascular smooth muscle cell function. *J Hypertens* 6:1921–1929.

Witteman JC, Kannel WB, Wolf PA et al. 1990. Aortic calcified plaques and cardiovascular disease (the Framingham Study). *Am J Cardiol* 66:1060–1064.

Yao J, van Sambeek MR, Dall'Agata A et al. 1998. Three-dimensional ultrasound study of carotid arteries before and after endarterectomy; analysis of stenotic lesions and surgical impact on the vessel. *Stroke* 29:2026–2031.

Ye GJ, Nesmith AP, Parker KK. 2014. The role of mechanotransduction on vascular smooth muscle myocytes cytoskeleton and contractile function. *Anat Rec* 297:1758–1769.

Yim P, Demarco K, Castro MA, Cebral J. 2005. Characterization of shear stress on the wall of the carotid artery using magnetic resonance imaging and computational fluid dynamics. *Stud Health Technol Inform* 113:412–442.

Yuan C, Oikawa M, Miller Z, Hatsukami T. 2008. MRI of carotid atherosclerosis. *J Nucl Cardiol* 15:266–275.

Zebda N, Dubrovskyi O, Birukov KG. 2012. Focal adhesion kinase regulation of mechanotransduction and its impact on endothelial cell functions. *Microvasc Res* 83:71–81.

Ziegler T, Bouzourène K, Harrison VJ, Brunner HR, Hayoz D. 1998. Influence of oscillatory and unidirectional flow environments on the expression of endothelin and nitric oxide synthase in cultured endothelial cells. *Arterioscler Thromb Vasc Biol* 18:686–692.

8

Red Blood Cell and Platelet Mechanics

S. Gekle and M. Bender

Contents

The two most abundant cell types in blood flow are red blood cells (RBCs) and platelets. Red blood cells perform a vital function in any higher organism by delivering oxygen to tissue cells, while platelets are essential to stop bleeding in case of vessel injuries. Compared with other constituents such as leukocytes, RBCs and platelets are extremely simple objects and do not even possess a cell nucleus. However, their mechanical properties are rather distinct: RBCs can be thought of as deflated elastic balloons filled with a viscous hemoglobin solution, which makes them extremely deformable and gives them the ability to squeeze through capillaries, which are even smaller than their equilibrium diameter. Platelets, unless activated, are rather rigid disc-like cells; these are substantially smaller than the RBCs.

8.1 Red Blood Cell Mechanics

8.1.1 Introduction

When subjected to an external flow, red blood cells (RBCs) are easily deformed by the surrounding flow. This flow, in turn, is influenced by the RBC representing a complex-shaped moving obstacle. This two-way coupling leads to a surprisingly rich dynamical behavior, even for such simple cases as a single RBC in a tube or shear flow (Fedosov et al. 2014, Viallat and Abkarian 2014). With the RBC interior being a simple Newtonian liquid, the decisive factor for RBC dynamics is the mechanical properties of the cell membrane, which we will describe in some detail in Sections 8.1.2 and 8.1.3.

In large vessels, RBCs occupy up to 45% of the total vessel volume, while in the microcirculation, this number can drop to around 20% (Popel and Johnson 2005). However, even these figures are easily large enough to allow for considerable hydrodynamic interactions between the flowing RBCs: any individual RBC "feels" the disturbance in the hydrodynamic flow field created by its neighbors. These mutual interactions create a highly coupled fluid-mechanical problem, in which the RBC dynamics can be very different than the RBC dynamics for isolated RBCs (Gompper and Fedosov 2016).

The hydrodynamics of RBC suspensions has been the subject of intense scientific research for decades. Unfortunately, because of the complexity of the problem, the insight that can be gained from analytical theories (i.e., models that are simple enough that they can be solved in closed form by using pen and paper) is limited. However, the ever-increasing power of supercomputers, together with advanced simulation techniques and improved biomechanical models, has led to considerable progress and insight into RBC dynamics (Freund 2014). On the experimental side, the main tool has been microscopic imaging, whose applicability is unfortunately somewhat limited by the fact that it only allows to visualize two-dimensional (2D) projections of the three-dimensional (3D) RBC shapes. Confocal imaging might represent a promising way to circumvent this problem in the near future.

8.1.2 Biophysical Components of Red Blood Cells

Red blood cells in a quiescent fluid possess a discocyte shape and have a diameter of about 8 µm, as illustrated in Figure 8.1. Their interior is filled with a hemoglobin solution, which is a Newtonian liquid with a viscosity about five times higher than that of blood plasma, the latter having about the same viscosity as water.

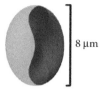

Figure 8.1 Illustration of the discocyte quiescent shape of a red blood cell.

The RBC membrane is about 100-nm thick, and its mechanics is determined by two essential components: the lipid bilayer and the spectrin network. The former is composed of thousands of chain-like lipid molecules, whose one end (the "head") is hydrophilic, while the other end (the "tail") is strongly hydrophobic. In water, such molecules spontaneously assemble into a bilayer structure, as illustrated in Figure 8.2. To minimize their interaction energy with the surrounding water, the hydrophilic heads are arranged such that they are in direct contact with the water, while the tails are buried in the bilayer interior. Lipid bilayers are a common theme in cell membranes, and they also form the outermost shell of the RBC membrane.

The spectrin layer is a network of elongated proteins biochemically crosslinked with each other. This highly porous scaffold structure is relatively easy to deform by external forces, but as soon as the forces are removed, it moves back elastically and regains its original shape.

Two more membrane components are relevant for the biological function of RBCs, but they do not strongly influence its mechanics and will therefore not be considered further in the following text: (1) transmembrane proteins, which pierce the membrane and allow for the exchange of liquid and other substances between the interior and the surrounding fluid; and (2) the glycocalyx, which is a set of biomolecules anchored to the outside of the lipid bilayer.

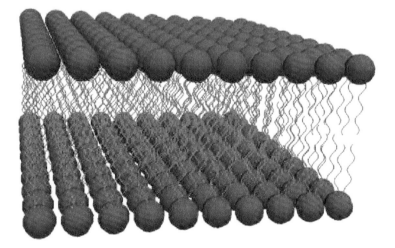

Figure 8.2 A lipid bilayer composed of hydrophilic heads (red) and hydrophobic tails (blue) forms the outer part of the red blood cell membrane.

8.1.3 Membrane Mechanics

Given that the RBC membrane is only about 100-nm thick but occupies an area in the micrometer range, the most common approach for a mechanical description is the so-called thin-shell theory (Møllmann 1981, Steigmann 1999, Pozrikidis 2001, Deserno 2015, Guckenberger and Gekle 2017). The essential idea of thin-shell theory is to exclusively focus on the lateral variations of any quantity and to neglect its variation across the membrane (to be precise, one considers vertically averaged quantities). One starts by covering the membrane surface with a 2D coordinate system, as illustrated in Figure 8.3. Any point on the surface is thus assigned a unique label by a specific combination of two values (η and ξ), which it retains even if the membrane is deformed. To describe the RBC shape, one then utilizes a vectorial function $\mathbf{x}(\eta, \xi)$. The reference shape shall be called $\mathbf{x}_0$, while we shall name the deformed shape simply $\mathbf{x}$. The deformation is the difference $\mathbf{u} = \mathbf{x}_0 - \mathbf{x}$. The goal of thin-shell theory is now to compute the mechanical stress $\tau(\eta, \xi)$ for a given deformation $\mathbf{u}(\eta, \xi)$. The stress τ is a tensorial quantity (roughly speaking, it is a 3×3 matrix). In the reference state $\mathbf{x}_0$, the stress vanishes. For an overview of the considerable mathematics involved in thin-shell theory, we refer the reader to the recent excellent review (Deserno 2015).

An RBC in flow experiences a hydrodynamic force from the surrounding fluid, which creates mechanical deformation $\mathbf{u}(\eta, \xi)$. This deformation, in turn, creates mechanical stresses, which try to "work against" the imposed deformation. These stresses (or, more precisely, the resulting forces that are gradients of the stress) act back on the fluid and modify the hydrodynamic flow. In a nutshell, this circular interaction is the origin of the two-way coupling between hydrodynamics and membrane mechanics, alluded to in the introduction.

Owing to their different biophysical composition, the mechanical properties of the spectrin network and the lipid bilayer differ largely: the former provides resistance to in-plane shear deformations, while the latter resists bending deformation and area dilatation. Nevertheless, for the mathematical description, both components will be considered as a unified surface $\mathbf{x}(\eta, \xi)$, as will be described in the following subsection.

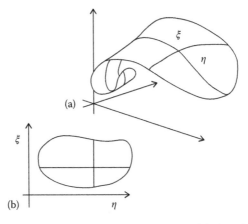

Figure 8.3   Description of the thin membrane shape embedded in three-dimensional space shown in (a) using a local coordinate system η, ξ as illustrated in (b).

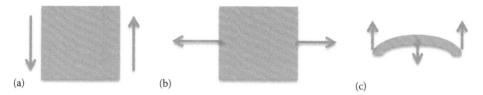

Figure 8.4   Illustration of (a) shear deformation, (b) area dilatation, and (c) bending.

8.1.3.1 Shear Resistance

The chemical crosslinking between the spectrin molecules tightly connects each of them with its surrounding neighbors. A shear deformation stretches these connections, leading to a mechanical stress acting against the deformation (see Figure 8.4a). In the regime of small deformations, the stresses are directly proportional to the deformation gradients, as they are in a normal Hookean 3D elastic solid:

$$\tau = C\nabla\mathbf{u}$$

where C is a matrix containing the elastic constants, such as Young's modulus and Poisson ratio (Bower 2010). However, in the case of larger deformations, the stresses increase nonlinearly with the deformation, and in the case of even-larger stresses, the chemical crosslinks between the spectrin molecules would eventually break. This behavior is termed strain hardening. Mathematically, it can be described by empirical laws, whose most widely used representative in the case of RBCs is the one proposed by Skalak (Skalak et al. 1973, Freund 2014). Here, the stress–strain relationship for the 2D membrane can be derived from a strain energy function of the form:

$$W = \frac{\kappa_s}{4}\left(\frac{1}{2}I_1^2 + I_1 - I_2\right) + \frac{\kappa_a}{8}I_2^2 \tag{8.1}$$

The first constant κ_s is the shear modulus, which for RBCs is in the range of 5 N/m.[1] The quantities I_1 and I_2 identify the first and second invariants, respectively, of the strain tensor (Skalak et al. 1973, Freund 2014).

The second modulus κ_a is related to area dilatation resistance, which we will describe in Section 8.1.3.2.

8.1.3.2 Area Dilatation Resistance

The lipid molecules that make up the lipid bilayer are tightly held together by the hydrophobic interactions introduced earlier in the chapter. Therefore, one requires very large forces to increase (stretch) or decrease (compress) the area of the bilayer, as illustrated in Figure 8.4b. These forces are much larger than hydrodynamic forces typically occurring in blood flow, and thus, to a very good approximation, the total

---

[1] Since κ_s is a surface elastic modulus, its units are N/m, in contrast to the more commonly known 3D elastic moduli, which are measured in Pa, that is, N/m². Its value can be determined by, for example, cell stretching and micropipette aspiration experiments.

surface area of an RBC can be considered a fixed quantity, which does not change even when the RBC shape is strongly deformed by the hydrodynamic flow.

In mathematical modeling, it is possible to rigorously enforce this constant-area constraint by using the method of Lagrange multipliers (Farutin et al. 2014). However, a simpler and more often used route employs the Skalak law given in Equation 8.1. The second term in this equation involves the surface area modulus κ_a. Taking κ_a to be very large (compared with its shear counterpart κ_s) results in the creation of large stresses, effectively opposing any but the tiniest area expansions or compressions. Typical values for κ_a are in the range of 1000–10,000 κ_s; however, many computer simulations use somewhat-smaller values for reasons of numerical stability (Freund 2014).

8.1.3.3 Bending Resistance

The final component of mechanical resistance described herein is again related to the lipid bilayer (Guckenberger et al. 2016, Guckenberger and Gekle 2017). Considering Figure 8.4c, any bending of the bilayer requires a stretching of the outer monolayer and a corresponding compression of the inner monolayer. These deformations being highly unfavorable, as described in the preceding subsection, the bilayer strongly resists bending deformations. Similar to the Skalak law, the mathematical description of bending resistance starts from an energy function that usually follows a form introduced by Helfrich (Helfrich 1973):

$$W_B = \int_S 2\kappa_b \left(H - H_0 \right)^2 dS$$

Here, H is the local membrane curvature, which is computed from the second derivative of the local shape, the so-called Laplace–Beltrami operator Δ_s (Guckenberger and Gekle 2017)

$$H(\mathbf{x}) = \frac{1}{2} \sum_{i=1}^{3} \left(\Delta_s x_i \right) n_i \left(\mathbf{x} \right)$$

with n being the local normal vector. The bending modulus κ_b is an empirical quantity that measures the "stiffness" of the membrane and needs to be determined from experiments or more sophisticated modeling efforts (Bassereau et al. 2014). Typical values for RBCs lie in the range 2–4 10^{-19} Nm. The quantity H_0 is called the spontaneous curvature, denoting the stress-free state: if $H(x) = H_0(x)$ everywhere, the bending energy and thus the resulting stresses vanish over the entire membrane.

8.1.3.4 Spontaneous Curvature and Stress-Free State

It has long been known that an RBC in a quiescent medium or on a substrate exhibits a discocyte shape, as depicted in Figure 8.1. One might thus naively assume that this also corresponds to the stress-free state, in which shear and bending stresses vanish. Then, the reference state x^R and the reference curvature H_0 would be precisely those given by the shape in Figure 8.1. However, this intuitive interpretation does not necessarily need to be true.

Physically, an equilibrium shape such as that depicted in Figure 8.1 is determined, such that the elastic energy is a local minimum and all forces mutually balance, resulting in zero net forces throughout the membrane. Accordingly, any deformation away from the equilibrium shape causes an increase in the elastic energy and, as a result, in a restoring force, driving the membrane back into its equilibrium position. However, since the elastic energy results from summing shearing, area deformation, and bending contributions, it is very conceivable that these contributions can precisely cancel each other. Then, the shape in Figure 8.1, while corresponding to an equilibrium minimum energy shape, is not stress-free. This prestress can have important implications for RBC mechanics.

Unfortunately, the reference states x^R and H_0 depend in a complex fashion on the biophysical composition of the lipid bilayer and the spectrin network. Their prediction is thus beyond the reach of purely mechanical models. At the same time, there exists virtually no experimental method that could measure mechanical stress. The question whether the discocyte is truly the stress-free state or just a local energy minimum resulting from counterbalancing shearing and bending forces has attracted considerable interest; however, it still remains largely unsettled.

8.1.4 Red Blood Cells in Flow

During its approximately 120-day life time, an RBC continuously flows through blood vessels of various sizes, ranging from large vessels, such as the aorta, to microcapillaries with a diameter of a few micrometers, possibly even smaller than the RBC equilibrium diameter (Freund 2013). In these small vessels, the concentration of RBCs is low and cells flow in single file. On the other hand, in larger vessels, RBCs continuously collide and collective phenomena such as the famous Fahræus and Fahræus–Lindqvist effects are dominant. Finally, although less important in vivo, a much-studied situation is an RBC in an externally imposed shear flow (Dupire et al. 2012).

8.1.4.1 Single Cells in Cylindrical Tubes

The probably simplest situation one could imagine is a long cylindrical tube through which a fluid is pushed by an externally imposed pressure gradient. This leads to the famous Poiseuille flow profile, in which the flow velocity v is unidirectional along the tube axis (here denominated by x), with a quadratic dependence on the radial position. The flow is given by

$$v(r) = V_0\left(1 - \left(\frac{r}{R}\right)^2\right)$$

where V_0 is the maximal velocity occurring in the channel center, R is the tube radius, and r is the radial position. In very small capillaries, where R is less than

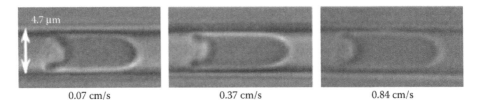

Figure 8.5   A red blood cell in a very narrow channel forms the so-called bullet shape. (From Tomaiuolo, G. et al., *Soft Matter.*, 5, 3736–3740, 2009.)

4 μm, that is, smaller than the RBC equilibrium radius, RBCs are known to deform into what has been called a bullet shape; see Figure 8.5. This shape retains the axisymmetry of the system. One of the two dimples that were originally present in the equilibrium shape forms the nose, while the other dimple forms the inner-most spot. The bullet shape is beneficial since it features a large contact area between the vessel wall and the RBC surface, which allows for efficient exchange of oxygen and carbon dioxide between the endothelial cells and the hemoglobin confined in the RBC interior. It has indeed been speculated (although never proven) that this might be one of the reasons why nature has decided to construct RBCs with a discocyte equilibrium shape. The bullet shape in these small vessels is largely independent of the flow velocity.

On slightly increasing the vessel size but still considering a single RBC, the behavior changes dramatically. First, one finds a pronounced dependence of the RBC shape on the flow velocity. Second, the axisymmetry can spontaneously be broken and nonaxisymmetric shapes can appear (Kaoui et al. 2009, Farutin and Misbah 2011). Third, dynamic states are observed, in which the membrane continuously rotates around the cell. Finally, some recent studies even pointed toward bistability, that is, for the same parameters, two different modes of motion can be observed, depending on the initial conditions (Farutin and Misbah 2014). Because of this complexity, a number of questions are still unresolved, even in this very simple system, and therefore, it remains an active area of study.

The flow velocity is typically measured by a nondimensional number called the elastic capillary number, Ca, which expresses the ratio between elastic shear forces and viscous drag:

$$Ca = \frac{\mu V_0}{a\kappa_s}$$

with a being the long RBC radius. Note that, sometimes, different conventions are used.

A second important parameter is the confinement, that is, the ratio $\chi = R/a$ between the channel radius, R, and the RBC radius, a. With these two parameters, one can construct a "phase diagram," that is, a two-dimensional plot, with Ca and χ denoting the two axes being filled with dots, where the color of each dot designates

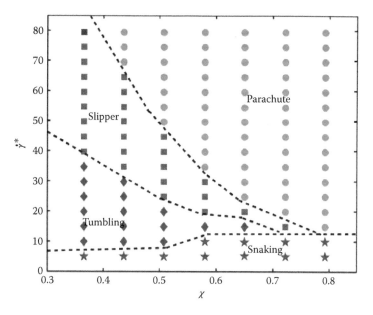

Figure 8.6 Phase diagram of a red blood cell in a cylindrical channel. (From Fedosov, D. A. et al., *Soft Matter.*, 10, 4258–4267, 2014.)

the mode of motion observed. An example phase diagram that has been determined by numerical simulations is shown in Figure 8.6.

We will now describe the main modes of motion that an RBC features in a Poiseuille flow inside a channel whose diameter is larger, but not much larger, than the RBC radius (4 μm < R < 12 μm):

1. *Tumbling*: Here, the velocities and thus the shear forces acting on the RBC membrane are so low that the cell only slightly deforms away from its equilibrium discocyte shape. Instead, the entire cell performs a tumbling motion around an axis perpendicular to the flow direction, as illustrated in Figure 8.7a.

2. *Snaking*: This mode is similar to tumbling but includes some rotation of the membrane.

3. *Slipper*: Here, the RBC attains a very characteristic shape that is best described by a "slipper." In the slipper shape, axisymmetry is broken and only a single plane of mirror symmetry remains, as shown in Figure 8.7b. Typically, the slipper RBC travels at a position that is slightly off-center and performs a tank-treading motion. The membrane continuously rotates around the cell interior, leading to periodic oscillations of the cell shape.

4. *Parachute*: The parachute is very similar to the bullet but less elongated. It is also axisymmetric.

5. *Croissant*: The croissant shape at the first sight looks very reminiscent of the parachute shape but exhibits one essential qualitative difference: it is no longer axisymmetric. This can be seen by the fact that the left-most ring is a perfect circle in the parachute shape but looks more like an indented curve in the croissant shape, as illustrated in Figure 8.7c. Croissant shapes possess two orthogonal planes of mirror symmetry. Since, in many cases, this indentation is small compared with the

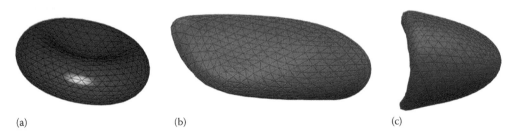

Figure 8.7   Illustration of some prototypical RBC shapes in a rectangular flow: (a) tumbling, (b) slipper, and (c) parachute/croissant. (Guckenberger, A. et al., *Soft Matter.*, 14, 2032–2043, 2018.)

> overall RBC dimension, some research works do not clearly distinguish between parachute and croissant and, in fact, also denote slightly nonaxisymmetric shapes as parachutes.

Besides the large variety of possible motions, there are two key difficulties in the accurate determination of the phase diagram. Experimentally, one is faced with the challenge of imaging truly 3D shapes. Typical microscopy set-ups work with 2D projections; this makes it impossible to unambiguously identify, for example, a slipper shape, which looks completely different depending on whether one views it from the side or from the top. Theoretically, the major challenge lies in the fact that the continuous flow creates a nonequilibrium situation, where familiar thermodynamic principles do not hold. While any equilibrium system would always attain the state of minimum energy, this principle cannot be applied to an RBC in an external flow. Accordingly, in the shapes described previously, the sum of shearing and bending elastic energy (see Section 8.1.3) is not minimal. At present, there is no such simple principle as energy minimization for a nonequilibrium situation.

Accordingly, many of the insights into single-RBC dynamics in Poiseuille flow rely on computer simulations, whose capabilities and reliability have continuously increased over the last years.

8.1.5 Collective Effects

While there is no fundamental principle of minimum energy, as just explained, a situation in which the RBC is not strongly deformed will still be favored over a situation with larger deformation. Large deformations are induced by shear forces, that is, forces that appear if the external flow pulls more strongly on one side of the RBC than on the other side. Considering the parabolic flow profile in a cylindrical tube, it is clear that shear forces are larger as one moves away from the center, with the largest shear appearing near the wall. Accordingly, RBCs, in general, prefer to flow in the vessel center (with some exceptions such as the nonaxisymmetric off-center slipper shapes mentioned earlier). This leads to the formation of a pronounced cell-free layer near the walls of the vessels. The width of this layer depends on the flow velocity and, most prominently, on the hematocrit (Zhang et al. 2009, Gekle 2016, Bächer et al. 2017).

8.2 Red Blood Cell Aggregation

8.2.1 Introduction

If a suspension of RBCs in plasma is standing quietly or flowing at very low speeds through a channel, one can observe that RBCs spontaneously start to form well-ordered stacks. These stacks are named by the French word *rouleaux* and are illustrated in Figure 8.8. The stacks are either straight or form branched structures. Red blood cell aggregation is directly connected to the presence of large molecules in the solvent. Washed RBCs in simple buffer solution do not show any aggregation. In full blood, the molecule thought to be responsible for RBC aggregation is fibrinogen. However, aggregation can be easily reinduced if large synthetic molecules, such as dextran, are added to a buffer solution.

The formation of rouleaux is physiologically relevant, as it strongly affects blood viscosity at low shear rates. If an RBC suspension containing rouleaux is driven through a blood vessel or microchannel at low flow speeds, the rouleaux are strong enough to withstand shearing forces and thus remain largely intact. Consequently, their relatively large size hinders blood flow, which manifests itself in a large macroscopic flow resistance and eventually in large values of the apparent viscosity. If shear rates are increased, the rouleaux gradually start to break apart, leading to a suspension containing more and more isolated RBCs. These individual cells can more easily slide past each other than the large rouleaux. Consequently, the flow resistance is lower and the apparent viscosity of blood diminishes on increasing the shear rate. In the language of non-Newtonian rheology, such behavior is termed shear thinning. By using appropriate phenomenological aggregation models, computer simulations are able to reproduce the effect of rouleaux breakup and shear thinning fairly well (Fedosov et al. 2011).

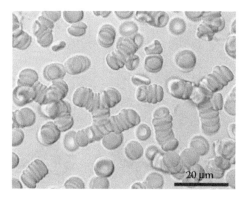

Figure 8.8 Rouleaux of red blood cells. (From Brust, M. et al., *Sci. Rep.*, 4, 4348, 2014.)

The intriguing fact about RBC aggregation is that, despite decade-long research efforts, its origin is still not fully understood. Two competing explanations exist: the bridging and the depletion models, both of which are described in the following sections. In the end, most likely, both effects contribute their share to RBC aggregation in physiologic situations.

8.2.2 Bridging Model

The idea of the bridging model is fairly simple. It is postulated that there exists some, at present unknown, mechanism by which fibrinogen, dextran, and other large molecules can adsorb to an RBC membrane. Once one end of the molecule is adsorbed to an RBC, the other end can adsorb to another RBC, thus forming a bridge between the two. This is illustrated in Figure 8.9. If bridges are built between a series of RBCs, a rouleau naturally forms.

8.2.3 Depletion Model

The depletion model is slightly more involved. It is motivated by the observation that RBC aggregation can be induced by a variety of biochemically very different molecules such as fibrinogen and dextran. It is thus speculated that a more fundamental physical mechanism might be at work. The central idea comes from colloidal physics, the discipline that studies the dynamical behavior of small (<1 μm) particles in fluids.

Colloids are small enough that they exhibit significant Brownian motion, that is, random position fluctuations induced by the thermal energy of the surrounding fluid. Accordingly, any colloid will, in the course of time, explore the entire space that is made available to it. The more the space available, the more favorable the situation for the colloids. Accordingly, a system with many colloids will always attempt to arrange itself in such a way that the colloids have the largest possible space available.

Bridging macromolecules

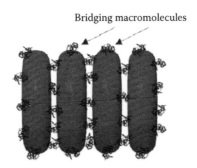

Figure 8.9 Illustration of the bridges formed between red blood cells by macromolecules. This bridging model is one possible explanation for rouleaux formation and RBC aggregation. (From Flormann, D., Physical characterization of red blood cell aggregation, PhD dissertation, Saarland University, 2017.)

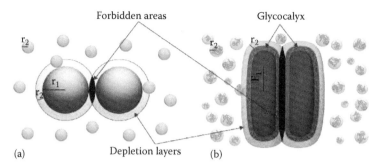

Figure 8.10 (a) Illustration of the depletion effect in a mixture of small and large rigid colloids. (b) Corresponding situation with red blood cells and fibrinogen. (From Flormann, D., *Physical characterization of red blood cell aggregation*, PhD dissertation, Saarland University, 2017.)

Thermodynamically speaking, the system maximizes its entropy. This behavior has dramatic consequences if one considers a mixture of large and small colloids. As illustrated in Figure 8.10a, each large colloid is surrounded by a small volume into which the small colloids cannot fully penetrate. Taking its center of mass as the position of a small colloid, the small colloid cannot approach the large one closer than half of its diameter. This forbidden area reduces the space available for the Brownian motion of the small colloids. As reasoned previously, in order to maximize its entropy, the system will strive to attain a configuration in which the total forbidden area (summed over all large colloids) is minimal. This is clearly achieved if the large colloids touch as much as possible, such that their respective forbidden areas overlap. If many small colloids surround a relatively small number of large colloids, the resulting entropic force driving aggregation of the large colloids can be considerable.

For RBC aggregation, a similar mechanism has been proposed and turned into quantitative models, for example (Neu and Meiselman 2002, Steffen et al. 2013), as illustrated in Figure 8.10b. Here, the role of the large colloids is played by the RBCs, while the small colloids correspond to fibrinogen or dextran. This physically motivated and very general mechanism provides an alternative or, most likely, additional pathway to explain RBC aggregation, besides the bridging model introduced previously.

8.3 Platelet Adhesion, Activation, and Aggregation

8.3.1 Introduction

The human body produces 10^{11} platelets daily (Branehog et al. 1975). Platelets are anucleated cells and the smallest cell type in the blood system, with a diameter of 1–2 µm in mice and 3–4 µm in humans. They can rapidly change their discoid shape to a spherical shape, with pseudopodia formation on activation with different ligands. The number of platelets in human blood is about 150,000–300,000/µL, whereas the count in mice is approximately 1,000,000/μL. These cells have only a short life span of about 5 days and 10 days in mice and humans, respectively, before the aged platelets are removed from the circulation. Platelets are derived from bone marrow mega-karyocytes, which are in proximity to sinusoidal blood vessels and extend long cyto-plasmic protrusions, the so-called proplatelets, from which they sequentially release platelets into the vasculature (Patel et al. 2005). Reorganization of the megakaryocyte cytoskeleton is essential for platelet production (Hartwig and Italiano 2003, Patel et al. 2005, Bender et al. 2010, Bender et al. 2015); however, the precise mechanisms involved remain poorly understood. Once in the bloodstream, platelets are essential players in hemostasis, as they "survey" the integrity of the vascular system. Upon vessel wall injury, they rapidly adhere to exposed extracellular matrix components and form a hemostatic plug that seals the wound. On the other hand, uncontrolled thrombus formation in pathological situations can lead to irreversible occlusion of the vessel, causing acute ischemic diseases, such as myocardial infarction and stroke (Jackson 2011, Nieswandt et al. 2011), which are the leading causes of disability and mortality worldwide (Lopez et al. 2006). To date, there is still a high demand for powerful yet safe antithrombotic drugs without side effects such as bleeding complications.

Platelet adhesion, activation, and aggregation together form a multistep process that requires multiple platelet receptor–ligand interactions, as shown in Figure 8.11. After damage to the vessel wall, circulating platelets undergo a rapid deceleration,

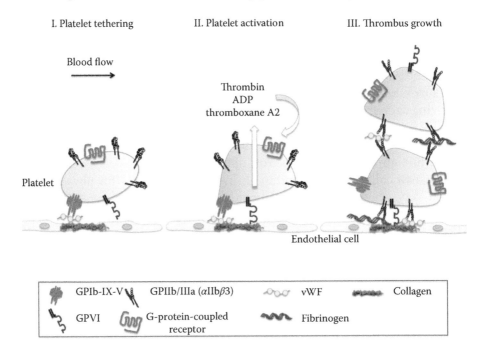

Figure 8.11 Simplified model of adhesion receptor involvement in thrombus formation. Platelet tethering is mediated by the GPIb–vWF interaction. This allows binding of GPVI to collagen and cellular activation, resulting in inside-out upregulation of integrin affinity and firm platelet adhesion. Released ADP and synthesis of thromboxane A2 (TxA2) amplify integrin activation on adherent platelets and mediate thrombus growth by activating additional platelets.

which is mainly mediated by the interaction of the platelet-specific glycoprotein (GP) Ib-V-IX complex and immobilized von Willebrand factor (vWF) bound to exposed collagen (Savage et al. 1998). However, the binding of GPIb to vWF has a fast off-rate and is therefore insufficient to mediate stable adhesion, but it rather maintains the platelet in close contact with the vessel wall. Finally, the translocating platelets establish contact with the thrombogenic protein collagen through the receptor glycoprotein VI (Dutting et al. 2012). This protein, though a low-affinity receptor for collagen and thus unable to mediate firm adhesion, triggers intracellular signaling, which results in a shift of platelet integrins from a low- to a high-affinity state. Subsequently, the platelet activation process is reinforced by the local production of thrombin and the release and synthesis, of the secondary mediators adenosine diphosphate (ADP) and thromboxane A2, respectively, which, in turn, activate G-protein-coupled receptors (Gq, Gi, and G12/13) (Offermanns 2006). These signaling pathways finally induce full platelet activation, resulting in shape change due to extensive cytoskeletal rearrangement, release of granule contents, and coagulant activity. The stabilization of a newly formed thrombus is essential to stop bleeding; therefore, the final thrombus is embedded in a fibrin network to withstand shear forces generated by the blood flow. In addition, outside-in signaling-mediated clot retraction through integrin αIIbβ3 plays a critical role in thrombus stabilization, and an increasing number of other receptors have been identified to be potentially involved in thrombus perpetuation as well as in limiting thrombus growth (Nieswandt et al. 2011). Recently, it was described that not all platelets in a thrombus are activated to the same extent, but platelet activation is rather heterogeneous. While some platelets undergo a full activation response, others display only minimal signs of activation. Thus, a thrombus consists of a core with fully activated, densely packed platelets, a shell of less activated and packed platelets, and a transition zone between these two layers (Stalker et al. 2014). A better understanding of the mechanisms involved in thrombus growth and the thrombus architecture will have important implications for the understanding of new and existing antiplatelet agents and their potential side effects.

In the following sections, the function of key adhesive surface proteins GPIb, GPVI and integrin αIIbβ3 in the multistep process of platelet aggregation will be discussed in more detail.

8.3.2 The Glycoprotein Ib-V-IX Complex

The GPIb-V-IX receptor complex is exclusively expressed on the megakaryocyte and platelet surfaces, with a ratio per platelet of 2:2:2:1 (with approximately 25,000 copies of GPIbα, GPIbβ, and GPIX and 12,500 copies of GPV) (Fox et al. 1988). The cytoplasmic domain of GPIbα contains binding sites for signaling molecules, such as 14-3-3ζ, and for the scaffold protein filamin A, which anchors the complex to the submembranous actin filament network (Canobbio et al. 2004). The N-terminal region of the subunit GPIbα binds to many ligands, including thrombin, vWF, P-selectin, and macrophage antigen 1 (Mac-1), and the coagulation factors XI and XII. Lack or dysfunction of human GPIb-V-IX causes the Bernard–Soulier syndrome, a rare autosomal recessive disorder characterized by a bleeding phenotype and macrothrombocytopenia (increased platelet size and reduced platelet count) (Nurden et al. 1983). Interestingly, mice lacking GPIbα (Ware et al. 2000) or GPIbβ (Kato et al. 2004) mirror the phenotype observed in humans, whereas no mutations in the Gp5 gene have been described in humans and mice that are associated with the Bernard–Soulier syndrome (Kahn et al. 1999). The interaction of platelet GPIbα and collagen-bound vWF is critical to slow down circulating platelets at high shear flow rates. However, the binding of these two proteins is only transient and induces a platelet rolling on the vWF layer (Savage et al. 1998). Interestingly, it was shown that at extremely high shear rates ($>10,000$ s^{-1}), platelet adhesion and aggregation are exclusively dependent on the GPIb–vWF interaction, without obvious requirement for full platelet activation (Ruggeri et al. 2006, Nesbitt et al. 2009). One suggestion is that the binding of GPIb to vWF induces weak intracellular signaling, resulting in integrin activation (Canobbio et al. 2004). Despite recent advances, details of the GPIb signaling cascade remain elusive to a large extent. The essential role of GPIb in arterial thrombus formation was revealed by in vivo studies by using GPIb mutant mice or blocking antibodies. Here, platelet adhesion was abolished, and consequently, occlusive arterial thrombus formation was prevented in various models with different vascular beds and types of injury (Bergmeier et al. 2006, Konstantinides et al. 2006). The antithrombotic potential of targeting the vWF–GPIb axis was also demonstrated in nonhuman primates (Cauwenberghs et al. 2000).

Although the GPIb complex was recognized as a platelet mechanosensor a long time ago (Kroll et al. 1996), how this receptor complex senses shear stress and converts this mechanical information into signaling has remained elusive until recently; this will be discussed in Section 8.4.

8.3.3 Glycoprotein VI

The activating platelet collagen receptor, GPVI, is a megakaryocyte-/platelet-specific transmembrane receptor; it is noncovalently associated with the FcR γ chain, which contains an immunoreceptor tyrosine-based activation motif. On ligand-induced GPVI clustering, this motif becomes tyrosine phosphorylated and initiates a series of phosphorylation events, finally resulting in full cellular activation (Figure 8.11) (Berlanga et al. 2007, Dutting et al. 2012). GPVI has been estimated to be expressed at 4000–6000 copies (Berlanga et al. 2007). Multiple studies have shown that only the dimeric form of the receptor binds exposed subendothelial collagen with high affinity (Miura et al. 2002). A few patients with GPVI-related defects (Arthur et al. 2007, Dumont et al. 2009, Hermans et al. 2009, Matus et al. 2013) have been reported so far, suffering merely from a mild bleeding tendency, but their platelets are unresponsive to collagen. It was revealed that GPVI is largely dispensable for normal hemostasis but has a predominant role in the formation of (experimental) arterial thrombi in vivo (Dutting et al. 2012).

8.3.4 Integrins α2β1 and αIIbβ3

Integrins are heterodimeric adhesion receptors formed by noncovalent association of different α and β chains and mediate platelet adhesion or platelet–platelet binding (Hynes 2002). Platelets express three $\beta 1$ integrins: $\alpha 5\beta 1$ (fibronectin receptor), $\alpha 6\beta 1$ (laminin receptor), and $\alpha 2\beta 1$ (collagen receptor). The $\beta 1$ integrins were revealed to have a supportive role in platelet adhesion rather than an essential role, since GPVI was established as the major activating collagen receptor on the platelet surface (Dutting et al. 2012). On the other hand, platelets express two $\beta 3$ integrins: $\alpha IIb\beta 3$ and $\alpha V\beta 3$ (binding to vitronectin, fibronectin, and osteopontin); the latter one is present only at very low levels. Integrin $\alpha IIb\beta 3$ (up to 100,000 per platelet) binds several ligands, such as fibrinogen, fibrin, vWF, fibronectin, thrombospondin, and vitronectin. It plays an essential role for firm platelet adhesion on the extracellular matrix and for thrombus formation by bridging of adjacent platelets via fibrinogen or, at high shear rates, vWF (Ruggeri et al. 1999). Inherited deficiency or dysfunction of this integrin in humans results in a disorder called Glanzmann thrombasthenia, characterized by defective platelet aggregation and a severe bleeding diathesis (Nurden 2006). Mice lacking either one subunit display a similar phenotype with defective platelet aggregation and bleeding (Hodivala-Dilke et al. 1999, Tronik-Le Roux et al. 2000). To ensure firm platelet adhesion exclusively at the sites of injury, $\alpha IIb\beta 3$ is present on the surface in a low-affinity state and shifts to a high-affinity state on cellular activation through inside-out signaling. This enables the integrin to bind tightly to its ligand, which, in turn, mediates outside-in signaling, leading to cytoskeletal rearrangement-dependent processes, such as platelet spreading (Figure 8.12a) and clot retraction (Figure 8.12b) (Ginsberg et al. 2005).

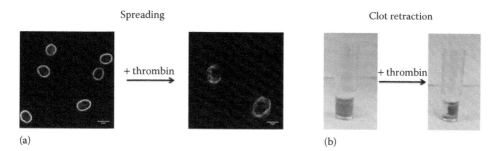

Spreading   Clot retraction

(a)   (b)

Figure 8.12 (a) Resting (nonactivated) mouse platelets or spread platelets on fibrinogen. α-tubulin in green, and F-actin in red. (b) Representative image of clot retraction of mouse platelets after activation with thrombin. Red blood cells (1 μL) were added to platelet suspension.

8.4 Platelet Mechanics

8.4.1 Introduction

During the last years, substantial progress has been made in understanding the molecular function of platelet receptors and associated signaling machineries and in dissecting their involvement in hemostatic plug formation and pathologic thrombus formation. However, the biophysical interaction of platelets and their microenvironment and, consequently, the generation and transmission of mechanical forces are less well characterized.

The platelet cytoskeleton consists of three major components: a spectrin-based skeleton adherent to the plasma membrane, microtubule coils (marginal band) along the perimeter, and the cytoplasmic actin network. Actin is the most abundant protein, with 2×10^6 molecules per platelet. Approximately 800,000 actin monomers assemble to form 2000–4000 actin filaments (Hartwig and DeSisto 1991). The crosslinker protein filamin A was shown to be important for controlling the distribution of the GPIb-V-IX receptor on the platelet surface and attaching it to the actin cytoskeleton (Nakamura et al. 2006). On activation, platelets rearrange their cytoskeleton with the help of cytoskeletal-regulatory proteins (such as gelsolin, cofilin, profilin, Arp2/3, Wiskott–Aldrich Syndrome protein (WASP), and CapZ), change their discoid form to spherical shape, and tether the integrin $\alpha IIb\beta 3$ to the underlying, newly assembled actin filaments. Finally, cytoplasmic myosin binds to actin polymers and applies contractile forces (Cove and Crawford 1975). In general, the platelet has turned out be a good model to study mechanobiological questions, since platelets are anucleated cells, have a high actin content, and highly express mechanical-relevant receptors, such as integrins ($\alpha IIb\beta 3$: 80,000 copies), on a small surface (Ciciliano et al. 2014).

8.4.2 Platelet Contraction and Clot Stiffening

Clot retraction (contraction, or shrinking of a blood clot) is necessary to promote wound closure, secure hemostasis, and prevent thrombotic occlusion of a vessel (Figure 8.12b). It was reported that clot retraction (duration in an in vitro assay: 20–120 min) is a multistep process that can be divided into three phases: initiation of contraction, linear contraction, and mechanical stabilization (Tutwiler et al. 2016). In Phase 1, the initiation of clot contraction is mediated by platelet activation (~2 min), fibrin network formation, platelet–fibrin binding, and start of platelet contraction. Phase 2 consists of the continuation of the latter, along with fibrin network remodeling. Finally, fibrin crosslinking via coagulation factor XIIIa causes mechanical stabilization (Phase 3). Taken together, thrombin, high platelet counts, platelet–fibrin binding, fibrin crosslinking, and platelet contraction support clot retraction, whereas high fibrinogen concentration, high hematocrit, and increased RBC mechanical interference limit clot retraction (Tutwiler et al. 2016). The importance of platelets in clot retraction is corroborated by a study in which the elasticities of platelet-rich clots and platelet-free clots were determined to be 600 Pa and 70 Pa, respectively (Jen and McIntire 1982, Carr 2003). Single platelets can generate high contraction forces, ranging from 1.5 to 79 nN, form adhesions stronger than 70 nN, have an elasticity of 10 kPa after contraction, and show an extensibility mean of about 1.57 before rupture from a fibrinogen-coated surface (Lam et al. 2011). However, it has to be noted that different adhesion force values can be obtained, depending on the coated matrix (Nguyen et al. 2016). Platelets can generate higher stall forces when exposed to a stiffer microenvironment. Thus, platelets can stiffen fibrin fibers, which contribute to the stiffening of the whole clot (Figure 8.13) (Lam et al. 2011). Moreover, considerable evidence has accumulated, suggesting that the actin–myosin complex is a crucial component for clot compaction. Platelets treated with the cell-permeable and selective drug Y-27632 to inhibit the Rho-associated, coiled-coil-containing protein kinase (ROCK), ML-7 to inhibit the myosin light-chain kinase (MLCK), and blebbistatin to inhibit the myosin ATPase activity generated strongly reduced platelet forces, as quantified by deflection of microposts (Feghhi et al. 2016). Similar observations were made using platelets from patients with the bleeding disorders Wiskott–Aldrich syndrome (WAS) and MYH9-related disease, in which the platelet cytoskeletal machinery is affected. Here, significantly lower contraction forces on soft and stiff environments were measured for platelets from patients than for platelets from healthy volunteers. Interestingly, a larger subpopulation of platelets from these patients showed almost no contractile force on the stiff environment (Myers et al. 2017). These data suggest that defects in mechanical properties of platelets can translate into increased bleeding risk.

Taken together, platelet forces are essential to stabilize the hemostatic clot. The integrin $\alpha IIb\beta 3$ serves as a bidirectional signaling protein and connector of the extracellular matrix to the platelet cytoskeleton, whereas the actin–myosin complex provides the contractile force.

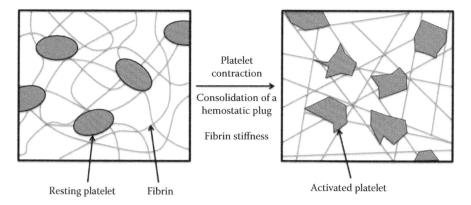

Figure 8.13   Activated platelets in a fibrin network. Platelet forces mediate fibrin stiffening and clot retraction.

8.4.3 Interaction Forces of Platelet Pairs

The binding strength between single platelets was analyzed to better understand the interaction forces of single platelets during activation and aggregation. Therefore, the dissipation work of platelet–platelet interaction was determined to better quantify the impact of all mediators between two platelets. A non/weakly activated platelet was attached to a non/weakly activated platelet (matrix: collagen), partially activated platelet (matrix: fibronectin), or activated platelet (matrix: poly-L-lysine), depending on the coated matrix. The dissipation work of platelet–platelet interaction was 1.40×10^{-16} J on collagen, 2.12×10^{-16} J on fibronectin, and 3.73×10^{-16} J on poly-L-lysine, demonstrating that the binding strength increases with the degree of platelet activation (Nguyen et al. 2016). The feasibility to measure interaction forces of platelets on different substances might provide an insight into a better understanding of the interplay between platelets, surfaces (biomaterial), and drugs.

8.4.4 Glycoprotein Ib-IX: The Platelet Mechanosensor

Studies using microstenosed channels resembling a vessel stenosis unveiled that at (very) high shear conditions or in regions of disturbed blood, rheology-dependent platelet aggregation of discoid platelets is exclusively mediated by the interaction of vWF and GPIb (Jackson et al. 2009, Nesbitt et al. 2009). Although GPIb was recognized to be a mechanosensor on the platelet surface a long time ago (Kroll et al. 1996), the exact mechanism by which this receptor senses shear stress and translates it into signaling has remained elusive. However, very recently, it was shown that vWF-mediated pulling (force: 5–20 pN) at the GPIbα receptor under shear induces the unfolding of a juxtamembrane mechanosensitive domain (Figure 8.14) (Zhang et al. 2015). The identification of this domain might explain platelet mechanosensing under dynamic conditions and GPIb-induced intracellular signaling. Moreover, it was described that the binding site on GPIbα for the crosslinker protein filamin A is essential for the transmission of cytoskeletal forces. These forces are important for binding to vWF, for strengthening of the catch bond, and, consequently, for platelet adhesion and aggregation (Feghhi et al. 2016).

    In summary, recent advances in understanding the function of the GPIb-V-IX complex have revealed that this receptor not only has a "simple" adhesive function but is now also accepted as a platelet mechanoreceptor sensing the mechanical environment and transmitting contractile forces. This might have functional consequences for platelets beyond adhesion and aggregation, as it was shown that

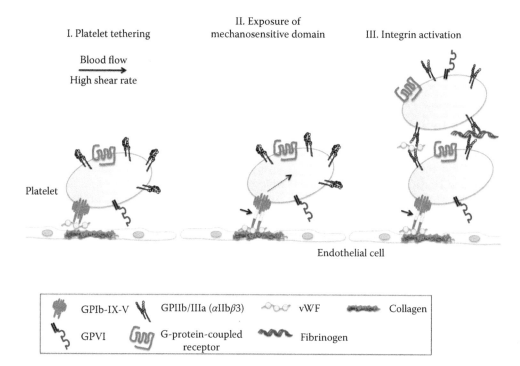

Figure 8.14 Proposed model of GPIb-dependent thrombus formation at high shear rates. Platelet tethering is mediated by the GPIb–vWF interaction, exposing the hidden mechanosensitive domain (indicated with small black arrow). This induces a signaling cascade (dashed black arrow), leading to inside-out activation of integrin activation and aggregation of discoid, not fully activated platelets.

shear-induced unfolding of the GPIbα mechanosensory domain leads to platelet clearance from the circulation (Deng et al. 2016).

8.4.5 Conclusion

While the role of platelets in preventing blood loss is well characterized from a biological perspective, the biomechanical aspects of interactions between platelets, platelet receptors, and the microenvironment are only at the beginning of being understood. A better comprehension of the underlying biophysical mechanisms might contribute to improved diagnosis and treatment of patients with bleeding complications. Existing and new technologies for force analysis will be key to address this relatively frequent clinical problem.

References

Arthur, J. F., S. Dunkley, and R. K. Andrews. 2007. Platelet glycoprotein VI-related clinical defects. *Br J Haematol* 139 (3): 363–372. doi:10.1111/j.1365-2141.2007.06799.x.

Bächer, C., L. Schrack, and S. Gekle. 2017. Clustering of microscopic particles in constricted blood flow. *Phys Rev Fluids* 2 (1). doi:10.1103/Physrevfluids.2.013102.

Bassereau, P., B. Sorre, and A. Levy. 2014. Bending lipid membranes: Experiments after W. Helfrich's model. *Adv Colloid Interface Sci* 208: 47–57. doi:10.1016/j.cis.2014.02.002.

Bender, M., A. Eckly, J. H. Hartwig, M. Elvers, I. Pleines, S. Gupta, G. Krohne et al. 2010. ADF/n-cofilin-dependent actin turnover determines platelet formation and sizing. *Blood* 116 (10): 1767–1775. doi:10.1182/blood-2010-03-274340.

Bender, M., J. N. Thon, A. J. Ehrlicher, S. Wu, L. Mazutis, E. Deschmann, M. Sola-Visner, J. E. Italiano, and J. H. Hartwig. 2015. Microtubule sliding drives proplatelet elongation and is dependent on cytoplasmic dynein. *Blood* 125 (5): 860–868. doi:10.1182/blood-2014-09-600858.

Bergmeier, W., C. L. Piffath, T. Goerge, S. M. Cifuni, Z. M. Ruggeri, J. Ware, and D. D. Wagner. 2006. The role of platelet adhesion receptor GPIbalpha far exceeds that of its main ligand, von Willebrand factor, in arterial thrombosis. *Proc Natl Acad Sci U S A* 103 (45): 16900–16905. doi:10.1073/pnas.0608207103.

Berlanga, O., T. Bori-Sanz, J. R. James, J. Frampton, S. J. Davis, M. G. Tomlinson, and S. P. Watson. 2007. Glycoprotein VI oligomerization in cell lines and platelets. *J Thromb Haemost* 5 (5): 1026–1033. doi:10.1111/j.1538-7836.2007.02449.x.

Bower, A. F. 2009. *Applied Mechanics of Solids*. Boca Raton, FL: CRC Press.

Branehog, I., B. Ridell, B. Swolin, and A. Weinfeld. 1975. Megakaryocyte quantifications in relation to thrombokinetics in primary thrombocythaemia and allied diseases. *Scand J Haematol* 15 (5): 321–332.

Brust, M., O. Aouane, M. Thiebaud, D. Flormann, C. Verdier, L. Kaestner, M. W. Laschke et al. 2014. The plasma protein fibrinogen stabilizes clusters of red blood cells in microcapillary flows. *Sci Rep* 4: 4348. doi:10.1038/srep04348.

Canobbio, I., C. Balduini, and M. Torti. 2004. Signalling through the platelet glycoprotein Ib-V-IX complex. *Cell Signal* 16 (12): 1329–1344. doi:10.1016/j.cellsig.2004.05.008.

Carr, M. E., Jr. 2003. Development of platelet contractile force as a research and clinical measure of platelet function. *Cell Biochem Biophys* 38 (1): 55–78. doi:10.1385/CBB:38:1:55.

Cauwenberghs, N., M. Meiring, S. Vauterin, V. van Wyk, S. Lamprecht, J. P. Roodt, L. Novak, J. Harsfalvi, H. Deckmyn, and H. F. Kotze. 2000. Antithrombotic effect of platelet glycoprotein Ib-blocking monoclonal antibody Fab fragments in nonhuman primates. *Arterioscler Thromb Vasc Biol* 20 (5): 1347–1353.

Ciciliano, J. C., R. Tran, Y. Sakurai, and W. A. Lam. 2014. The platelet and the biophysical microenvironment: lessons from cellular mechanics. *Thromb Res* 133 (4): 532–537. doi:10.1016/j.thromres.2013.12.037.

Cove, D. H., and N. Crawford. 1975. Platelet contractile proteins: separation and characterization of the actin and myosin-like components. *J Mechanochem Cell Motil* 3 (2): 123–133.

Deng, W., Y. Xu, W. Chen, D. S. Paul, A. K. Syed, M. A. Dragovich, X. Liang et al. 2016. Platelet clearance via shear-induced unfolding of a membrane mechanoreceptor. *Nat Commun* 7: 12863. doi:10.1038/ncomms12863.

Deserno, M. 2015. Fluid lipid membranes: From differential geometry to curvature stresses. *Chem Phys Lipids* 185: 11–45. doi:10.1016/j.chemphyslip.2014.05.001.

Dumont, B., D. Lasne, C. Rothschild, M. Bouabdelli, V. Ollivier, C. Oudin, N. Ajzenberg, B. Grandchamp, and M. Jandrot-Perrus. 2009. Absence of collagen-induced platelet activation caused by compound heterozygous GPVI mutations. *Blood* 114 (9): 1900–1903. doi:10.1182/blood-2009-03-213504.

Dupire, J., M. Socol, and A. Viallat. 2012. Full dynamics of a red blood cell in shear flow. *Proc Natl Acad Sci U S A* 109 (51): 20808–20813. doi:10.1073/pnas.1210236109.

Dutting, S., M. Bender, and B. Nieswandt. 2012. Platelet GPVI: A target for antithrombotic therapy?! *Trends Pharmacol Sci* 33 (11): 583–590. doi:10.1016/j.tips.2012.07.004.

Farutin, A., T. Biben, and C. Misbah. 2014. 3D numerical simulations of vesicle and inextensible capsule dynamics. *J Comput Phys* 275: 539–568. doi:10.1016/j.jcp.2014.07.008.

Farutin, A., and C. Misbah. 2011. Symmetry breaking of vesicle shapes in Poiseuille flow. *Phys Rev E* 84 (1). doi:10.1103/Physreve.84.011902.

Farutin, A., and C. Misbah. 2014. Symmetry breaking and cross-streamline migration of three-dimensional vesicles in an axial Poiseuille flow. *Phys Rev E* 89 (4). doi:10.1103/Physreve.89.042709.

Fedosov, D. A., W. Pan, B. Caswell, G. Gompper, and G. E. Karniadakis. 2011. Predicting human blood viscosity in silico. *Proc Natl Acad Sci U S A* 108 (29): 11772–11777. doi:10.1073/pnas.1101210108.

Fedosov, D. A., M. Peltomaki, and G. Gompper. 2014. Deformation and dynamics of red blood cells in flow through cylindrical microchannels. *Soft Matter* 10 (24): 4258–4267. doi:10.1039/c4sm00248b.

Feghhi, S., A. D. Munday, W. W. Tooley, S. Rajsekar, A. M. Fura, J. D. Kulman, J. A. Lopez, and N. J. Sniadecki. 2016. Glycoprotein Ib-IX-V complex transmits cytoskeletal forces that enhance platelet adhesion. *Biophys J* 111 (3): 601–608. doi:10.1016/j.bpj.2016.06.023.

Feghhi, S., W. W. Tooley, and N. J. Sniadecki. 2016. Nonmuscle myosin IIA regulates platelet contractile forces through rho kinase and myosin light-chain kinase. *J Biomech Eng* 138 (10). doi:10.1115/1.4034489.

Flormann, D. 2017. Physical characterization of red blood cell aggregation. PhD dissertation, Saarland University.

Fox, J. E., L. P. Aggerbeck, and M. C. Berndt. 1988. Structure of the glycoprotein Ib. IX complex from platelet membranes. *J Biol Chem* 263 (10): 4882–4890.

Freund, J. B. 2013. The flow of red blood cells through a narrow spleen-like slit. *Phys Fluids* 25 (11). doi:10.1063/1.4819341.

Freund, J. B. 2014. Numerical simulation of flowing blood cells. *Annu Rev Fluid Mech* 46: 67–95. doi:10.1146/annurev-fluid-010313-141349.

Gekle, S. 2016. Strongly accelerated margination of active particles in blood flow. *Biophys J* 110 (2): 514–520. doi:10.1016/j.bpj.2015.12.005.

Ginsberg, M. H., A. Partridge, and S. J. Shattil. 2005. Integrin regulation. *Curr Opin Cell Biol* 17 (5): 509–516. doi:10.1016/j.ceb.2005.08.010.

Gompper, G., and D. A. Fedosov. 2016. Modeling microcirculatory blood flow: Current state and future perspectives. *Wiley Interdiscip Rev Syst Biol Med* 8 (2): 157–168. doi:10.1002/wsbm.1326.

Guckenberger, A., and S. Gekle. 2017. Theory and algorithms to compute Helfrich bending forces: A review. *J Phys Condens Matter* 29: 203001. doi:10.1088/1361-648X/aa6313.

Guckenberger, A., M. P. Schraml, P. G. Chen, M. Leonetti, and S. Gekle. 2016. On the bending algorithms for soft objects in flows. *Comput Phys Commun* 207: 1–23. doi:10.1016/j. cpc.2016.04.018.

Hartwig, J. H., and M. DeSisto. 1991. The cytoskeleton of the resting human blood platelet: Structure of the membrane skeleton and its attachment to actin filaments. *J Cell Biol* 112 (3): 407–425.

Hartwig, J., and J. Italiano, Jr. 2003. The birth of the platelet. *J Thromb Haemost* 1 (7): 1580–1586.

Helfrich, W. 1973. Elastic properties of lipid bilayers: Theory and possible experiments. *Z Naturforsch C* 28 (11–1): 693–703.

Hermans, C., C. Wittevrongel, C. Thys, P. A. Smethurst, C. Van Geet, and K. Freson. 2009. A compound heterozygous mutation in glycoprotein VI in a patient with a bleeding disorder. *J Thromb Haemost* 7 (8): 1356–1363. doi:10.1111/j.1538-7836.2009.03520.x.

Hodivala-Dilke, K. M., K. P. McHugh, D. A. Tsakiris, H. Rayburn, D. Crowley, M. Ullman-Cullere, F. P. Ross, B. S. Coller, S. Teitelbaum, and R. O. Hynes. 1999. Beta3-integrin-deficient mice are a model for Glanzmann thrombasthenia showing placental defects and reduced survival. *J Clin Invest* 103 (2): 229–238. doi:10.1172/JCI5487.

Hynes, R. O. 2002. Integrins: bidirectional, allosteric signaling machines. *Cell* 110 (6): 673–687.

Jackson, S. P. 2011. Arterial thrombosis—insidious, unpredictable and deadly. *Nat Med* 17 (11): 1423–1436. doi:10.1038/nm.2515.

Jackson, S. P., W. S. Nesbitt, and E. Westein. 2009. Dynamics of platelet thrombus formation. *J Thromb Haemost* 7 Suppl 1: 17–20. doi:10.1111/j.1538-7836.2009.03401.x.

Jen, C. J., and L. V. McIntire. 1982. The structural properties and contractile force of a clot. *Cell Motil* 2 (5): 445–455.

Kahn, M. L., T. G. Diacovo, D. F. Bainton, F. Lanza, J. Trejo, and S. R. Coughlin. 1999. Glycoprotein V-deficient platelets have undiminished thrombin responsiveness and do not exhibit a Bernard-Soulier phenotype. *Blood* 94 (12): 4112–4121.

Kaoui, B., G. Biros, and C. Misbah. 2009. Why do red blood cells have asymmetric shapes even in a symmetric flow? *Phys Rev Lett* 103 (18). doi:10.1103/Physrevlett.103.188101.

Kato, K., C. Martinez, S. Russell, P. Nurden, A. Nurden, S. Fiering, and J. Ware. 2004. Genetic deletion of mouse platelet glycoprotein Ibbeta produces a Bernard-Soulier phenotype with increased alpha-granule size. *Blood* 104 (8): 2339–2344. doi:10.1182/blood-2004-03-1127.

Konstantinides, S., J. Ware, P. Marchese, F. Almus-Jacobs, D. J. Loskutoff, and Z. M. Ruggeri. 2006. Distinct antithrombotic consequences of platelet glycoprotein Ibalpha and VI deficiency in a mouse model of arterial thrombosis. *J Thromb Haemost* 4 (9): 2014–2021. doi:10.1111/j.1538-7836.2006.02086.x.

Kroll, M. H., J. D. Hellums, L. V. McIntire, A. I. Schafer, and J. L. Moake. 1996. Platelets and shear stress. *Blood* 88 (5): 1525–1541.

Lam, W. A., O. Chaudhuri, A. Crow, K. D. Webster, T. D. Li, A. Kita, J. Huang, and D. A. Fletcher. 2011. Mechanics and contraction dynamics of single platelets and implications for clot stiffening. *Nat Mater* 10 (1): 61–66. doi:10.1038/nmat2903.

Lopez, A. D., C. D. Mathers, M. Ezzati, D. T. Jamison, and C. J. Murray. 2006. Global and regional burden of disease and risk factors, 2001: Systematic analysis of population health data. *Lancet* 367 (9524): 1747–1757. doi:10.1016/S0140-6736(06)68770-9.

Matus, V., G. Valenzuela, C. G. Saez, P. Hidalgo, M. Lagos, E. Aranda, O. Panes et al. 2013. An adenine insertion in exon 6 of human GP6 generates a truncated protein associated with a bleeding disorder in four Chilean families. *J Thromb Haemost* 11 (9): 1751–1759. doi:10.1111/jth.12334.

Miura, Y., T. Takahashi, S. M. Jung, and M. Moroi. 2002. Analysis of the interaction of platelet collagen receptor glycoprotein VI (GPVI) with collagen. A dimeric form of GPVI, but not the monomeric form, shows affinity to fibrous collagen. *J Biol Chem* 277 (48): 46197–46204. doi:10.1074/jbc.M204029200.

Møllmann, H. 1981. *Introduction to the Theory of Thin Shells*. Chichester, UK: Wiley.

Myers, D. R., Y. Qiu, M. E. Fay, M. Tennenbaum, D. Chester, J. Cuadrado, Y. Sakurai et al. 2017. Single-platelet nanomechanics measured by high-throughput cytometry. *Nat Mater* 16 (2): 230–235. doi:10.1038/nmat4772.

Nakamura, F., R. Pudas, O. Heikkinen, P. Permi, I. Kilpelainen, A. D. Munday, J. H. Hartwig, T. P. Stossel, and J. Ylanne. 2006. The structure of the GPIb-filamin A complex. *Blood* 107 (5): 1925–1932. doi:10.1182/blood-2005-10-3964.

Nesbitt, W. S., E. Westein, F. J. Tovar-Lopez, E. Tolouei, A. Mitchell, J. Fu, J. Carberry, A. Fouras, and S. P. Jackson. 2009. A shear gradient-dependent platelet aggregation mechanism drives thrombus formation. *Nat Med* 15 (6): 665–673. doi:10.1038/nm.1955.

Neu, B., and H. J. Meiselman. 2002. Depletion-mediated red blood cell aggregation in polymer solutions. *Biophys J* 83 (5): 2482–2490. doi:10.1016/S0006-3495(02)75259-4.

Nguyen, T. H., R. Palankar, V. C. Bui, N. Medvedev, A. Greinacher, and M. Delcea. 2016. Rupture Forces among Human Blood Platelets at different Degrees of Activation. *Sci Rep* 6: 25402. doi:10.1038/srep25402.

Nieswandt, B., I. Pleines, and M. Bender. 2011. Platelet adhesion and activation mechanisms in arterial thrombosis and ischaemic stroke. *J Thromb Haemost* 9 Suppl 1: 92–104. doi:10.1111/j.1538-7836.2011.04361.x.

Nurden, A. T. 2006. Glanzmann thrombasthenia. *Orphanet J Rare Dis* 1:10. doi:10.1186/1750-1172-1-10.

Nurden, A. T., D. Didry, and J. P. Rosa. 1983. Molecular defects of platelets in Bernard-Soulier syndrome. *Blood Cells* 9 (2): 333–358.

Offermanns, S. 2006. Activation of platelet function through G protein-coupled receptors. *Circ Res* 99 (12): 1293–1304. doi:10.1161/01.RES.0000251742.71301.16.

Patel, S. R., J. H. Hartwig, and J. E. Italiano, Jr. 2005. The biogenesis of platelets from megakaryocyte proplatelets. *J Clin Invest* 115 (12): 3348–3354. doi:10.1172/JCI26891.

Patel, S. R., J. L. Richardson, H. Schulze, E. Kahle, N. Galjart, K. Drabek, R. A. Shivdasani, J. H. Hartwig, and J. E. Italiano, Jr. 2005. Differential roles of microtubule assembly and sliding in proplatelet formation by megakaryocytes. *Blood* 106 (13): 4076–4085. doi:10.1182/blood-2005-06-2204.

Popel, A. S., and P. C. Johnson. 2005. Microcirculation and hemorheology. *Annu Rev Fluid Mech* 37: 43–69. doi:10.1146/annurev.fluid.37.042604.133933.

Pozrikidis, C. 2001. Interfacial dynamics for Stokes flow. *J Comput Phys* 169 (2): 250–301. doi:10.1006/jcph.2000.6582.

Ruggeri, Z. M., J. A. Dent, and E. Saldivar. 1999. Contribution of distinct adhesive interactions to platelet aggregation in flowing blood. *Blood* 94 (1): 172–178.

Ruggeri, Z. M., J. N. Orje, R. Habermann, A. B. Federici, and A. J. Reininger. 2006. Activation-independent platelet adhesion and aggregation under elevated shear stress. *Blood* 108 (6): 1903–1910. doi:10.1182/blood-2006-04-011551.

Savage, B., F. Almus-Jacobs, and Z. M. Ruggeri. 1998. Specific synergy of multiple substrate-receptor interactions in platelet thrombus formation under flow. *Cell* 94 (5): 657–666.

Skalak, R., A. Tozeren, R. P. Zarda, and S. Chien. 1973. Strain Energy Function of Red Blood-Cell Membranes. *Biophys J* 13 (3): 245–280.

Stalker, T. J., J. D. Welsh, and L. F. Brass. 2014. Shaping the platelet response to vascular injury. *Curr Opin Hematol* 21 (5): 410–417. doi:10.1097/MOH.0000000000000070.

Steffen, P., C. Verdier, and C. Wagner. 2013. Quantification of depletion-induced adhesion of red blood cells. *Phys Rev Lett* 110 (1): 018102. doi:10.1103/PhysRevLett.110.018102.

Steigmann, D. J. 1999. Fluid films with curvature elasticity. *Arch Ration Mech Anal* 150 (2): 127–152. doi:10.1007/s002050050183.

Tomaiuolo, G., M. Simeone, V. Martinelli, B. Rotoli, and S. Guido. 2009. Red blood cell deformation in microconfined flow. *Soft Matter* 5 (19): 3736–3740. doi:10.1039/b904584h.

Tronik-Le Roux, D., V. Roullot, C. Poujol, T. Kortulewski, P. Nurden, and G. Marguerie. 2000. Thrombasthenic mice generated by replacement of the integrin alpha(IIb) gene: Demonstration that transcriptional activation of this megakaryocytic locus precedes lineage commitment. *Blood* 96 (4): 1399–1408.

Tutwiler, V., R. I. Litvinov, A. P. Lozhkin, A. D. Peshkova, T. Lebedeva, F. I. Ataullakhanov, K. L. Spiller, D. B. Cines, and J. W. Weisel. 2016. Kinetics and mechanics of clot contraction are governed by the molecular and cellular composition of the blood. *Blood* 127 (1): 149–159. doi:10.1182/blood-2015-05-647560.

Viallat, A., and M. Abkarian. 2014. Red blood cell: from its mechanics to its motion in shear flow. *Int J Lab Hematol* 36 (3): 237–243. doi:10.1111/ijlh.12233.

Ware, J., S. Russell, and Z. M. Ruggeri. 2000. Generation and rescue of a murine model of platelet dysfunction: the Bernard-Soulier syndrome. *Proc Natl Acad Sci U S A* 97 (6): 2803–2308. doi:10.1073/pnas.050582097.

Zhang, J. F., P. C. Johnson, and A. S. Popel. 2009. Effects of erythrocyte deformability and aggregation on the cell free layer and apparent viscosity of microscopic blood flows. *Microvasc Res* 77 (3): 265–272. doi:10.1016/j.mvr.2009.01.010.

Zhang, W., W. Deng, L. Zhou, Y. Xu, W. Yang, X. Liang, Y. Wang, J. D. Kulman, X. F. Zhang, and R. Li. 2015. Identification of a juxtamembrane mechanosensitive domain in the platelet mechanosensor glycoprotein Ib-IX complex. *Blood* 125 (3): 562–569. doi:10.1182/blood-2014-07-589507.

9

Aortic Valve Mechanics

J. Dallard, M. Boodhwani, and M. R. Labrosse

Contents

9.1 Introduction

The aortic valve (AV), located between the left ventricle and the aorta, is one of the four valves of the heart (see Chapter 1). It opens during systole (i.e., left ventricular contraction) to let blood flow into the aorta and closes to prevent backflow in diastole (i.e., left ventricular relaxation). The AV opens and closes about 103,000 times a day (Thubrikar, 1989). During a lifetime, the normal functioning AV experiences at least three billion open–close cycles; as a result, the AV has evolved into a highly specialized structure (Stella and Sacks, 2007). The first interest in the AV, and most specifically in the sinuses of Valsalva, seems to date back to the Renaissance, with descriptions and drawings by Leonardo da Vinci (Reid, 1970).

The emphasis in this chapter will be placed on biomechanical and surgical aspects, with relevance to AV treatment solutions. We will start with a general description of the biological structure, including histological aspects, and then describe the AV dynamic function. More detailed dimensional quantification will follow, to serve as background to biomechanical modeling and reference values for normal valves. Then, clinically relevant issues will be discussed, with a focus on AV anatomical malformations and their failure mechanisms, using anatomical and functional descriptions and classifications. As a natural next step, we will describe the most commonly used surgical procedures to better understand the philosophy of AV surgery in treating the various failure mechanisms introduced earlier. Next, biomechanical experimental data about AV that allow for tissue and functional characterization will be presented. Finally, after a brief theoretical introduction to finite element (FE) modeling, we will review mechanical modeling approaches for native AVs and AV surgery. This will highlight the complementary nature of biomechanical and surgical aspects, the high potential of surgical mechanical modeling, and various knowledge gaps and technical limitations that are worth addressing in the future.

9.1.1 General Description

The AV is classically divided into different structures to make the description easier (Berdajs, 2015). The so-called aortic root is the biological structure at the transition between the left ventricular outflow tract and the ascending aorta. This transition is a complex and mixed structure, both part of the left ventricle from a physiological point of view and part of the aorta from a morphological point of view. The aortic root is mainly composed of the three sinuses of Valsalva located between the ventriculoaortic junction (VAJ) and the sinotubular junction (STJ). The three sinuses of Valsalva are outwardly ballooned regions of the aortic wall (Figure 9.1a), with an approximately hemispherical shape (Thubrikar, 1989). Two of these sinuses include orifices for the coronary arteries. There is a leaflet or cusp inside each sinus of Valsalva (Sauren et al., 1980).

A normal AV is composed of three cusps (Figure 9.1b): the right coronary cusp (RC), the left coronary cusp (LC), and the noncoronary cusp (NC). The base of each

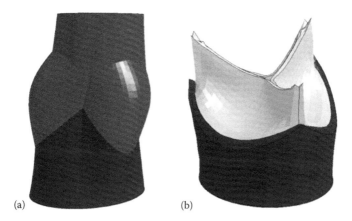

(a)   (b)

Figure 9.1 Three-dimensional schematic representation of the aortic valve (a) with aortic root (brown) and left ventricular outflow tract (red), and (b) with aortic sinuses and ascending aorta removed to show the three cusps of a normal tricuspid aortic valve.

cusp is inserted into the aortic root and is also fused with the adjacent cusps on its lateral sides. The commissures are formed by the mural regions, where two cusps insert side by side along parallel lines (Thubrikar, 1989). From the aortic root point of view, the sinuses of Valsalva also merge with one another at the commissures and continue across the sinus rim distally into the aorta.

9.1.2 Anatomical and Histological Description

The three sinuses are composed of three layers that are also typical of arterial vessels: the intima, the media, and the adventitia (Thubrikar, 1989). The intima, the innermost layer in contact with blood, is the thinnest layer and is composed of endothelial cells. Although biochemically very important, this very thin layer does not have a significant contribution to the mechanical properties of the aortic root wall (Holzapfel et al., 2000). The media, the middle layer, is also the thickest (Thubrikar, 1989). It is composed of alternate layers of smooth muscle, elastin, and collagen fibers. The orientation and interconnection between these different components constitute a fibrous helix (Holzapfel et al., 2000). The media is mainly responsible for the elasticity of the sinuses and is mechanically the most important layer. Finally, the adventitia, the outermost layer, is composed of fibrous connective tissue, with insertion of thick bundles of collagen fibrils, which are arranged in helical structures and serve to reinforce the aortic wall (Holzapfel et al., 2000).

The reader is referred to Chapter 2 for a detailed description of the histology of AV cusps. Briefly, the cusps also have a multilayered structure composed of the ventricularis, the spongiosa, and the fibrosa (Stella and Sacks, 2007; Sun et al., 2014). The fibrosa faces the aorta, the ventricularis faces the left ventricle, and the spongiosa is situated in between the layers. In terms of composition, the fibrosa is globally made of type I collagen fibers arranged in a dense network forming large structures and well aligned with the free margin of the cusp. The ventricularis is made of a dense network of elastin and collagen fibers. Finally, the spongiosa is composed of connective tissue and includes fibrous structures; it has an important role as a connection between the other two layers (Stella and Sacks, 2007; Buchanan and Sacks, 2014). The cusp insertions into the aortic wall, which can be considered transition areas, are composed almost exclusively of dense collagenous tissue (Thubrikar, 1989).

9.1.3 Aortic Valve Dynamic Function

The AV is a one-directional valve or check valve (Nishimura, 2002). During the cardiac cycle, blood pressure increases when the left ventricle contracts (systole). The AV opens when blood pressure is greater than the pressure in the aorta, allowing blood to flow from the left ventricle into the aorta. When the left ventricle relaxes (diastole), blood pressure in the left ventricle decreases and the higher pressure in the aorta forces the valve to close.

As the valve closes, the cusps collapse against each other, until they make enough contact to find an equilibrium configuration against the difference in blood pressure between the aorta and the left ventricle (Figure 9.2). The contact surface is called coaptation surface. In a healthy closed AV, the three cusps are well aligned (Nishimura, 2002) and coapt at the center of the AV orifice. This prevents any backflow of blood into the left ventricle (Boodhwani and El Khoury, 2014). The cusps typically coapt at the mid-distance between the VAJ and STJ levels (Boodhwani et al., 2009b). Overall, the AV experiences typical variations in blood pressure, from 80 mmHg in diastole to 120 mmHg in systole.

This initial description highlights the complexity of the AV structure in terms of function and anatomy; it is complemented by a more detailed and quantitative description of the AV dimensions in the next section.

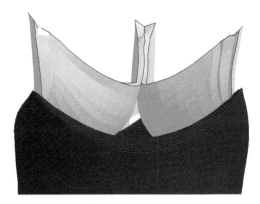

Figure 9.2 Three-dimensional schematic representation of cusps coaptation in diastole. One cusp was removed to better see the other pair.

9.2 Aortic Valve Dimensions and Performance Measures

9.2.1 Aortic Valve Dimensions

In this section, we describe a set of dimensions that can be used to describe the geometry of the normal or tricuspid aortic valve (TAV). Although variations can be observed between the dimensions of the three cusps, their normal geometry is expected to be similar enough to be described by a general approach (Sun et al., 2014). Such AV idealization was proposed in Swanson and Clark (1974) and Thubrikar (1989).

We begin with the geometry of insertion of a cusp into the aortic wall, known as the attachment line. The attachment line can be divided into two different parts: the proximal part, involving the insertion of one cusp into the aortic root, and the distal part (or commissure), involving the merging of two adjacent cusps and the aortic wall (Figure 9.3). From a modeling perspective, the proximal part of the attachment line can be idealized as a conic section (Thubrikar, 1989). Landmarks to construct conic sections for all three cusps are the proximal commissural points and the nadirs of the cusps. The commissures are defined by the lines between the proximal and distal commissural points (in green in Figure 9.3), separated by commissural height, H_S.

Based on these first definitions, we can describe the idealized aortic root. The STJ is defined in the plane passing through the three distal commissural points (Figure 9.3). Since the structure of the STJ can be considered circular (Berdajs, 2015), its diameter is commonly quantified as the diameter of the circle fitted through the three distal commissural points. Similarly, the VAJ can be defined in the plane passing through the nadirs of the three cusps (Figure 9.3). The shape of the VAJ appears to be an ellipse in many individuals or may be simplified into a circle (Aicher and Schäfers, 2012). Therefore, the VAJ can be described by two dimensions in the axes of the ellipse or by one equivalent diameter based on surface area or averaged dimensions of the axes. In the clinical literature, the term *basal ring* is also often used, instead of VAJ, as explained in de Kerchove et al. (2015). Finally, the height of the sinuses of Valsalva can be defined as the distance between the VAJ and STJ planes along the AV axis (Figure 9.3).

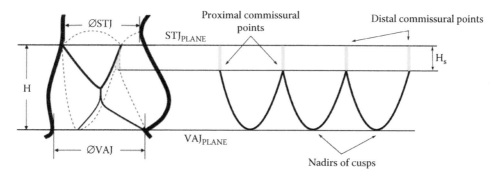

Figure 9.3 Definition of the cusp attachment lines and commissures. STJ: sinotubular junction; VAJ: ventriculoaortic junction; H_S: commissural height.

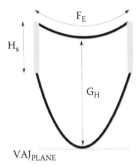

Figure 9.4 Definition of the cusp main dimensions. F_E: free edge (or margin) length; G_H: geometric height; VAJ: ventriculoaortic junction; H_S: commissural height.

The geometry of the cusps can be idealized by a few dimensions. The free margin or free edge F_E of the cusp is defined as the curvilinear distance between the two distal commissural points of a cusp (Figure 9.4). The geometric height G_H of the cusp is defined as the curvilinear distance between its nadir and the middle point of the free edge. The cusp sweep angle θ is defined as the angle formed by the two commissures and is measured from the centerline of the AV. In a perfectly symmetrical TAV, the cusp sweep angle would be 120 degrees.

The set of dimensions described previously is particularly well suited to healthy AVs. However, for diseased AVs, especially with malformations involving geometric variations, additional dimensions should be used as needed.

9.2.2 Geometric Measures of Aortic Valve Performance

Specific geometrical measures have also been proposed in the literature to evaluate the AV performance (Schäfers et al., 2006) and have been adapted to the clinical routine (Vahanian et al., 2012). For instance, one criterion is the geometric orifice area (GOA), which quantifies the projected opening area of the valve in systole. This measure describes how much blood can flow through the valve. A similar approach can be applied to represent how much backflow can occur through a leaky valve in diastole; one will then be interested in the geometric regurgitant orifice area (GROA). Both GOA and GROA have their clinical counterparts established by using ultrasound imaging and planimetry (effective orifice area, EOA) and ultrasound imaging and various methods involving echo-Doppler and processing of the regurgitant jet (effective regurgitant orifice area, EROA), respectively. These measures are helpful for cardiologists and surgeons to quantify the AV malfunction in different valvular diseases (Garcia and Kadem, 2006). Cusp coaptation can also be related to AV performance (Thubrikar, 1989). Indeed, functional levels of coaptation are expected to prevent any backflow. One measure of coaptation in healthy valves is the central height of coaptation Xs (Figure 9.5). A new measure has recently been proposed for healthy and regurgitant (leaky) valves, to evaluate the performance of each cusp (Schäfers et al., 2006). The measure, so-called effective height (eH), is the projected

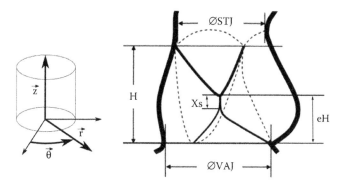

Figure 9.5 Definition of cusp coaptation measures. Xs: central height of coaptation; eH: effective height. The valve has dimensions defined by STJ (sinotubular junction) diameter, VAJ (ventriculoaortic junction) diameter, and height H.

distance along the longitudinal axis of the valve between the central point of the free edge of a cusp and its nadir (Figure 9.5). Additional measures of coaptation have been proposed in the literature, such as the cusp flexion angle (Thubrikar, 1989) and the coaptation surface area (Sohmer et al., 2013).

9.2.3 Dimensional Studies

Many dimensional studies of the AV can be found in the literature (Kunzelman et al., 1994; Labrosse et al., 2006; Bierbach et al., 2010; de Kerchove et al., 2015). To provide the reader with orders of magnitude regarding AV dimensions, Tables 9.1 and 9.2 summarize available measurements from a nonexhaustive list of clinical and biomechanical sources. Table 9.1 describes the aortic root geometry through the classical dimensions previously defined in this chapter: STJ diameter, VAJ diameter, and height H of the sinuses of Valsalva.

As can be seen from Table 9.1, various approaches have been used in the literature to carry out measurements in AVs, from transesophageal echocardiography in healthy volunteers (Bierbach et al., 2010) and patients (de Kerchove et al., 2015) to intraoperative measurements (Schäfers et al., 2013), in vitro measurements (Kunzelman et al., 1994), and measurements using silicone rubber molds (Labrosse et al., 2006). Overall, in healthy subjects, VAJ diameters in the range of 21–24 mm, STJ diameters in the range of 19–25 mm, and sinus heights in the range of 21–23 mm have been observed. As expected, AVs in children (age = 5.8 ± 3 years) presented with lower dimensions, with 14, 15, and 14 mm, respectively, for the VAJ diameter, the STJ diameter, and the sinus height (Bierbach et al., 2010). Patients affected by aortic root dilatation exhibited a range of 24–30 mm for the VAJ diameter and 32–41 mm for the STJ diameter (Schäfers et al., 2013; de Kerchove et al., 2015).

Table 9.2 describes the cusp geometry through the classical dimensions previously defined in this chapter: cusp geometric height (G_H), free-edge length (F_E), and effective height (eH).

TABLE 9.1 Aortic Root Dimensions

Source	Subjects	Measurement Method	Valve Type	Condition of Valve	Age (yrs)	n	VAJ (mm)	STJ (mm)	H (mm)
Bierbach et al. (2010)	Healthy adults	TEE	TAV	Pressurized, diastole	33.8 ± 14	100	21 ± 2.8	25 ± 3.7	22.4 ± 4.2
	Healthy children	TEE	TAV	Pressurized, diastole	5.8 ± 3	30	13.9 ± 2	15.4 ± 2.9	13.7 ± 2.4
Kunzelman et al. (1994)	Healthy adults	In vitro study	TAV	Unpressurized	39 ± 12	10	23.4 ± 1.2	18.9 ± 0.9	
Labrosse et al. (2006)	Healthy adults	Silicone rubber molds	TAV	Pressurized, diastole		15	24.6	22.9	21.7
de Kerchove et al. (2015)	Subcommissural annuloplasty patients	TEE	TAV	Pressurized	61 ± 15	146	24 ± 3	32 ± 7	
	Valve-sparing reimplantation patients	TEE	TAV	Pressurized	53 ± 16	154	27 ± 4	40 ± 8	
Schäfers et al. (2013)	Patients	Intraoperative	TAV	Unpressurized	60.4 ± 13.2	329	27.6 ± 2.8	34.5 ± 7.1	
	Patients	Intraoperative	BAV	Unpressurized	46.6 ± 13.4	286	29.7 ± 3.2	31.0 ± 5.8	

TEE: transesophageal echocardiography; TAV: tricuspid aortic valve; BAV: bicuspid aortic valve.

TABLE 9.2 Aortic Valve Cusp Dimensions

Source	Subjects	Measurement Method	Valve Type	Condition of Valve	Age (yrs)	n	eH (mm)	G_H (mm)			F_E (mm)		
								RC	LC	NC	RC	LC	NC
Bierbach et al. (2010)	Healthy adults	TEE	TAV	Pressurized, diastole	33.8 ± 14	100	Average = 9.5 ± 1.4						
	Healthy children	TEE	TAV	Pressurized, diastole	5.8 ± 3	30	Average = 6.2 ± 1.3						
Kunzelman et al. (1994)	Healthy adults	In vitro study	TAV	Unpressurized	39 ± 12	10		13.3 ± 0.6	13.9 ± 0.8	13.7 ± 0.4	33 ± 1.4	31.5 ± 1.4	32.7 ± 1.3
Labrosse et al. (2006)	Healthy adults	Silicone rubber molds	TAV	Pressurized, diastole		15		Average = 13.4			Average = 31		
Schäfers et al. (2013)	Patients	Intraoperative	TAV	Unpressurized	60.4 ± 13.2	329		20 ± 2.1	20 ± 2.1	20.7 ± 2.2			
	Patients	Intraoperative	BAV	Unpressurized	46.6 ± 13.4	286		Nonfused: 23.8 ± 2					

TEE: transesophageal echocardiography; TAV: tricuspid aortic valve; BAV: bicuspid aortic valve.

As shown in Table 9.2, free edge lengths of cusps in the range of 31–33 mm (Kunzelman et al., 1994; Labrosse et al., 2006) and effective heights of cusps of about 10 mm have been observed in healthy adults (Bierbach et al., 2010). According to surgeons, the effective height of a functional valve should be in the range of 8–10 mm (Schäfers et al., 2006). For geometric heights of cusps, we notice two different orders of magnitude in the literature: 13–14 mm (Kunzelman et al., 1994; Labrosse et al., 2006) and around 20 mm (Schäfers et al., 2013). The difference can be explained by the significant pull exerted on the cusp before measurements were taken in the latter case. Additional cusp measurements may include the attached length, 47.4 mm, and the surface area of the cusps, 304 mm^2, performed during an in vitro study on 10 subjects (Kunzelman et al., 1994).

Finally, the thickness of cusps, including their different layers, has also been studied in detail (Sahasakul et al., 1988; McDonald et al., 2002). Generally on the order of 0.5 mm, the AV cusp thickness varies with location and increases with age.

The idealized geometry detailed so far allows one to relatively easily model the AV under the assumption of sufficient symmetry and regularity, which may not be compatible with the complex and real shape of the valve. However, this approach provides a valuable common framework for both biomedical engineers and surgeons.

9.3 Aortic Valve Diseases

9.3.1 Aortic Stenosis

Aortic stenosis (AS) refers to the narrowing of the AV opening during systole (Nishimura, 2002), producing an obstruction of the left ventricular outflow (Ketelsen et al., 2010). It can be caused by a congenital abnormality of the valve or by progressive calcification (Nishimura, 2002; ACC/AHA, 2006). The decrease in the GOA of the AV induces an overload for the left ventricle. Aortic stenosis is associated with elevated pressures in the left ventricle during systole, as the left ventricle attempts to produce the same cardiac output, despite the reduced GOA. This results in a hypertrophic process, whereby the left ventricular wall thickens (for more muscle), while the left ventricular volume is maintained.

9.3.2 Aortic Insufficiency

One common AV lesion is aortic insufficiency (AI), also known as aortic regurgitation, in which the valve does not close completely in diastole (EROA > 0), allowing blood to flow in the reverse direction (leak). There are several causes for AI, including, but not limited to, aortic dilatation, congenital abnormality of the valve, and calcification (ACC/AHA, 2006). The blood reflux from the aorta into the left ventricle increases the ventricular workload through pressure and volume overloads (ACC/AHA, 2006; Ketelsen et al., 2010). In turn, these overloads trigger a hypertrophic dilatation of the left ventricle.

9.3.3 Aortic Valve Malformations

Congenital malformations represent different cases involving various numbers of cusps, from one to five (Table 9.3). Some of these cusps can be fused with a raphe (Figure 9.6). The term *raphe* defines the conjoined area between two underdeveloped cusps that turns into a malformed commissure (Sievers and Schmidtke, 2007). Different types of conjoined area can be observed, involving complete or incomplete fusions of the cusps (Koenraadt et al., 2016). The raphe often attaches to the cusp base in the form of a pseudocommissure. Compared with a true commissure between two regular cusps, a pseudocommissure generally occupies a greater proportion of the

TABLE 9.3   Anatomical and Functional Classifications of the Main Aortic Valve Malformations

Anatomical description	Number of cusp	1	2	3			4	5
	Number of commissure	0	2	2	1	3	4	5
	Number of raphe	0	0	1	2	0	0	0
Functional description	Number of cusp	1	2		1	3	4	5
		Unicuspid Acommissural	Bicuspid Type 0	Type 1	Unicuspid unicommissural	Tricuspid	Quadricuspid	Pentacuspid
Schematic representation	Main							
	Subcategories							

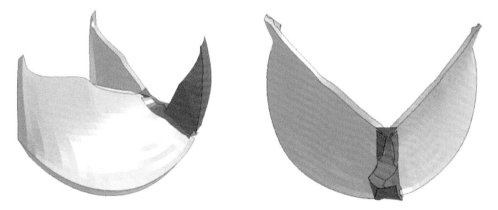

Figure 9.6   Illustration of the fusion of two anatomical cusps into a functional cusp with a raphe (in brown).

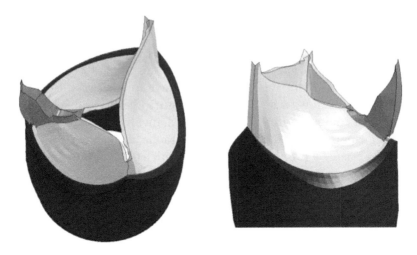

Figure 9.7   Three-dimensional illustration of a type 1 bicuspid aortic valve.

valve circumference and has a lower height (Boodhwani et al., 2010b). Once fused, two anatomical cusps (or three) become a single cusp from a functional point of view (Figure 9.6). Therefore, an important distinction must be made between the anatomical and functional number of cusps.

The normal AV or TAV involves three anatomical and functional leaflets with three normal commissures (Figure 9.1). According to the malformations involved, these cusps can be modified, involving fusions with raphes or divisions.

One of the most common variants involves a single fusion of two cusps with a single raphe (Figure 9.7) and two normal commissures, resulting in a bicuspid aortic valve with two functional cusps. Other variants can also be found, with two fusions (involving two distinct raphes) having only one normal commissure, usually NC or LC (Aicher and Schäfers, 2012); they result into unicuspid valves, with only one functional cusp.

Alternatively, divisions of cusps can be observed. One division produces a four-cusp or quadricuspid aortic valve (QAV). The QAVs involve four functional cusps and four commissures. The rarest malformation may involve two divisions and five cusps, resulting into a pentacuspid aortic valve (PAV) (Cemri et al., 200). Only about 10 cases of PAVs have been reported (Ozyilmaz et al., 2015). A PAV may exhibit normal left and right cusps and three small cusps that are divided by well-developed commissures (Kuroki et al., 2012), along with severe regurgitation.

Some patients present BAVs with two symmetric cusps, with two normal commissures and no median raphe. Finally, some AVs feature only one cusp without any commissure, owing to a central opening.

9.3.4 Functional Classification of Malformed Valves

According to functional criteria, different classifications have been proposed in the literature. The main criterion is generally the number of functional cusps. For instance, the BAV category is composed of two functional cusps (Ridley et al., 2016) and includes both AVs with two anatomical cusps, the so-called type 0 BAV, and AVs with three anatomical cusps, among which two are fused, leaving two functional leaflets, the so-called type 1 BAV (Figure 9.7). However, BAVs can exist anywhere along a spectrum between types 0 and 1 (El Khoury and de Kerchove, 2013). The BAV is the most common congenital cardiac malformation associated with AI, with an estimated prevalence of 1%–2% in the general population (Fedak et al., 2002; Kuroki et al., 2012; Mathieu et al., 2015), which represents about half a million people in Canada. The majority of BAV patients develop complications that require treatment, and a large proportion of them require surgical intervention (Michelena et al., 2008; Tzemos et al., 2008). Type 0 configuration is present in a minority of cases and usually does not require surgical treatment. Type 1 BAV is significantly more prevalent (Boodhwani et al., 2010b) and is of high surgical relevance. The unicuspid aortic valve (UAV) is composed of one functional cusp (Mookadam et al., 2010). This category includes AVs that have three anatomical cusps with two fusions (two raphes), resulting in one functional leaflet and one commissure, the so-called unicommissural UAV. This category also includes AVs featuring one anatomical cusp and no commissure, the so-called acommissural UAV, whose estimated prevalence is 0.02% of the general population (Aicher et al., 2013).

The QAV and PAV categories have the same definitions, whether from an anatomical or a functional point of view. The incidence of QAVs is far less than that of BAVs, at approximately 0.003%–0.033% of the general population (Cemri et al., 2000; Kuroki et al., 2012).

Beyond the various cases presented earlier, new cases that do not fit within the existing classifications (anatomically and/or functionally) are reported on a regular basis. Furthermore, anomalous cord-like extensions sometimes connect the raphe of the conjoint cusp near its free margin to the wall of the ascending aorta (Vowels et al., 2014).

9.3.5 Failure Mechanisms of the Aortic Valve with Aortic Insufficiency

Classifications of AI failure mechanisms have been proposed to provide cardiac surgeons with a better understanding of the diseased AV and help them guide the approach to be used for treatment (Haydar et al., 1997; Lansac et al., 2008; Boodhwani et al., 2009a). Because stenotic valves cannot usually be surgically repaired (they need to be replaced instead), more efforts have been devoted to regurgitant AVs. Existing classifications are generally based on the distinction between two underlying causes for AI, issues with the aortic root, and issues with the cusps (Boodhwani and El Khoury, 2014). All the mechanisms described here directly affect the coaptation performance and generate a regurgitant orifice and a regurgitant jet through that orifice. Patients may have single or multiple lesions contributing to their AI and exhibit one or multiple AI mechanisms (Boodhwani et al., 2009a) (Figure 9.8).

Following the classification in Boodhwani et al. (2009a), the first type is for regurgitation associated with normal motion of cusps. The majority of such cases involve dilatation of specific locations of the aortic root, enlargement of the STJ (type Ia), dilatation of the sinuses of Valsalva and the STJ (type Ib), and dilatation of the VAJ (type Ic).

AI class	Type I Normal cusp motion with FAA dilatation or cusp perforation				Type II Cusp Prolapse	Type III Cusp Prolapse
	la	lb	lc	ld		
Mechanism	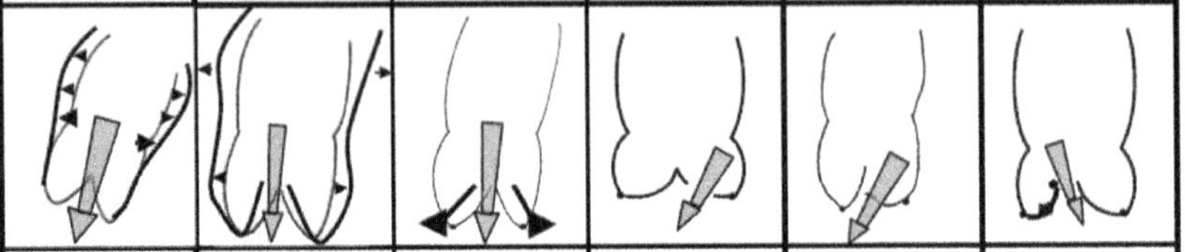					
Repair techniques (primary)	STJ remodeling *Ascending aortic graft*	Aortic valve sparing: *Reimplantation or Remodeling with SCA*	SCA	Patch repair *Autologous or bovine pericardium*	Prolapse repair *Plication Triangular resection Free margin Resuspension Patch*	Leaflet repair *Shaving Decaßcißcatio Patch*
(Secondary)	SCA		STJ Annuloplasty	SCA	SCA	SCA

Figure 9.8 Repair-oriented functional classification of aortic insufficiency (AI), with description of disease mechanisms and repair techniques used. FAA: functional aortic annulus; STJ: sinotubular junction; SCA: subcommissural annuloplasty. (Reprinted with permission from Boodhwani et al., 2009a.)

Type Id is due to cusp perforation, without a primary functional aortic lesion. This type can also be found in another classification according to the criterion of aortic root nondilatation (Lansac et al., 2008). Any dilatation affecting the aortic root will increase the distance between the commissures and may result in an incompetent AV function (Berdajs, 2015). For example, a type Ib AI involving a dilatation of the sinus of Valsalva will generate a central regurgitant jet (Figure 9.9) (Boodhwani and El Khoury, 2014).

Types II and III of the classification are determined based on the major cusp-failure mechanisms. Type II describes cusp prolapse (Figure 9.10), as the consequence of tissue redundancy (Haydar et al., 1997; Aicher and Schäfers, 2012) or commissural disruption (Boodhwani et al., 2009a). Cusp prolapse is defined as the displacement of the free edge of a cusp down to below the coaptation area of other normal cusps (Boodhwani et al., 2009b). Cusp prolapse is well known to be one of the mechanisms responsible for AI (de Kerchove et al., 2009). In terms of diagnostic by cardiologists, cusp prolapse is the consequence of tissue redundancy in the free edge and can be suspected in the presence of an eccentric jet, in the opposite direction of the prolapsing cusp, on echocardiography (Boodhwani et al., 2009b; Aicher and Schäfers, 2012). Conversely, type III designates cusp restriction (Haydar et al., 1997), whereby cusp mobility is reduced as a result of malformation, calcification, thickening, or fibrosis of the cusp (Boodhwani et al., 2009b).

Malformations such as BAVs affect not only the cusps but also the whole aortic root. Type II AI is frequently observed in BAVs and commonly involves the fused cusp but may also be present in the normal nonfused cusp (Aicher and Schäfers, 2012). Furthermore, in malformed AVs featuring a cusps fusion, the raphe may affect cusp

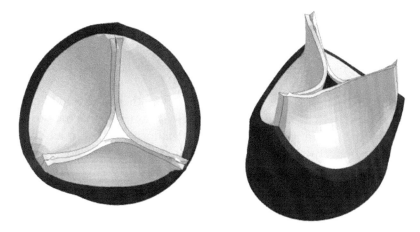

Figure 9.9 Three-dimensional illustration of a regurgitant aortic valve with a central opening.

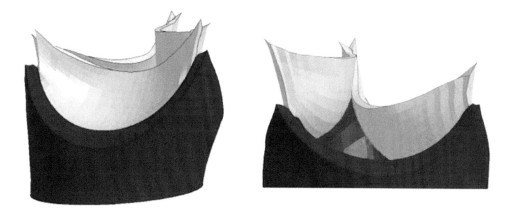

Figure 9.10 Three-dimensional illustration of a regurgitant aortic valve with prolapse of two cusps.

motion in various ways (El Khoury and de Kerchove, 2013). It can be restrictive and decrease cusp motion during the cardiac cycle, generating a restriction (type III AI). Such a raphe would be described in the surgical literature as "rigid" (El Khoury and de Kerchove, 2013). Alternatively, the raphe may be nonrestrictive, with no significant influence on cusp motion, and may be associated with prolapsing cusps (type II AI).

9.3.6 Discussion

There is obviously a large variability in terms of AV abnormalities and failure mechanisms. Comprehension and assessment of the native valve geometry, dynamics, and pathology are the first challenges of the surgeon (Schäfers et al., 2006). Quantification of AI can also be challenging, especially the quantification of the degree of cusp prolapse (Boodhwani et al., 2009b, 2010). These preoperative steps are generally based on medical imaging. The surgical treatment of AV pathologies can be very challenging, and surgeons need as much information as possible to better understand the patient's pathology before entering the operative room.

With regard to Section 9.2 on dimensional aspects, there is a need to enrich existing geometric descriptions of the AV with new landmarks and measures that are able to capture the specific features of various malformed AVs. In addition, from a biomechanical perspective, it would be relevant to seek a better understanding of the dynamic function of malformed AVs, especially AVs involving restrictive or nonrestrictive raphes. This would be expected to possibly broaden the use of AV repair procedures, which are discussed in the next section on AV surgery.

9.4 Aortic Valve Surgery

9.4.1 Surgical Options

There are mostly two surgical approaches to the treatment of AV disease: the first one being the replacement of the original whole valve with a prosthetic valve, and the second one being the repair of the original valve by leaving as much original tissue in place as possible, while addressing the failure mechanism(s).

Available prosthetic valves can be classified into mechanical and bioprosthetic valves (Zhao et al., 2016). The majority of the aortic valve replacements (AVRs) involve a mechanical valve: out of 120,000 valves implanted each year in the United States, 60% are mechanical valves (Alemu and Bluestein, 2007). Contemporary mechanical valves commonly feature two leaflets and are mostly made from pyrolytic carbon (Rajashekar, 2015). However, because the rigid structure of mechanical heart valves damages red blood cells and induces blood clotting, the patients who receive mechanical heart valves need to be treated with life-long anticoagulation therapy.

On the other hand, bioprosthetic valves are derived from porcine or bovine AVs, after tissue-fixation treatment to destroy any living cells and avoid rejection by the patient's immune system. Without living cells, the tissues of the implanted valves cannot repair themselves, as normal living tissues do, and as a result, bioprosthetic valves degrade over time (10–15 years) and present risks of calcification and tears (Vesely, 2003; Johnston et al., 2015).

Aortic valve replacement is the definitive therapy for severe AS (Vahanian et al., 2012); it typically involves open-chest surgery. Although a less invasive procedure, the transcatheter aortic valve implantation (TAVI) is increasingly recognized as a viable therapeutic option for a wider range of patients with severe AS (Masson et al., 2009). This procedure allows a bioprosthetic valve implantation by using a long narrow tube called a catheter. The bioprosthetic valve is delivered on a catheter through the femoral artery or the left ventricular apex (Smith et al., 2011). The TAVI devices include a rigid frame, for example, cobalt–chromium alloy, on which are sown cusps, manufactured from, for example, bovine pericardium (Bailey et al., 2016).

In current practice, AVR remains the most widely used surgical technique because of its relative ease and the high prevalence of AS. However, in the case of AI, the proportion of valve repair procedures is increasing in experienced centers (Vahanian et al., 2012). Indeed, in the case of AI, valve repair has emerged as a viable alternative to replacement with a bioprosthetic valve, because both methods enjoy similar durability and safety (Ashikhmina et al., 2010). Valve repair presents important benefits for patients with valvular regurgitation, because it avoids or minimizes the risks associated with prosthetic valve replacement, including long-term anticoagulation-related hemorrhage, structural deterioration, clot formation, and valve infection late after surgery (Boodhwani and El Khoury, 2014). The goal of repair is not to restore the anatomy but the valve function; this is typically done by transforming the native diseased valve into a functional configuration.

9.4.2 Aortic Valve Repair Techniques

Aortic valve repair techniques can be divided into aortic root procedures and cusp corrections (Rankin and Gaca, 2011).

The main goal of aortic root procedures is the correction of the different types of aortic root dilatations (types Ia to Ic in terms of failure mechanisms). Various aortic root procedures have been proposed, whose common goal is to retain the original AV cusps of the patient while repairing, replacing, or stabilizing the aortic root components (Hopkins, 2003). The David procedure and the Yacoub procedure are the most common aortic root procedures (Soncini et al., 2009). Both involve a Dacron® tube graft to replace the biological tissues of the original aortic root, including all three sinuses of Valsalva (Hopkins, 2003; Vojáček et al., 2017). In addition, in both cases, the aortic root is cut away (resected) and a residual sewing margin of 3–5 mm is kept along the cusps' attachment lines. The David procedure, the so-called "reimplantation," consists of suturing the tube graft along the VAJ. Then, the original commissures are resuspended inside the tube graft. The Yacoub procedure, the so-called "remodeling," consists of suturing the tube graft along the residual sewing margin. When progressive postoperative dilatation of the VAJ is a concern, subcommissural annuloplasty can be performed to stabilize the dimensions of the VAJ (Boodhwani et al., 2009b; Vojáček et al., 2017).

In addition to an aortic root procedure (or in isolation, if the original root is not dilated), cusp correction may be needed. The main goal of cusp repair is the correction of prolapsing cusps (type II AI), as prolapse is the most frequent cusp pathology (Boodhwani and El Khoury, 2014). Two surgical techniques commonly used are resuspension and plication; they share the goal of reducing the free margin of the cusp (Boodhwani et al., 2010a; Labrosse et al., 2011). A free-margin resuspension involves a continuous suture (Figure 9.11) running the entire length of the cusp margin. The free margin is then reduced by applying traction on the continuous suture, and its length is stabilized. In the cusp plication technique (Figure 9.11), the quantity of excess free margin is folded (plicated) on the aortic side by tying a suture. The plication can be central or commissural. Furthermore, cusp plication can be used in conjunction with free-margin resuspension.

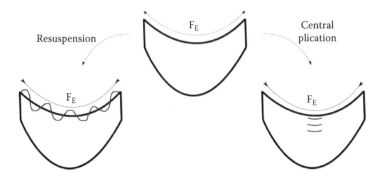

Figure 9.11 Cusp correction techniques: cusp free-margin resuspension (left) and cusp central plication (right).

9.4.3 More Advanced Aortic Valve Repair Techniques

Malformed valves (e.g., BAVs and UAVs) that have become diseased may need replacement, but sometimes, they can be repaired. Again, repair of such valves is intended to transform the native valve into a functional configuration. Depending on the native valve configuration, repair includes different surgical approaches.

One approach consists of creating normal functional commissures (Schäfers et al., 2008) by substituting a raphe with an appropriately sized patch. This approach can be applied to type 1 BAVs to tricuspidize the diseased valves or to unicommissural UAVs to bicuspidize them. Another approach consists of totally removing a false commissure. This approach can be used in type 1 BAVs to turn them into functional type 0 BAVs. These procedures are typically combined with aortic root remodeling or reimplantation, allowing surgeons to reorient the commissures and maximize functionality of the valve. In addition, cusp correction is performed as needed.

The choice between different approaches is directly related to the geometry of the native diseased AV. A common criterion used by surgeons is the sweep angle of the native nonfused cusp. For a native sweep angle greater than 140 degrees, surgeons will likely turn the BAV into a type 0, while for a sweep angle less than 140 degrees, they will likely tricuspidize the valve.

9.4.4 How to Intraoperatively Assess a Repaired Valve?

The intraoperative assessment of the quality of AV repair is based on the quality of the functionality restored in a valve and the likelihood of long-term durability of the repair (Schäfers et al., 2006; de Waroux et al., 2009). Different measurements can be taken during surgery toward this assessment. For example, the effective height of the new configuration is a valuable parameter to measure during AV repair, so as to ensure a suitable value of 8–10 mm (Schäfers et al., 2006). Intraoperative medical imaging is also used to detect and quantify any residual regurgitant jet after surgical repair. If the original AI has not been fixed by the repair, a prosthetic valve may be used as a last resort.

These different surgical treatments require rigorous and regular follow-ups for many years after surgery (ACC/AHA, 2006; Vahanian et al., 2012). Again, medical imaging is used to detect and monitor the emergence of any regurgitant jet, which would be a symptom pointing to the development of one, or several, new AI failure mechanisms.

9.4.5 Discussion

Especially in the case of AI repair, the choice and application of an appropriate surgical approach, and the associated surgical technique, require the surgeon's thorough understanding of the AV failure mechanism(s) at play (Boodhwani and El Khoury, 2014). Indeed, to repair heart valves, cardiac surgeons must single-handedly master the complex interplay of shape, material properties and function of their components.

As discussed, several criteria are used by surgeons, such as the cusp sweep angle (for aortic root reconstruction) and the degree of prolapse (for cusp correction). Still, the quantification of the degree of cusp prolapse can be challenging, with the risk of undercorrection (leaving prolapse) or overcorrection (leading to restriction) (Boodhwani et al., 2010a). Furthermore, the long-term assessment of AV repair is challenging. Currently, no tool is available to predict the long-term performance of repaired AVs.

From the biomechanical modeling perspective, the wide range of surgical procedures available, along with the variability in execution between surgeons, makes even the coarsest predictions of functional outcomes very challenging. Although computational simulations (as will be discussed in Section 9.6.2) can provide specific insights into the value of one procedure over another, some standardization will eventually be required in terms of surgical implementation, such that most surgeons perform a given procedure in the same manner.

However, before turning to computational modeling aspects, it is important to consider experimental aspects of characterization of the AV, from the tissue to the organ levels, as discussed in next section.

9.5 Experimental Aspects

9.5.1 Tissue Characterization

As mentioned earlier, the multilayered structures of the aortic root and cusps are complex. In addition, owing to the high proportion of type I collagen fibers, these tissues exhibit strong anisotropic mechanical properties, whereby deformations are different in different directions. As discussed in greater detail in Chapter 5, biaxial mechanical testing is commonly used to characterize anisotropic tissues (Billiar and Sacks, 2000; Stella and Sacks, 2007; Gundiah et al., 2008; Azadani et al., 2012; Martin and Sun, 2012; Alavi et al., 2013; Labrosse et al., 2016). For logistical reasons (e.g., difficulty in accessing human tissues), cusps from various animals, such

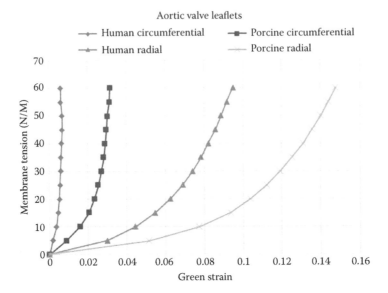

Figure 9.12 Results of equibiaxial tests on human and porcine aortic valve cusps in the circumferential and radial directions. (Digitized and redrawn from Martin, C., and Sun, W., *J. Biomed. Mater. Res. A*, 100, 1591–1599, 2012.)

as ovine and porcine, have been characterized to complement the scarce data from humans. Figure 9.12 shows experimental biaxial results adapted from (Martin and Sun, 2012) for human and porcine cusps in the radial and circumferential directions. The biaxial tests on human tissues were performed on samples from 10 subjects who were 80.6 years old on average. As expected, highly nonlinear stress–strain relationship and a strong anisotropic effect between the radial and circumferential directions could be observed (Alavi et al., 2013). Figure 9.12 also shows that cusp tissues have significant differences between animal and aged human sources (Sun et al., 2014). It appears that the 1-year-old ovine and the 6- to 9-month-old porcine may not be representative of the typical aged human patient; in all cases, the aged human tissues are significantly stiffer. A biaxial testing study compared various cusp replacement biomaterials with porcine cusps and concluded that CardioCel®, PeriGuard®, and Supple Peri-Guard® patches were the closest replacements in terms of elasticity and anisotropy (Labrosse et al., 2016).

Flexural testing has also been performed on porcine cusps (Mirnajafi et al., 2006). The commissural regions of the cusps were found to exhibit compliant properties. The authors estimated the commissural regions to be about three times more compliant than the belly region. These results may be linked to the collagen fiber networks in porcine cusps, as imaging analysis revealed a denser fiber network in the belly region (Mega et al., 2016).

Figure 9.13 reproduces biaxial testing results from human aortic sinus and ascending aorta samples in both circumferential and longitudinal directions (Azadani et al., 2012). The samples were obtained from 14 subjects who were 47 years old on average. Again, the strong nonlinear stress–strain response of these tissues can be appreciated

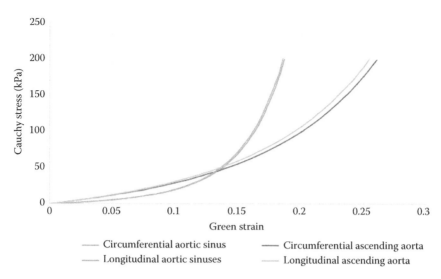

Figure 9.13   Results of equibiaxial tests on human aortic sinus and ascending aorta in the circumferential and longitudinal directions. (Digitized and redrawn from Azadani, A.N. et al., *Ann. Thorac. Surg.*, 93, 87–94, 2012.)

in both directions. It is important to note that, under the physiological stress range, the ascending aorta is significantly more compliant than the aortic sinuses, both in the circumferential and longitudinal directions. Aged human aortic sinuses (81 years old) were also much stiffer than porcine aortic sinuses (Azadani et al., 2012). Regional differences between the sinuses were also noted: the left coronary sinus was found to be more compliant than the right and noncoronary sinuses (Gundiah et al., 2008). The circumferential direction was also found to be more compliant than the longitudinal direction for the left and right coronary sinuses, but no significant difference between directions was observed in the noncoronary sinus.

Although restrictive raphe material has been described as "rigid" by surgeons (Boodhwani and El Khoury, 2014), there does not seem to be any reports of mechanical characterization of raphe tissue in the literature (Jermihov et al., 2011). Information on the constituents of the raphe is also strikingly scarce (Roberts, 1970; Pomerance, 1972). Histological sections have shown that the raphe may or may not contain elastic fibers, depending on location and its congenital or acquired nature. There is also a general lack of information regarding the mechanical properties of cusps in malformed valves.

9.5.2 Organ-Level Characterization of the Dynamics of the Aortic Root and Valve

A few studies describe the dynamics of the aortic valve and the movements of the cusps (Thubrikar et al., 2000; Handke et al., 2003; Saikrishnan et al., 2012; Szeto et al., 2013).

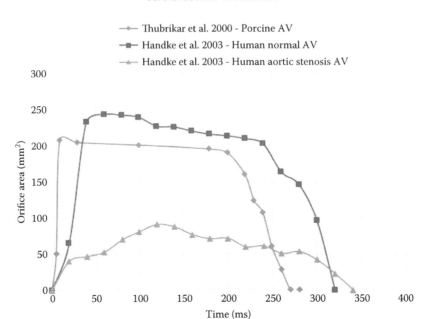

Figure 9.14   Changes in valve orifice area during systole in porcine (Thubrikar et al., 2000) and healthy humans and aortic stenosis subjects (Handke et al., 2003).

During systole, the AV opens and the area of AV orifice left open by the cusps increases. The orifice changes in shape and can be stellate, circular, or triangular or may exhibit an intermediate shape. Using ultrasound imaging in 31 normal subjects, Handke et al. (2003) observed 9 circular, 10 triangular, and 12 intermediate orifices at the time of maximum AV opening. Figure 9.14 provides orders of magnitude for AV orifice area during systole in porcine AVs (Thubrikar et al., 2000), healthy human AVs, and human stenotic AVs (Handke et al., 2003).

It is important to note that the experiments by Thubrikar et al. used a left-heart simulator, whereas the data in Handke et al. relied on three-dimensional (3D) echo-cardiography. Regardless, the cusp movement in normal AVs can be divided into three steps: rapid opening to the maximum opening area, followed by a quasiconstant opening area with a slow decrease, and a rapid end-systolic valve closure. The strong influence of AS on the orifice area can be observed in Figure 9.14. In BAVs, the shape of the orifice is commonly described as a "fish mouth" (Figure 9.15) (Saikrishnan et al., 2012).

Strains developing in the AV can be studied across the cardiac cycle in left-heart simulators (Yap et al., 2009; Szeto et al., 2013). Experiments performed on porcine TAV yielded values for the radial and circumferential stretches in the cusps during diastole. Their findings support the assumption of rather spatially uniform surface pressure (Yap et al., 2009). Then, during systole, the stretches transformed into radial elongation and circumferential compression. Szeto et al. evaluated the cusp strains in surgically created BAVs and TAVs involving porcine tissues. According to the authors, the fused cusp of BAVs experienced significantly more strain during systole

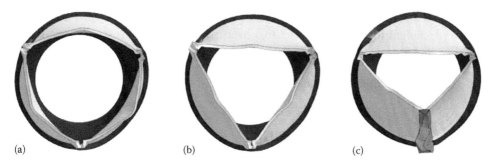

Figure 9.15 Illustrations of AV opening during systole: (a) healthy TAV with a circular opening, (b) healthy TAV with a triangular opening, (c) BAV with a typical "fish mouth" opening.

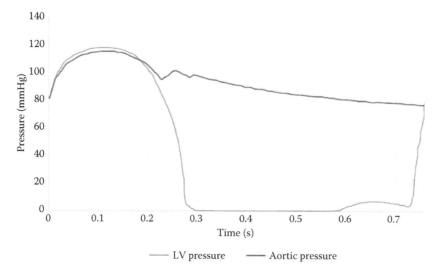

Figure 9.16 Typical pressure pulses in left ventricle (blue) and aorta (orange) during a cardiac cycle (mmHg). (Digitized and redrawn data from Kim, H. et al., *Ann. Biomed. Eng.*, 36, 262–275, 2008.)

when fully open than the TAV cusps (Szeto et al., 2013). These differences were most important in the radial direction.

The classic pressure curves in healthy AVs are drawn in Figure 9.16 for the left ventricle and the aorta during a cardiac cycle (20 mmHg ≈ 2.7 kPa).

9.5.3 Summary

Experiments have shown some differences between the mechanical responses of the aortic sinuses and the ascending aorta. In addition, although porcine AV tissues exhibit material properties similar to young human AV tissues, they are much more compliant than the aged human tissues, which are most often dealt with during surgery. Replacement biomaterials have also been shown to be anisotropic, and careful consideration should be given to their preferred direction to match those of the native tissues.

There is very little information available on the mechanical properties of diseased and malformed cusps, in general, and raphe material, in particular. Additional knowledge will be critical to the development of biomechanical models of clinically relevant valves. The fundamentals of biomechanical models are discussed in the next section.

9.6 Finite Element Modeling of the Aortic Valve

As discussed in Chapter 6, several computational approaches could potentially be used toward the modeling of the AV function. As blood flows through the valve, it induces pressures (varying in time and space) on the different components of the valve. In turn, these components are deformed by these pressures and affect the blood flow. While computational fluid dynamics (CFD) would typically handle blood flow in a rigid conduit, it is the fluid–structure interaction (FSI) studies that would normally be required for fully detailed biomechanical analyses of the AV. Fluid–structure interaction means that both the fluid and the structure (i.e., the aortic valve components) are modeled in detail. This, although feasible (e.g., Joda et al., 2016), comes at a considerable computational expense. However, interestingly, several studies have independently shown that spatial (as opposed to temporal) variations in the distribution of blood pressure on the valve components have a minimal influence on the AV dynamics (Howard et al., 2003; Soncini et al., 2009; Koch et al., 2010; Labrosse et al., 2010). Of course, FSI is indispensable if one is after the coupling between the mitral valve, the left ventricle, and the AV (Mao et al., 2017) or if one is interested in determining the shear stresses on the AV cusps (Cao and Sucosky, 2017). However, dry models (i.e., pressure-driven only; no fluids) can be valuable tools to assess native AV cusps kinematics and stresses and to simulate AV surgical procedures; however, it has been argued that they might not be the best choice for prosthetic valves (Luraghi et al., 2017). As such, the focus in the rest of this section will be placed on structural FE analysis of the AV, unless noted otherwise.

9.6.1 A Brief Introduction to the Finite Element Method for Structural Analyses

The FE approach is a general way of solving partial differential equations on a discretized geometric domain. The discretization is the operation of dividing a domain into smaller sections (elements) that are interconnected by common points (nodes). In mechanical simulations, inputs are the geometry of the domain, the boundary conditions (e.g., attachment conditions), the known external loads (e.g., pressure, forces, and/or imposed stretches), and the material properties. Outputs obtained from specific solvers include the displacements of the nodes and the mechanical stresses and strains in the elements. To study the dynamic behavior of a structure, the following global equation needs to be solved for each time t:

$$M\ddot{u}(t) + C\dot{u}(t) + Ku(t) = R(t),$$

where M, C, and K are the mass matrix, the damping matrix, and the stiffness matrix of the system, respectively, and $\ddot{u}$, $\dot{u}$, and u are the vectors of nodal accelerations, velocities, and displacements, respectively. Finally, $R(t)$ is the vector of external forces on the structure (Banks et al., 2011).

Locally, let X be the position vector of a particle in the structure in its reference configuration (say, unloaded), and let $x = X + u$ be the position vector of the same particle in the current loaded configuration (which is a function of time). These first definitions allow one to define the transformation gradient tensor, as:

$$F = \frac{\partial x}{\partial X}$$

The right Cauchy–Green tensor $C = F^T . F$ can then be defined as a measure of deformation. The principal invariants associated with the right Cauchy–Green tensor are as follows:

$$I_1 = tr(C) = \lambda_1^2 + \lambda_2^2 + \lambda_3^2$$

$$I_2 = \frac{1}{2}\left[(trC)^2 - tr\left(C^2\right) \right] = \lambda_1^2 \lambda_2^2 + \lambda_2^2 \lambda_3^2 + \lambda_3^2 \lambda_1^2$$

$$I_3 = \det C = \lambda_1^2 \lambda_2^2 \lambda_3^2$$

These tensor invariants are expressed in terms of the principal stretches $\{\lambda_i\}_{i=1,2,3}$. The third invariant I_3 describes the change of volume of the material and is also noted J^2.

Given applications with biological soft tissues, nonlinear elasticity and, most specifically, hyperelasticity are important concepts. A hyperelastic material is one for which a strain energy density function W exists; it represents a measure of the energy stored in the material as a result of deformation (Banks et al., 2011). The strain energy density function gives access to the Cauchy stress tensor σ as:

$$\sigma = \frac{2}{J} F . \frac{\partial W}{\partial C} . F^T - pI.$$

Lagrange multiplier p (with I the identity tensor) is associated with the near-incompressibility of the materials, given their high (~70%) water content. This term can be enforced as a penalty contribution to ensure the material's near-incompressibility. Finally, the tangent tensor D used to evaluate stress increments between load steps can be expressed in function of the strain energy function through:

$$D = 4 \frac{\partial^2 W}{\partial C \partial C}.$$

Although various strain energy function can be found in the literature (Boyce and Arruda, 2000), we will focus only on the most relevant hyperelastic models relevant to cardiovascular tissue modeling. One of the most commonly used hyperelastic constitutive equation is the Fung material model (Sun et al., 2014):

$$W_{\text{Fung}} = \frac{c}{2}\left(e^Q - 1\right)$$

Q was originally proposed as a quadratic function, including material parameters and Green strain tensor components (Fung et al., 1979), but various other forms can be found in the literature (Howard et al., 2003; Conti et al., 2010b).

Another hyperelastic material model is based on a power-law formulation; this was proposed by Rivlin (Boyce and Arruda, 2000). In its general formulation, with material constants C_{pq}:

$$W = \sum_{p,q=0}^{n} C_{pq}(I_1 - 3)^p (I_2 - 3)^q + \sum_{m=1}^{M} \frac{1}{D_m}(J - 1)^{2m}$$

This expression is suitable to various isotropic hyperelastic models, for example, the neo-Hookean model, defined by $p = 1$, $q = 0$, and the Mooney–Rivlin model, defined by $p = 1$, $q = 1$. To describe the preferential directions due to collagen fibers, different anisotropic contributions can be added to this general expression to model as many families of fibers as needed:

$$W = W_{iso} + \sum_{i=0}^{n} W_{ani} + W_{vol}$$

This expression distinguishes between W_{iso}, the isotropic contribution from the extracellular matrix; W_{ani}, the anisotropic contribution from each family of fibers; and W_{vol}, the contribution related to nearly-incompressible effects. One common expression for arteria tissue is the so-called Holzapfel–Gasser–Ogden (HGO) model (Holzapfel et al., 2000):

$$W_{HGO} = C_{10}\left(I_1 - 3\right) + \frac{k_1}{2k_2} \sum_{i=4,6} (e^{k_2(I_i - 1)^2} - 1)$$

In this expression, the isotropic contribution comes from a neo-Hookean model, and for each family fibers (here two family to model the fibrous helix in the aorta) an exponential Fung-type contribution involves invariants $I_{4,6}$ characterizing the preferred anisotropic directions (see Chapter 6 for more details).

In the following section, applications of the modeling approaches discussed previously are described, as they relate to FE simulations of native AVs and of surgical procedures.

9.6.2 Finite Element Simulations of Aortic Valves

Computational studies have focused on native healthy AVs (Gnyaneshwar et al., 2002; Howard et al., 2003; Conti et al., 2010b; Koch et al., 2010; Labrosse et al., 2010, 2015) and diseased AVs (Grande et al., 2000; Conti et al., 2010a; Jermihov et al., 2011; Labrosse et al., 2011). For example, Figure 9.17 illustrates the FE distributions of von Mises stresses in systole and diastole. The von Mises stresses conveniently summarize in one number the stress values present in different directions of the material at one location. Models of healthy AVs, based on average geometric models (Conti et al., 2010b) or patient-specific dimensions and age-dependent material properties (Labrosse et al., 2015), aim at better understanding the function of AVs from a mechanical point of view. More specifically, cusp kinematics and cusp coaptation mechanisms are of interest, especially as they are among the functional criteria used by surgeons. Computational studies have confirmed the experimental and clinical findings that the cusp-opening mechanism is a combination of aortic root dilatation (expansion in the radial direction of the commissures) and movement of the cusp in the direction of blood flow (Howard et al., 2003).

Computational studies of diseased TAVs have investigated the influence of calcification on the reduction in orifice area during systole, and according to their authors, sites of strain concentrations were correlated to sites of calcification (Halevi et al., 2015). With stiffening of the aortic root, the cusps were shown to experience delayed and reduced opening (Howard et al., 2003). On the other hand, aortic root dilatation was shown to decrease cusp coaptation in diastole and to markedly increase cusp stresses and strains (Grande et al., 2000). In a study of prolapsing cusps, increases of 2 and 4 mm of the STJ diameter produced mild and severe AIs, respectively, in a healthy TAV (Labrosse et al., 2011).

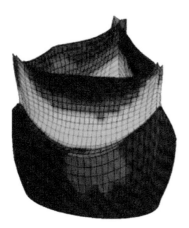 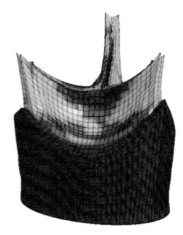

Figure 9.17 Von Mises stress distributions obtained from finite element analysis in dynamics of a TAV during systole (left) and diastole (right). The warmer the color, the higher the stress.

Few investigations have been conducted on malformed AVs. One can mention FE studies (Conti et al., 2010a; Jermihov et al., 2011) or FSI studies (Weinberg and Mofrad, 2008; Chandra et al., 2012; Chandran and Vigmostad, 2013) that aim to decipher the function of BAVs (Conti et al., 2010a). The cusps were noted to open asymmetrically during systole, and the fused cusp were observed to generate a large occlusion of the valve orifice. Higher stresses were observed in the central region of the fused cusps. The authors also highlighted the influence of the raphe on the stress distribution in this region (Conti et al., 2010a). In addition, FSI studies have shown the influence of malformed cusps in BAVs on the blood flow in terms of shear stresses (Chandra et al., 2012).

Regarding surgical procedures, many computational studies have focused on the widely used valve replacement (Sun et al., 2014), including TAVI deployment into a patient-specific aortic root (Bailey et al., 2016) and stentless aortic valve implant deployment (Auricchio et al., 2011), not to mention FSI studies of mechanical valves (Alemu and Bluestein, 2007). From these studies, it appears that the increase in the prosthesis diameter leads to a decrease in effective height, while increasing the cusp coaptation surface area.

With the mounting interest in the surgical repair of AVs, computational studies have also addressed it (Sun et al., 2014). Various valve-sparing procedures, including the David and Yacoub procedures, have been modeled (Soncini et al., 2009; Tasca et al., 2017). According to a comparative study between these procedures, both were noted to be able to restore cusp coaptation; however, they altered cusps kinematics, with more evident alterations observed after the David procedure, owing to stiffer support from the neoaortic root. The influence of various graft shapes, especially grafts involving artificial sinuses of Valsalva, was studied using FSI (Katayama et al., 2008). According to the authors, vortex formation in the pseudosinuses during the early phase of ejection facilitates the smooth closure of the valve. Cusp correction techniques have also been studied using FE analyses. It was found that the cusp resuspension technique induced more moderate stresses in the cusps compared with central plication (Labrosse et al., 2011). Commissural plication was deemed the worst because of very high stresses induced at the commissures, and surgeons have mostly abandoned this technique. It was also determined that when replacing an original cup with a pericardium patch, the patch should be sized larger in both width and height compared with the original cusp to properly achieve valve closure (Hammer et al., 2012).

9.6.2.1 Aortic Valve Geometric Modeling

The geometry and dimensions of the AV can be obtained using medical images and segmentation tools (Grande et al., 2000; Auricchio et al., 2011; Heyden et al., 2015), following manual or automatic approaches. Such models are inherently patient-specific from the geometric perspective. Importantly, in vivo medical imaging yields geometric information about a pressurized configuration of the AV, and this does not meet the requirement of establishing an unloaded, stress-free reference configuration before an accurate determination of stresses and strains can be made in a structure that experiences large deformations (with respect to this reference configuration), as the AV does. For this reason, which has not always been fully appreciated in the modeling

community, and yet other reasons, many studies have been based on idealized geometric models (Gnyaneshwar et al., 2002; Howard et al., 2003; Koch et al., 2010; Soncini
et al., 2009; Conti et al., 2010b; Labrosse et al., 2010, 2011; Hammer et al., 2012; Morganti
et al., 2015; Oomen et al., 2016). Idealized geometric models are based on the approach
described in Section 9.2.1; these include models generated from average unpressurized
dimensions and subjects-specific models generated from measurements made from
medical imaging. In the latter case, a parameterized idealized model of the AV lends
itself well to individual and directional scaling of the dimensions of the pressurized AV
components, whereas direct shrinking by arbitrary scaling of the pressurized geometry, as obtained from segmentation, is not effective (Labrosse et al., 2015).

The geometric modeling of malformed AVs has been limited. In particular, the
raphe has received little attention. It has been approximated as an extra thickness
(e.g., four times the cusp thickness) on the fused cusps (Conti et al., 2010a).

9.6.2.2 Materials Properties

The complex multilayered structure of the aortic root and cusps is generally modeled as a unique homogeneous layer to make computational studies tractable (Koch
et al., 2010; Sun et al., 2014). Indeed, a full representation of the different layers would
require specific constitutive equations and corresponding material parameters for
each layer. These data are mostly out of reach for now; however, one group considered
multilayered cusps in an FSI approach (Weinberg and Mofrad, 2007, 2008).

Early studies used linear elasticity for the cusps, generally involving Young's modulus $E = 1$ MPa and a Poisson's ratio of $\nu = 0.3$–0.45. To account for the nonlinear
behavior of the cusps, the majority of more recent models use hyperelastic models.
While the isotropic Mooney–Rivlin model is sometimes used (Morganti et al., 2015),
most cusp hyperelastic models are based on Fung material model, which involves an
exponential form associated with polynomial Q. Different forms of Q have been used,
including a two-dimensional (2D) version expressed as:

$$Q = A_1 E_{11}^2 + A_2 E_{22}^2 + 2 A_3 E_{11} E_{22} + A_4 E_{12}^2 + 2 A_5 E_{11} E_{12} + 2 A_6 E_{22} E_{12}$$

Hammer et al. (2012) proposed values for normal human cusps based on equibiaxial
test, such that $c = 9.7$ kPa; $A_1 = 49.56$; $A_2 = 5.29$; $A_3 = -3.12$; $A_4 = 16.03$; $A_5 = -0.004$;
and $A_6 = -0.02$. This 2D approach does not involve the transverse shears in the 13 and
23 directions (Sun et al., 2014). Alternatively, Labrosse et al. (2010, 2011, 2015) have
used a 3D version of Q:

$$Q = A_1 E_{11}^2 + A_2 \left(E_{22}^2 + E_{33}^2 + E_{23}^2 + E_{32}^2 \right) + A_3 \left(E_{12}^2 + E_{13}^2 + E_{31}^2 + E_{21}^2 \right)$$

Polynomial Q has also been defined as (Conti et al., 2010b; Oomen et al., 2016):

$$Q = C_1 (I_1 - 3)^2 + C_2 (I_4 - 1)^2.$$

The material parameters associated with these various constitutive equations are
determined by inverse method to fit experimental data. Stress–strain data from

biaxial tests performed on porcine tissues from (Billiar and Sacks, 2000) are commonly used. However, an age-dependent approach was also proposed based on the linear interpolation of reconstructed experimental biaxial data (Labrosse et al., 2015).

The aortic root also exhibits a nonlinear anisotropic behavior, and the same approaches as with cusps have generally been used. Earlier models used linear elasticity for the aortic root and cusps or introduced nonlinear elasticity for the cusps. They employed Young's modulus values $E = 1.2$–2.0 MPa and Poisson's ratio values $\nu = 0.45$–0.4999. In more recent models, hyperelastic material models have been used for the aortic root.

The presence of calcific deposits in diseased cusps has been modeled using linear elasticity with a comparatively large Young's modulus $E = 1$ GPa (Halevi et al., 2015). Regarding the material properties of the raphe in BAVs, the same properties as the cusps have been considered (Conti et al., 2010a) or with an arbitrary increase of 25% has been considered for more stiffness (Chandran and Vigmostad, 2013). A linear material model has also been used, with $E = 2$ MPa, $\nu = 0.15$, and a mass density $\rho = 2200$ kg/m^3 (Jermihov et al., 2011).

Biomaterials used during surgery, such as valve implants (Bailey et al., 2016), cusps patches (Hammer et al., 2012), Dacron® synthetic grafts (Soncini et al., 2009), and sutures (Labrosse et al., 2011), form an integral part of the modeling of surgical procedures and need attention. Table 9.4 summarizes the most commonly used surgical biomaterials and the constitutive behaviors used to represent them. Used in valve-sparing procedures, Dacron® synthetic graft is stiffer than the native aortic biological tissues and may be modeled via linear elasticity, with Young's modulus $E = 7.84$ MPa (Soncini et al., 2009). Valve replacement prostheses and patches for cusps repair or

TABLE 9.4 Modeling Surgical Procedures and Materials in the Literature

Surgical Procedure	Source	Description	Constitutive Equation	Material Parameters
TAVI deployment	Bailey et al. (2015)	TAVI manufactured from bovine pericardium	Ogden	
Stentless valve	Auricchio et al. (2011)	Two cusps manufactured from bovine pericardium	Mooney–Rivlin	$C_{10} = 552$ kPa; $C_{01} = 138$ kPa
David and Yacoub valve-sparing procedures	Soncini et al. (2009)	Dacron® synthetic graft	Linear elasticity	$E = 7.84$ MPa; $\nu = 0.3$
Cusp replacement	Hammer et al. (2012)	Bovine pericardium	Fung-type model	$c = 3056$; $A_1 = 25.46$; $A_2 = 12.10$; $A_3 = 5.07$; $A_4 = 25.99$; $A_5 = 0$; $A_6 = 0$
Cusp correction	Labrosse et al. (2011)	6-0 Polypropylene suture	Element type *SEATBELT in LS-DYNA (LSTC, Livermore, CA)	

tricuspidization (or also bicuspidization) are commonly made of the same materials, most specifically bovine pericardium (Table 9.4).

Owing to the marked nonlinear stress–strain behavior of bovine pericardium, it is commonly modeled using a hyperelastic material model, with or without anisotropic representation (Ogden model [Bailey et al., 2016], Mooney–Rivlin model [Auricchio et al., 2011], and Fung-type model [Hammer et al., 2012]). Depending on the surgical procedure of interest, suture modeling may be an important aspect of FE simulations. To represent stitches, Labrosse et al. (2011) used one-dimensional elements connecting two nodes at a time. The elements were instructed to shrink by a controlled amount at the onset of the simulation to make the nodes almost coincident, thereby mimicking sutures. In the rest of the simulation, the elements behaved according to linear elasticity, based on the material properties and characteristics of the suture line employed.

Another important aspect in the computational simulation of biological tissues relates to their near-incompressibility. The most common approach to enforce near-incompressibility is to split the strain energy into deviatoric and volumetric (or hydrostatic) components (Boyce and Arruda, 2000); however, this is fully justified only for isotropic materials and can lead to serious problems with anisotropic materials (Annaidh et al., 2013; Nolan et al., 2014). One of the most commonly used hydrostatic strain energy formulation W_{VOL} is expressed as:

$$W_{VOL} = \frac{1}{D}(J-1)^2.$$

Many AV models feature nearly incompressible formulations. It is worth mentioning that models featuring 2D Fung-type formulations cannot enforce incompressibility, and the through-thickness deformation is then unrelated to in-plane deformations.

9.6.2.3 Loads, Boundary Conditions, and Contact Management

Quasistatic models generally model AV closure by applying a uniform pressure to a geometry resembling that of the AV in diastole (Auricchio et al., 2011; Bailey et al., 2016). On the other hand, dynamic models use spatially uniform time-dependent pressures on the inner wall of the valve and can simulate the AV function across the cardiac cycle (Labrosse et al., 2010, 2011, 2015; Conti et al., 2010b). The region below the cusps is loaded with the left ventricular pressure, while the region above the leaflets is loaded with the aortic pressure. The cusps are usually subjected to the pressure differential between aortic and left ventricular pressures (Figure 9.17), because loading the aortic side of the cusp with aortic pressure and the left ventricular side of the cusp with left ventricular pressure may lead to the unrealistic flattening of the FEs making up the cusp. It is also interesting to note that dynamic AV simulations that do not include damping (which would normally come from the presence and viscosity of blood) can be affected by unrealistic vibrations (Sun et al., 2014). To mitigate this effect, Kim et al. introduced damping based on a physiological representative damping constant (Kim et al., 2008).

Ideally, the boundary conditions of the AV model should be as physiological as possible and include some radial timewise variation of the VAJ dimensions. Instead of controlling the VAJ, a practical approach consists of lengthening the left ventricular outflow tract and of fixing its proximal end in all directions. The elasticity of the left ventricular outflow tract can then be adjusted, such that physiological variations of the VAJ are obtained (in combination with the function of the rest of the valve). In addition, a longitudinal stretch (on the order of 1.2 in young adults) should be applied to the ascending aorta (Han and Fung, 1995).

The simulation of contact in dynamics can be performed using a penalty method. Hammer et al. (2012) used a contact stiffness of $k = 10$ N/m. Some authors have modeled contact to occur without friction or with a friction coefficient of 0.05. In the absence of more specific experimental data, this value, characterizing contact between soft and wet surfaces (similar to those found in cusps) may be used (Soncini et al., 2009). However, according to the literature, a friction coefficient variation within the range of 0–0.5 negligibly affects numerical solutions (Soncini et al., 2009). This is confirmed by the experimental observation that the cusps do not slip with respect to each during coaptation, and therefore, no tangential forces related to friction have the opportunity to develop.

9.6.2.4 Model Verification and Validation

One of the first verifications to run on a computational model is a mesh sensitivity analysis (Koch et al., 2010). It is also good practice to verify that materials that are supposed to behave incompressibly during static or dynamic simulations. Regarding validation, several options are available; however, they are somewhat limited in detail.

As previously discussed, dimensional measurements obtained from medical imaging usually pertain to a pressurized configuration. Therefore, if one is after simulating patient-specific cases, one needs to make sure that the unpressurized geometry is such that, once pressurized, it matches the geometry observed from medical imaging. Different authors have proposed optimization procedures to produce and validate such models, based on the verification of a certain number of key parameters (Conti et al., 2010b; Labrosse et al., 2015).

Additional model validation can be performed through comparisons with experimental data. Labrosse et al. (2010) used experimental GOA versus time data to validate their simulation of the dynamics of a porcine valve. In their study of cusp replacements with bovine pericardium patches, Hammer et al. (2012) used a surgically modified porcine AV air pressurized to 80 mmHg and CT imaging to validate their model against experimentally measured central coaptation heights. Kim et al. (2008) quantitatively compared their numerically predicted strain distributions with the experimentally measured data under corresponding pressure loads on the cusps.

A comprehensive verification and validation method for computational simulations is yet to establish. Ideally, in native AVs, such method would compare the detailed timewise 3D kinematics of the cusps and aortic root (i.e., the dynamic function of the valve), as obtained from four-dimensional medical imaging, with the same information available from simulations. This is a tall order, as tools to carry out such timewise point-to-point comparisons are still lacking. For surgically modified valves, similar ideas could be applied using medical imaging data acquired from left-heart simulators and/or animal models as references.

9.7 Conclusions

In many respects, computational simulations of AV mechanics represent the culmination of many efforts, including geometric modeling, material characterization, and the implementation of accurate solution processes. While significant strides have been made regarding these aspects in the recent decades, each aspect needs further refinement to achieve the precision, reliability, and dependability required in clinical decision-making. Indeed, although proofs of concept have been established regarding the analysis of native AVs as well as some AV surgical procedures, such as TAVI deployment, valve-sparing procedures, and cusp free-margin correction, the models have typically not been fully validated over large sample sizes. As a result, clinical applicability is still extremely limited, despite promising results. Experimental data that can be used toward the material characterization of human AVs are also extremely scarce. More fundamentally, little experimental insight is available as to how the malformed geometry of AVs impacts the AV function and cusp kinematics and how it can be surgically improved. The UAV and BAV surgical repair procedures are very challenging, and advances in their simulation would carry a lot of impact, as approximately 50% of AV patients in the operating room present with such valves. Still, the feasibility of simulating specific techniques has never been assessed in malformed AVs repair (e.g., commissural removal, bicuspidization, and tricuspidization).

Ultimately, as it will most likely be impossible to make all sources of simulation errors disappear, one practical approach may lie in the assessment of uncertainty associated with simulations and the determination of how much uncertainty in the simulation outputs can be tolerated while still producing valuable information for clinicians. For example, in the case of AV repair surgery, simulations may suggest reducing the free margin of a cusp by 4 mm to eliminate a prolapse. What is the simulation error on this value, given the uncertainty on the geometry, material properties, loads and boundary conditions, and, perhaps, limited accuracy of solvers? Then, how sensitive is the clinical outcome to this value? In other words, would a 3-mm cusp reduction not produce the desired effect? Now, if 4 mm is the target value, can a surgeon reliably implement a controlled 4-mm free-margin correction? These questions (and others) will require careful analyses and answers that will depend on the different surgical procedures under investigation. Again, this is part of the price of making engineering simulations clinically relevant, and it requires the active involvement of surgeons and engineers.

Interestingly, efforts to improve engineering simulations of open-chest heart valve surgeries will also benefit the simulations of minimally invasive, catheter-based, or laparoscopic valvular surgeries, whose numbers are rapidly growing. Cardiologists are welcome to participate and help toward these goals.

References

Aicher D, Bewarder M, Kindermann M, Abdul-Khalique H, Schäfers HJ. Aortic valve function after bicuspidization of the unicuspid aortic valve. *The Annals of Thoracic Surgery* 2013;95(5):1545–1550.

Aicher D, Schäfers HJ. Aortic valve repair—current status, indications, and outcomes. *Seminars in Thoracic and Cardiovascular Surgery* 2012;24(3):195–201.

Alavi SH, Ruiz V, Krasieva T, Botvinick EL, Kheradvar A. Characterizing the collagen fiber orientation in pericardial leaflets under mechanical loading conditions. *Annals of Biomedical Engineering* 2013;41(3):547–561.

Alemu Y, Bluestein D. Flow-induced platelet activation and damage accumulation in a mechanical heart valve: Numerical studies. *Artificial organs* 2007;31(9):677–688.

American College of Cardiology, American Heart Association Task Force on Practice Guidelines. ACC/AHA 2006 guidelines for the management of patients with valvular heart disease: A report of the American College of Cardiology/American Heart Association Task Force on Practice Guidelines (Writing Committee to Revise the 1998 Guidelines for the Management of Patients With Valvular Heart Disease): Developed in collaboration with the Society of Cardiovascular Anesthesiologists: Endorsed by the Society for Cardiovascular Angiography and Interventions and the Society of Thoracic Surgeons. *Circulation* 2006;114(5):e84.

Annaidh AN, Destrade M, Gilchrist MD, Murphy JG. Deficiencies in numerical models of anisotropic nonlinearly elastic materials. *Biomechanics and Modeling in Mechanobiology* 2013;12(4):781–791.

Ashikhmina E, Sundt TM, Dearani JA, Connolly HM, Li Z, Schaff HV. Repair of the bicuspid aortic valve: A viable alternative to replacement with a bioprosthesis. *The Journal of Thoracic and Cardiovascular Surgery* 2010;139(6):1395–1401.

Auricchio F, Conti M, Morganti S, Totaro P. A computational tool to support preoperative planning of stentless aortic valve implant. *Medical Engineering and Physics* 2011;33(10):1183–1192.

Azadani AN, Chitsaz S, Matthews PB, Jaussaud N, Leung J, Tsinman T, Ge L, Tseng EE. Comparison of mechanical properties of human ascending aorta and aortic sinuses. *The Annals of Thoracic Surgery* 2012;93(1):87–94.

Bailey J, Curzen N, Bressloff NW. Assessing the impact of including leaflets in the simulation of TAVI deployment into a patient-specific aortic root. *Computer Methods in Biomechanics and Biomedical Engineering* 2016;19(7):733–744.

Banks HT, Hu S, Kenz ZR. A brief review of elasticity and viscoelasticity for solids. *Advances in Applied Mathematics and Mechanics* 2011;3(1):1–51.

Berdajs DA. Aortic root morphology: A paradigm for successful reconstruction. *Interactive Cardiovascular and Thoracic Surgery* 2015;22(1):85–91.

Bierbach BO, Aicher D, Issa OA, Bomberg H, Gräber S, Glombitza P, Schäfers HJ. Aortic root and cusp configuration determine aortic valve function. *European Journal of Cardio-Thoracic Surgery* 2010;38(4):400–406.

Billiar KL, Sacks MS. Biaxial mechanical properties of the natural and glutaraldehyde treated aortic valve cusp—part I: Experimental results. *Journal of Biomechanical Engineering* 2000;122(1):23–30.

Boodhwani M, de Kerchove L, Glineur D, El Khoury G. A simple method for the quantification and correction of aortic cusp prolapse by means of free margin plication. *The Journal of Thoracic and Cardiovascular Surgery* 2010a;139(4):1075–1077.

Boodhwani M, de Kerchove L, Glineur D, Poncelet A, Rubay J, Astarci P, Verhelst R, Noirhomme P, El Khoury G. Repair-oriented classification of aortic insufficiency: Impact on surgical techniques and clinical outcomes. *The Journal of Thoracic and Cardiovascular Surgery* 2009a;137(2):286–294.

Boodhwani M, de Kerchove L, Glineur D, Rubay J, Vanoverschelde JL, Noirhomme P, El Khoury G. Repair of regurgitant bicuspid aortic valves: A systematic approach. *The Journal of Thoracic and Cardiovascular Surgery* 2010b;140(2):276–284.

Boodhwani M, El Khoury G. Aortic valve repair: Indications and outcomes. *Current Cardiology Reports* 2014;16(6):490.

Boodhwani M, Glineur D, Noirhomme P, El GK. Repair of aortic valve cusp prolapse. *Multimedia Manual of Cardiothoracic Surgery: MMCTS* 2009b;2009(702):mmcts-2008.

Boyce MC, Arruda EM. Constitutive models of rubber elasticity: A review. *Rubber Chemistry and Technology* 2000;73(3):504–523.

Buchanan RM, Sacks MS. Interlayer micromechanics of the aortic heart valve leaflet. *Biomechanics and Modeling in Mechanobiology* 2014;13(4):813–826.

Cao K, Sucosky P. Aortic valve leaflet wall shear stress characterization revisited: Impact of coronary flow. *Computer Methods in Biomechanics and Biomedical Engineering* 2017;20(5):468–470.

Cemri M, Cengel A, Timurkaynak T. Pentacuspid aortic valve diagnosed by transoesophageal echocardiography. *Heart* 2000;84(4):e9–.

Chandra S, Rajamannan NM, Sucosky P. Computational assessment of bicuspid aortic valve wall-shear stress: Implications for calcific aortic valve disease. *Biomechanics and Modeling in Mechanobiology* 2012;11(7):1085–1096.

Chandran KB, Vigmostad SC. Patient-specific bicuspid valve dynamics: Overview of methods and challenges. *Journal of Biomechanics* 2013;46(2):208–216.

Conti CA, Della Corte A, Votta E, Del Viscovo L, Bancone C, De Santo LS, Redaelli A. Biomechanical implications of the congenital bicuspid aortic valve: A finite element study of aortic root function from in vivo data. *The Journal of Thoracic and Cardiovascular Surgery* 2010a;140(4):890–896.

Conti CA, Votta E, Della Corte A, Del Viscovo L, Bancone C, Cotrufo M, Redaelli A. Dynamic finite element analysis of the aortic root from MRI-derived parameters. *Medical Engineering and Physics* 2010b;32(2):212–221.

de Kerchove L, Boodhwani M, Glineur D, Poncelet A, Rubay J, Watremez C, Vanoverschelde JL, Noirhomme P, El Khoury G. Cusp prolapse repair in trileaflet aortic valves: Free margin plication and free margin resuspension techniques. *The Annals of Thoracic Surgery* 2009;88(2):455–461.

de Kerchove L, Mastrobuoni S, Boodhwani M, Astarci P, Rubay J, Poncelet A, Vanoverschelde JL, Noirhomme P, El Khoury G. The role of annular dimension and annuloplasty in tricuspid aortic valve repair. *European Journal of Cardio-Thoracic Surgery* 2015;49(2):428–438.

de Waroux JB, Pouleur AC, Robert A, Pasquet A, Gerber BL, Noirhomme P, El Khoury G, Vanoverschelde JL. Mechanisms of recurrent aortic regurgitation after aortic valve repair: predictive value of intraoperative transesophageal echocardiography. *JACC: Cardiovascular Imaging* 2009;2(8):931–939.

El Khoury G, de Kerchove L. Principles of aortic valve repair. *The Journal of Thoracic and Cardiovascular Surgery* 2013;145(3):S26–S29.

Fedak PW, Verma S, David TE, Leask RL, Weisel RD, Butany J. Clinical and pathophysiological implications of a bicuspid aortic valve. *Circulation* 2002;106(8):900–904.

Fung YC, Fronek K, Patitucci P. Pseudoelasticity of arteries and the choice of its mathematical expression. *American Journal of Physiology-Heart and Circulatory Physiology* 1979;237(5):H620–H631.

Garcia D, Kadem L. What do you mean by aortic valve area: geometric orifice area, effective orifice area, or gorlin area? *Journal of Heart Valve Disease* 2006;15(5):601.

Gnyaneshwar R, Kumar RK, Balakrishnan KR. Dynamic analysis of the aortic valve using a finite element model. *The Annals of Thoracic Surgery* 2002;73(4):1122–1129.

Grande KJ, Cochran RP, Reinhall PG, Kunzelman KS. Mechanisms of aortic valve incompetence: Finite element modeling of aortic root dilatation. *The Annals of Thoracic Surgery* 2000;69(6):1851–1857.

Gundiah N, Kam K, Matthews PB, Guccione J, Dwyer HA, Saloner D, Chuter TA, Guy TS, Ratcliffe MB, Tseng EE. Asymmetric mechanical properties of porcine aortic sinuses. *The Annals of Thoracic Surgery* 2008;85(5):1631–1638.

Halevi R, Hamdan A, Marom G, Mega M, Raanani E, Haj-Ali R. Progressive aortic valve calcification: Three-dimensional visualization and biomechanical analysis. *Journal of Biomechanics* 2015;48(3):489–497.

Hammer PE, Chen PC, Pedro J, Howe RD. Computational model of aortic valve surgical repair using grafted pericardium. *Journal of Biomechanics* 2012;45(7):1199–1204.

Han HC, Fung YC. Longitudinal strain of canine and porcine aortas. *Journal of Biomechanics* 1995;28(5):637–641.

Handke M, Heinrichs G, Beyersdorf F, Olschewski M, Bode C, Geibel A. In vivo analysis of aortic valve dynamics by transesophageal 3-dimensional echocardiography with high temporal resolution. *The Journal of Thoracic and Cardiovascular Surgery* 2003;125(6):1412–1419.

Haydar HS, He GW, Hovaguimian H, McIrvin DM, King DH, Starr A. Valve repair for aortic insufficiency: Surgical classification and techniques. *European Journal of Cardio-Thoracic Surgery* 1997;11(2):258–265.

Heyden S, Nagler A, Bertoglio C, Biehler J, Gee MW, Wall WA, Ortiz M. Material modeling of cardiac valve tissue: Experiments, constitutive analysis and numerical investigation. *Journal of Biomechanics* 2015;48(16):4287–4296.

Holzapfel GA, Gasser TC, Ogden RW. A new constitutive framework for arterial wall mechanics and a comparative study of material models. *Journal of Elasticity and the Physical Science of Solids* 2000;61(1–3):1–48.

Hopkins RA. Aortic valve leaflet sparing and salvage surgery: Evolution of techniques for aortic root reconstruction. *European Journal of Cardio-Thoracic Surgery* 2003; 24(6):886–897.

Howard IC, Patterson EA, Yoxall A. On the opening mechanism of the aortic valve: Some observations from simulations. *Journal of Medical Engineering & Technology* 2003;27(6):259–266.

Jermihov PN, Jia L, Sacks MS, Gorman RC, Gorman JH, Chandran KB. Effect of geometry on the leaflet stresses in simulated models of congenital bicuspid aortic valves. *Cardiovascular Engineering and Technology* 2011;2(1):48–56.

Joda A, Jin Z, Haverich A, Summers J, Korossis S. Multiphysics simulation of the effect of leaflet thickness inhomogeneity and material anisotropy on the stress–strain distribution on the aortic valve. *Journal of Biomechanics* 2016;49(12):2502–2512.

Johnston DR, Soltesz EG, Vakil N, Rajeswaran J, Roselli EE, Sabik JF, Smedira NG, Svensson LG, Lytle BW, Blackstone EH. Long-term durability of bioprosthetic aortic valves: Implications from 12,569 implants. *The Annals of Thoracic Surgery* 2015;99(4):1239–1247.

Katayama S, Umetani N, Sugiura S, Hisada T. The sinus of Valsalva relieves abnormal stress on aortic valve leaflets by facilitating smooth closure. *The Journal of Thoracic and Cardiovascular Surgery* 2008;136(6):1528–1535.

Ketelsen D, Fishman EK, Claussen CD, Vogel-Claussen J. Computed tomography evaluation of cardiac valves: A review. *Radiologic Clinics* 2010;48(4):783–797.

Kim H, Lu J, Sacks MS, Chandran KB. Dynamic simulation of bioprosthetic heart valves using a stress resultant shell model. *Annals of Biomedical Engineering* 2008;36(2):262–275.

Koch TM, Reddy BD, Zilla P, Franz T. Aortic valve leaflet mechanical properties facilitate diastolic valve function. *Computer Methods in Biomechanics and Biomedical Engineering* 2010;13(2):225–234.

Koenraadt WM, Grewal N, Gaidoukevitch OY, DeRuiter MC, Gittenberger-de Groot AC, Bartelings MM, Holman ER, Klautz RJ, Schalij MJ, Jongbloed MR. The extent of the raphe in bicuspid aortic valves is associated with aortic regurgitation and aortic root dilatation. *Netherlands Heart Journal* 2016;24(2):127–133.

Kunzelman KS, Grande KJ, David TE, Cochran RP, Verrier ED. Aortic root and valve relationships: Impact on surgical repair. *The Journal of Thoracic and Cardiovascular Surgery* 1994;107(1):162–170.

Kuroki H, Hirooka K, Ohnuki M. Pentacuspid aortic valve causing severe aortic regurgitation. *The Journal of Thoracic and Cardiovascular Surgery* 2012;143(2):e11–e12.

Labrosse MR, Beller CJ, Boodhwani M, Hudson C, Sohmer B. Subject-specific finite-element modeling of normal aortic valve biomechanics from 3D+t TEE images. *Medical Image Analysis* 2015;20(1):162–172.

Labrosse MR, Beller CJ, Robicsek F, Thubrikar MJ. Geometric modeling of functional trileaflet aortic valves: Development and clinical applications. *Journal of Biomechanics* 2006;39(14):2665–2672.

Labrosse MR, Boodhwani M, Sohmer B, Beller CJ. Modeling leaflet correction techniques in aortic valve repair: A finite element study. *Journal of Biomechanics* 2011;44(12):2292–2298.

Labrosse MR, Lobo K, Beller CJ. Structural analysis of the natural aortic valve in dynamics: from unpressurized to physiologically loaded. *Journal of Biomechanics* 2010; 43(10):1916–1922.

Lansac E, Di Centa I, Raoux F, Attar NA, Acar C, Joudinaud T, Raffoul R. A lesional classification to standardize surgical management of aortic insufficiency towards valve repair. *European Journal of Cardio-Thoracic Surgery* 2008;33(5):872–880.

Luraghi G, Wu W, De Gaetano F, Matas JF, Moggridge GD, Serrani M, Stasiak J, Costantino ML, Migliavacca F. Evaluation of an aortic valve prosthesis: Fluid-structure interaction or structural simulation? *Journal of Biomechanics* 2017;58:45–51.

Mao W, Caballero A, McKay R, Primiano C, Sun W. Fully-coupled fluid-structure interaction simulation of the aortic and mitral valves in a realistic 3D left ventricle model. *PLoS One* 2017;12(9):e0184729.

Martin C, Sun W. Biomechanical characterization of aortic valve tissue in humans and common animal models. *Journal of Biomedical Materials Research Part A* 2012;100(6):1591–1599.

Masson JB, Kovac J, Schuler G, Ye J, Cheung A, Kapadia S, Tuzcu ME, Kodali S, Leon MB, Webb JG. Transcatheter aortic valve implantation: Review of the nature, management, and avoidance of procedural complications. *JACC: Cardiovascular Interventions* 2009;2(9):811–820.

Mathieu P, Bossé Y, Huggins GS, Corte AD, Pibarot P, Michelena HI, Limongelli G et al. The pathology and pathobiology of bicuspid aortic valve: State of the art and novel research perspectives. *The Journal of Pathology: Clinical Research* 2015;1(4):195–206.

McDonald PC, Wilson JE, McNeill S, Gao M, Spinelli JJ, Rosenberg F, Wiebe H, McManus BM. The challenge of defining normality for human mitral and aortic valves: Geometrical and compositional analysis. *Cardiovascular Pathology* 2002;11(4):193–209.

Mega M, Marom G, Halevi R, Hamdan A, Bluestein D, Haj-Ali R. Imaging analysis of collagen fiber networks in cusps of porcine aortic valves: Effect of their local distribution and alignment on valve functionality. *Computer Methods in Biomechanics and Biomedical Engineering* 2016;19(9):1002–1008.

Michelena HI, Desjardins VA, Avierinos JF, Russo A, Nkomo VT, Sundt TM, Pellikka PA, Tajik AJ, Enriquez-Sarano M. Natural history of asymptomatic patients with normally functioning or minimally dysfunctional bicuspid aortic valve in the community. *Circulation* 2008;117(21):2776–2784.

Mirnajafi A, Raymer JM, McClure LR, Sacks MS. The flexural rigidity of the aortic valve leaflet in the commissural region. *Journal of Biomechanics* 2006;39(16):2966–2973.

Mookadam F, Thota VR, Garcia-Lopez AM, Emani UR, Alharthi MS, Zamorano J, Khandheria BK. Unicuspid aortic valve in adults: a systematic review. *Journal of Heart Valve Disease* 2010;19(1):79–85.

Morganti S, Auricchio F, Benson DJ, Gambarin FI, Hartmann S, Hughes TJ, Reali A. Patient-specific isogeometric structural analysis of aortic valve closure. *Computer Methods in Applied Mechanics and Engineering* 2015;284:508–520.

Nishimura RA. Aortic valve disease. *Circulation* 2002;106(7):770–772.

Nolan DR, Gower AL, Destrade M, Ogden RW, McGarry JP. A robust anisotropic hyperelastic formulation for the modelling of soft tissue. *Journal of the Mechanical Behavior of Biomedical Materials* 2014;39:48–60.

Oomen PJ, Loerakker S, Van Geemen D, Neggers J, Goumans MJ, Van Den Bogaerdt AJ, Bogers AJ, Bouten CV, Baaijens FP. Age-dependent changes of stress and strain in the human heart valve and their relation with collagen remodeling. *Acta biomaterialia* 2016;29:161–169.

Ozyilmaz S, Akgul O, Guzeltas A, Ozyilmaz I. Diagnosis of pentacuspid aortic valve with severe regurgitation using three-dimensional transesophageal echocardiography. *Echocardiography* 2015;32(2):393–394.

Pomerance A. Pathogenesis of aortic stenosis and its relation to age. *British Heart Journal* 1972;34(6):569.

Rajashekar P. Development of mechanical heart valves-an inspiring tale. *Journal of the Practice of Cardiovascular Sciences* 2015;1(3):289.

Rankin JS, Gaca JG. Techniques of aortic valve repair. *Innovations: Technology and Techniques in Cardiothoracic and Vascular Surgery* 2011;6(6):348–354.

Reid K. The anatomy of the sinus of Valsalva. *Thorax* 1970;25(1):79–85.

Ridley CH, Vallabhajosyula P, Bavaria JE, Patel PA, Gutsche JT, Shah R, Feinman JW, Weiss SJ, Augoustides JG. The Sievers classification of the bicuspid aortic valve for the perioperative echocardiographer: The importance of valve phenotype for aortic valve repair in the era of the functional aortic annulus. *Journal of Cardiothoracic and Vascular Anesthesia* 2016;30(4):1142–1151.

Roberts WC. The congenitally bicuspid aortic valve: A study of 85 autopsy cases. *The American Journal of Cardiology* 1970;26(1):72–83.

Sahasakul Y, Edwards WD, Naessens JM, Tajik AJ. Age-related changes in aortic and mitral valve thickness: Implications for two-dimensional echocardiography based on an autopsy study of 200 normal human hearts. *American Journal of Cardiology* 1988;62(7):424–430.

Saikrishnan N, Yap CH, Milligan NC, Vasilyev NV, Yoganathan AP. In vitro characterization of bicuspid aortic valve hemodynamics using particle image velocimetry. *Annals of Biomedical Engineering* 2012;40(8):1760–1775.

Sauren AA, Kuijpers W, Van Steenhoven AA, Veldpaus FE. Aortic valve histology and its relation with mechanics—preliminary report. *Journal of Biomechanics* 1980;13(2):97–104.

Schäfers HJ, Aicher D, Riodionycheva S, Lindinger A, Rädle-Hurst T, Langer F, Abdul-Khaliq H. Bicuspidization of the unicuspid aortic valve: A new reconstructive approach. *The Annals of Thoracic Surgery* 2008;85(6):2012–2018.

Schäfers HJ, Bierbach B, Aicher D. A new approach to the assessment of aortic cusp geometry. *The Journal of Thoracic and Cardiovascular Surgery* 2006;132(2):436–438.

Schäfers HJ, Schmied W, Marom G, Aicher D. Cusp height in aortic valves. *The Journal of Thoracic and Cardiovascular Surgery* 2013;146(2):269–274.

Sievers HH, Schmidtke C. A classification system for the bicuspid aortic valve from 304 surgical specimens. *The Journal of Thoracic and Cardiovascular Surgery* 2007;133(5):1226–1233.

Sohmer B, Hudson C, Atherstone J, Lambert AS, Labrosse M, Boodhwani M. Measuring aortic valve coaptation surface area using three-dimensional transesophageal echocardiography. *Canadian Journal of Anesthesia/Journal canadien d'anesthésie* 2013;60(1):24–31.

Smith CR, Leon MB, Mack MJ, Miller DC, Moses JW, Svensson LG, Tuzcu EM, Webb JG, Fontana GP, Makkar RR, Williams M. Transcatheter versus surgical aortic-valve replacement in high-risk patients. *New England Journal of Medicine* 2011;364(23):2187–2198.

Soncini M, Votta E, Zinicchino S, Burrone V, Mangini A, Lemma M, Antona C, Redaelli A. Aortic root performance after valve sparing procedure: A comparative finite element analysis. *Medical Engineering and Physics* 2009;31(2):234–243.

Stella JA, Sacks MS. On the biaxial mechanical properties of the layers of the aortic valve leaflet. *Journal of Biomechanical Engineering* 2007;129(5):757–766.

Sun W, Martin C, Pham T. Computational modeling of cardiac valve function and intervention. *Annual Review of Biomedical Engineering* 2014;16:53–76.

Swanson WM, Clark RE. Dimensions and geometric relationships of the human aortic value as a function of pressure. *Circulation Research* 1974;35(6):871–882.

Szeto K, Pastuszko P, Álamo JC, Lasheras J, Nigam V. Bicuspid aortic valves experience increased strain as compared to tricuspid aortic valves. *World Journal for Pediatric and Congenital Heart Surgery* 2013;4(4):362–326.

Tasca G, Selmi M, Votta E, Redaelli P, Sturla F, Redaelli A, Gamba A. Aortic root biomechanics after Sleeve and David sparing techniques: A finite element analysis. *The Annals of Thoracic Surgery* 2017;103(5):1451–1459.

Thubrikar MJ. *The Aortic Valve*. Boca Raton, FL: CRC Press, 1989.

Thubrikar MJ, Gong GG, Konstantinov IE, Selim GA, Fowler BL, Robicsek F. Influence of sizing and subcoronary implantation technique on the function of porcine aortic homografts. *Journal of Medical Engineering & Technology* 2000;24(4):173–180.

Tzemos N, Therrien J, Yip J, Thanassoulis G, Tremblay S, Jamorski MT, Webb GD, Siu SC. Outcomes in adults with bicuspid aortic valves. *JAMA* 2008;300(11):1317–1325.

Vahanian A, Alfieri O, Andreotti F, Antunes MJ, Barón-Esquivias G, Baumgartner H, Borger MA, Carrel TP, De Bonis M, Evangelista A. Guidelines on the management of valvular heart disease (version 2012) The Joint Task Force on the Management of Valvular Heart Disease of the European Society of Cardiology (ESC) and the European Association for Cardio-Thoracic Surgery (EACTS). *European Heart Journal* 2012;33(19):2451–2496.

Vesely I. The evolution of bioprosthetic heart valve design and its impact on durability. *Cardiovascular Pathology* 2003;12(5):277–286.

Vojáček J, Žáček P, Dominik J. Aortic valve repair and valve sparing procedures. *Cor et Vasa* 2017;59(1):e77–e84.

Vowels TJ, Gonzalez-Stawinski GV, Ko JM, Trachiotis GD, Roberts BJ, Roberts CS, Roberts WC. Anomalous cord from the raphe of a congenitally bicuspid aortic valve to the aortic wall producing either acute or chronic aortic regurgitation. *Journal of the American College of Cardiology* 2014;63(2):153–157.

Weinberg EJ, Mofrad MR. Transient, three-dimensional, multiscale simulations of the human aortic valve. *Cardiovascular Engineering* 2007;7(4):140–155.

Weinberg EJ, Mofrad MR. A multiscale computational comparison of the bicuspid and tricuspid aortic valves in relation to calcific aortic stenosis. *Journal of Biomechanics* 2008;41(16):3482–3487.

Yap CH, Kim HS, Balachandran K, Weiler M, Haj-Ali R, Yoganathan AP. Dynamic deformation characteristics of porcine aortic valve leaflet under normal and hypertensive conditions. *American Journal of Physiology-Heart and Circulatory Physiology* 2009;298(2):H395–H405.

Zhao DF, Seco M, Wu JJ, Edelman JB, Wilson MK, Vallely MP, Byrom MJ, Bannon PG. Mechanical versus bioprosthetic aortic valve replacement in middle-aged adults: A systematic review and meta-analysis. *The Annals of Thoracic Surgery* 2016;102(1):315–327.

10

Mitral Valve Mechanics

A. Tran, T. G. Mesana, and V. Chan

Contents

10.1 Anatomy, Geometry, and Properties of Normal Mitral Valve

The mitral valve is a bicuspid structure separating the left atrium and ventricle. It serves as a unidirectional valve, allowing blood to fill the ventricle during diastole and aiding antegrade ejection of blood through the aorta during systole. The essential components of the mitral valve include the fibrous annulus, the anterior and posterior mitral leaflets, the chordae tendinae, and the papillary muscles. Collectively, these are known as the mitral valve apparatus. Dysfunction of any one of these components can lead to pathology.

During embryonic development, the atrioventricular canals form by the fusion of the superior and inferior endocardial cushions. The interatrial and interventricular septa separate the left and right hearts. The mitral valve develops in the left atrioventricular canal. Initially, the microscopic dissection of embryonic hearts found that very little of the septal leaflet consisted of endocardial cushion tissue. This led to the hypothesis that the cushions played a lesser role in the development of the valve [1,2]. Further investigation revealed that the septal (anterior) leaflet derives from the superior and inferior endocardial cushions. At the site of endocardial cushions, endothelial cells migrate and invade the cardiac jelly and differentiate into mesenchymal cells [3]. These cells continue to proliferate, allowing the formation of thin fibrous valve tissue. The mural (posterior) leaflet of the mitral valve develops from a mesenchymal cushion that is laterally located. The leaflets are further defined by undermining of the myocardium, leaving behind trabeculated structures corresponding to chordae tendinae. The leaflets comprise connective tissue, namely collagen, elastin, and glycosaminoglycans, collectively known as an extracellular matrix. Delamination of the valve gives way to the anterior and posterior leaflets. The delamination process ends at the commissures. Still, the precise mechanism of heart valve development remains poorly understood. Overall, it is a complex and intricate process, potentially governed by a network of signaling pathways [4,5].

The mitral annulus is part of a flexible, collagenous skeleton that serves as the framework for the mitral valve. The leaflets attach to the annulus and myocardium by both elastic and collagenous fibers [6]. A fibrous scaffold extends out from the annulus to form the "backbone" of the leaflets [7]. Ranganathan et al. studied 50 human hearts at autopsy and described the leaflets in detail [8]. The valve consists of anterior and posterior leaflets—a bicuspid valve. The posterior (mural) leaflet typically possesses three scallops defined by small indentations, with secondary chordal insertions into the cleft. Necroscopy has revealed varying numbers of scallops in the minority of patients [8]. Small commissural leaflets for bridge between the leaflets. The existence and function (if any) of these "accessory" leaflets have been debated for some time and have even given rise to the concept of a quadricuspid valve [9,10]. However, the lack of fibrous tissue suggests a less significant role in valve function, suggesting that accessory leaflets may be present for a full range of leaflet motion, aiding in coaptation on valve closure [11]. Accessory leaflets are traceable by following the papillary muscles and commissural chordae that fan out at the transition between the anterior and posterior leaflets [8,12]. The free margin of the leaflets has thickened tissue, referred to as the rough zone, where primary chordae insert. The remainder of the leaflet is termed the translucent zone. The average height of the anterior leaflet is 2.1–2.4 cm in males and females, while a greater overall leaflet width is found in men (3.6–3.7 cm) than in women (2.9–3.3 cm) [8,13,14]. The middle scallop of the posterior leaflet is largest in both height and width, ranging from 1.3 to 1.4 cm in height and from 2.3 to 3.3 cm in width. Anterolateral and posteromedial scallops are smaller and are typically 0.9–1.1 cm in height and 1.1–1.6 cm in width. Males tend to have larger dimensions overall [8,13,14]. The posterior leaflet has a larger overall area than the anterior leaflet; however, because of annular geometry, the anterior leaflet plays a more significant role in valve competency [15]. The leaflets are composed of layers of connective tissue. The leaflets consist of a fibrous tissue containing primarily types I and III collagen [16]. As described by Gross in 1931, a thin layer of endothelial cells coats the atrial and ventricular surfaces of the leaflets. Layers of the leaflets include the lamina spongiosa, the fibrosa, and the ventricularis. The fibrosa provides structural strength to the leaflet and emanates from the auricularis [7,17]. The leaflets themselves have also been found to possess nerve structures radiating down to the atrial surface, as summarized by Misfield and Sievers [6]. Coupled with nervous tissue emanating from the papillary muscles, innervation and alteration of nervous tissue over time may play a role in valve disease.

Chordae tendinae are fibrous strands originating at the papillary muscle or ventricular wall and inserting into the valve apparatus. They consist of an inner layer of tightly bound collagen intertwined with elastin fiber and aligned in the direction of tension. An outer looser layer of collagen and elastic fibers surrounds the core [18,19]. Using porcine hearts, Ritchey et al. described longitudinal vessels running from papillary muscle, through the chordae, into the mitral valve. Strut chordae were found to have the highest number of vessels [19]. There have been several proposed classification systems for chordal structures [12,18,19]. More modern definitions have separated chords based on insertion point and function. Lam et al. examined the morphology of 50 normal mitral valves and described three types of chordae [12].

Their classification included chordae inserting into the rough zone, leaflets (including clefts), and commissures. The anterior and posterior mitral leaflets have different configurations of chordal attachment. The chordae of the anterior leaflet insert into the apex, at the thicker free edge of leaflets termed the rough zone. In addition, there are typically two thicker chordae that insert into the ventricular surface of the valve at the posteromedial and anterolateral regions of the anterior leaflet, away from the free margin; these are known as strut chordae and have been measured to be on average 1.86 ± 0.43 cm in length and 1.24 ± 0.51 cm in thickness. For comparison, rough zone chordae were 1.75 ± 0.25 cm and 0.84 ± 0.28 cm in length and thickness, respectively [12]. The posterior leaflet possesses more defined scallops than the anterior leaflet. In addition to rough zone chordae, there are also basal chordae, which may originate from the wall of the ventricle or trabeculae carneae and insert into the annulus. Two cleft chordae, with insertions into the free margin of the cleft on the leaflet, are also present. Together, they aid in defining the three scallops of the posterior leaflet [12]. Lam et al. also described chordae fanning out at the commissure in the anterolateral and posteromedial regions, with some chords extending as far as the base of the scallop. Average length and diameter of chordae, measured by Lam et al., were found to be lower in the posterior leaflet chordae than in the anterior leaflet chordae.

Rusted and colleagues studied 200 normal hearts and reported that 70% of the anterolateral papillary muscle tended to be single, with a small groove at the apex, and were typically found in close relation to the commissures. However, posterolateral papillary muscles had two or three separate "heads" in more than 60% of cases [14]. Displacement of the papillary muscle plays an essential role in the development of valvular dysfunction, and is explored later in this chapter. Vascular supply to the papillary muscles is varied and may originate from either the left or right coronary system, based on dominant circulation [18,20].

10.2 Diseases of the Mitral Valve

A population-based study by Nkomo et al. found an increased prevalence of valvular heart disease with age [21]. Specifically, the prevalence of mitral valve diseased exponentially grew in their study population from the fifth decade of life onward, along with significantly decreased survival over time. Valvular heart disease remains a relevant cause of morbidity and mortality today.

At least 5 mm of anterior and posterior leaflet coaptation is necessary for a competent mitral valve and functioning mitral apparatus. Disease of either the mitral structures or the myocardium of the heart can result in a dysfunctional valve. This section will focus on acquired mitral disease. Mitral pathology can be degenerative or functional. Functional mitral disease is secondary to extravalvular pathology, as the valve is considered morphologically "normal." In the case of degenerative disease, pathology occurs at both the gross and histological levels. Manifestations of degenerative disease may be in the form of restricted or excessive leaflet motion, producing stenosis and regurgitation, respectively. Clinical assessment may reveal signs and symptoms of murmurs, arrhythmias, embolic disease, or evidence of heart failure. Echocardiography is the gold standard for diagnosing and characterizing valve disease.

Carpentier classified mitral regurgitation based on function and described three types [22]. Type I dysfunction occurs in the setting of normal leaflet motion, as seen in annular dilation or calcification. Type II dysfunction results from an increased leaflet motion such as prolapsed leaflets and flail segments. Type III dysfunction is secondary to leaflet restriction and is further broken down into type IIIa, occurring throughout the valve cycle, and type IIIb, occurring predominately during the systolic phase.

Degenerative disease can be secondary to a combination of pathological processes, including myxomatous infiltration, fibroelastic deficiency, and alteration of collagen, resulting into segmental to total billowing of the valve, as seen in Barlow disease [7,23]. Decreased production of connective tissue is seen in fibroelastic deficiency. The leaflet tissue appears thin, with areas of translucency, and this is common in the elderly population. At the histological level, deficient components include collagen, elastin, and proteoglycans [7]. Fibroelastic deficiency is a distinct phenomenon from myxomatous degeneration and Barlow disease. In this form of degenerative valve pathology, mitral valves show thinning of affected leaflets, resulting in a type IIIa Carpentier lesion [7,24]. In contrast, Barlow disease demonstrates extensive myxoid infiltration, affecting all layers of the leaflet tissue and resulting in "billowing" of the mitral leaflets (type I or type II Carpentier classification) secondary to diffusely redundant and thickened tissue. Leaflet or annular calcification is more commonly present in the setting of Barlow disease, whereas this is typically absent in fibroelastic deficiency [25]. In addition, echocardiographic findings reveal a leaflet thickness of more than 3 mm and an elevated anterior leaflet height of more than 3.8 cm [24,25]. Care should be taken when selecting the appropriate annuloplasty device and repair technique, as functional mitral stenosis can develop in patients who have undergone mitral repair and can thus impact the quality of life and patient outcomes [26,27]. Currently, a prospective, multicenter randomized clinical trial by Chan et al. compared repair with leaflet resection versus preservation and the long-term impact of functional stenosis in the Canadian Mitral Research Alliance (CAMRA) CardioLing-2 trial [28].

Other causes of valve degeneration are secondary to infective etiologies. The introduction of antibiotic treatment has decreased the incidence and prevalence of rheumatic valve disease in the Western world. Worldwide, rheumatic heart disease remains a significant burden, with an estimated prevalence of more than 30 million affected individuals and nearly 350,000 attributable deaths [29]. Infection with Group A streptococcus sets the stage for an inflammatory and autoimmune response [29,30]. Carditis involving the myocardium and endothelium produces scarring of the endothelium. The mitral valve is almost always affected [31]. Activation of the inflammation response and autoimmunity, summarized in a review by Yanagawa, lead to valvular damage and, eventually, stenosis [32]. An important aspect of the natural history of rheumatic valve disease is its chronicity, which leads to scarring of the leaflet [33,34]. Treatment of the initial infection is done with penicillin antibiotics.

Individuals progressing to clinically significant valvular dysfunction require surgical intervention. Valve repair in experienced centers is durable and safe and yields promising long-term results [35–37]. It is important to note that although mitral stenosis has become synonymous with rheumatic fever, not all patients with mitral stenosis have had rheumatic fever. Other causes of stenosis include degenerative disease, congenital abnormalities, and metabolic syndromes, all of which have the potential to promote chronic inflammation of the valve tissue and can lead to nodularity of the valve, calcification, thickening, and scallop fusion [38,39]. Typically, patients become symptomatic when mitral valve area is 1.5 cm^2 of less (normal 4–5 cm^2) [40–42]. As the effective orifice area decreases, there is a larger pressure gradient across the valve during diastolic filling and increased left atrial pressures. Patients develop pulmonary hypertension, pulmonary edema, arrhythmias, left atrial dilatation, and, eventually, right heart strain and hypertrophy [40–43]. Separate from rheumatic valve disease, other infections of the valve can result in infective endocarditis. The causal organisms vary; however, streptococci and staphylococcus species comprise the majority of organisms [44]. Here, bacteria circulating through the cardiovascular system colonize native valve tissue or prosthetic valves and lead to a build-up of debris known as vegetation, posing an embolic risk to the patient [45,46]; moreover, organisms secret destructive enzymes, leading to valvular damage and incompetence [47]. Typically, the treatment consists of excision and replacement of the valve, as it is often not amenable to repair [48].

Ischemic cardiomyopathy can impair normal mitral valve function. Indeed, damage to the ventricular wall results in segmental or global dysfunction and remodeling of the cardiac chamber, which is often accompanied by annular dilatation. Displacement of the papillary muscle(s) and annular enlargement result in tethering of the leaflets and, ultimately, poor coaptation, corresponding to type IIIa or IIIb Carpentier classification [49]. The sequela is mitral regurgitation in the setting of normal leaflet tissue. Consequences of regurgitation are left atrial and ventricular dilatation, pulmonary hypertension, and dysrhythmias. The pathophysiology is cyclical. Subvalvular apparatus dysfunction produces regurgitation, exacerbating ventricular dilatation. Per Laplace's law of tension, there is an increased wall stress, restricting perfusion, furthering the ischemic insult, and perpetuating the cycle [49]. As pointed out by Anyanwu et al., although the leaflets are considered "normal," close inspection of autopsy specimens reveal morphological differences; these include an alteration to collagen composition and leaflet structure, reported by Grand-Allen and colleagues [50]. Their study describes thinner and stiffer leaflets with reduced extensibility in transplant recipient hearts with either dilated or ischemic cardiomyopathy. Patients with ischemic mitral regurgitation are secondary to tethering of one or both mitral leaflets from left ventricular (LV) dilation. The tethering disrupts coaptation in either symmetrical or asymmetric fashion, thus allowing for regurgitation [51,52]. The Cardiothoracic Surgery Network (CTSNet) trial was a randomized multicenter study that compared mitral valve repair and mitral valve replacement in patients with severe ischemic mitral regurgitation [53]. Although the study investigators concluded that patients with repair had more frequent recurrent regurgitation and serious adverse events, it is important to realize that those patients who had repair without recurrent regurgitation demonstrated far better reverse remodeling (decrease in the LV systolic index) than those with replacements or those with recurrent mitral regurgitation.

10.3 Computational Simulation of Mitral Valve

Echocardiography remains the gold standard for investigation of valve structure and function. Advancement to three-dimensional (3D) and four-dimensional (4D) echocardiography has allowed for detailed analysis of the mitral valve. Levine et al. described nonplanarity of the mitral valve on 3D echocardiography, with an ascension of 1.4 ± 0.3 cm in 15 normal mitral valves, not previously seen on two-dimensional (2D) echocardiography [54]. Detailed preoperative valvular assessment now consists of high-definition, multislice computed tomography and magnetic resonance imagining (MRI). A study by Delgado et al. investigated 151 patients by using a 64-slice multislice computed tomographic scan to evaluate valve anatomy and the geometric effects leading to valve deformation in the setting of heart failure and LV dysfunction [55]. They documented high variability in the subvalvular apparatus and were able to characterize the degree of papillary muscle displacement as well as asymmetrical tethering of the mitral leaflets. Chandra and colleagues reported their series of 3D echocardiography-assessed mitral valves and found that 57 of the 77 patients had degenerative valve pathology [56]. They concluded that 3D echocardiography and detailed valve assessment were able to differentiate between normal and abnormal valves. Detailed morphological assessment has played an important role in distinguishing fibroelastic deficiency from Barlow pathology. To date, the intraoperative valve assessment under direct visualization has remained a crucial element before deciding on repair or replacement. However, new technology and high-definition imaging may aid in detailed assessment and preoperative planning.

Technological advancements have led to improved ways for preoperative assessment of valvular disease. Computational simulation and modeling may eventually aid in planning surgical repair and predicting the consequences of the repair method. Finite element analysis is a mathematical method for assessing how objects or materials react to applied forces. The mathematical details are beyond the scope of this chapter. However, finite element analysis is commonly used as a method of predicting stress, deformation, and response of materials to environmental forces and has been applied to cardiac mechanics [57]. Kunzelman et al. developed a finite element model of the mitral valve and subvalvular apparatus [58]. Through their analysis, they were able to identify the stress points on the valve and found that the direction of stress was in line with the orientation of the collagen fibers. More importantly, their model demonstrated that bioengineering methods could be applied in a way to detail the interaction of materials with real-world forces and potentially aid in planning for surgical repair or replacement. In conjunction with high-definition computed tomographic imaging and 3D echocardiography, computed models have become more accurate. For example, the mitral valve annulus was once assumed to be flat. With better imaging, it was later determined to possess a "saddle" shape with varying thickness, as previously mentioned. Incorporating these changes into the algorithm produces more accurate modeling, as demonstrated by other groups. One example is the research done by Prot and colleagues, who used porcine valves as models [59]. By incorporating the saddle annular shape and secondary chordal structures, they produced a finite element model and found that secondary chordae carried approximately 29% of stress on the mitral leaflets and played an important role in valve competence. They also stated that annular shape in their model (albeit only 2 mm of height difference in comparison with 9 mm in other studies) did not significantly alter chordal force distribution. Interestingly, they recognized that native mitral valves had variations in leaflet thickness, as described earlier, particularly in the rough zone, where primary chords attach. However, they simplified this problem by creating two models with either 0.5-mm or 1-mm homogenously thick leaflets. They found that thinner valves experienced greater stress and required lesser force (30 mmHg) for coaptation. Votta et al. used healthy subjects and analyzed their mitral valve by using 4D ultrasound [60]. They were able to construct a finite element model of the mitral valve. Their study outlined several limitations that should be corrected or explored in future models, including the inclusion of basal chordae, incorporation of variable leaflet thickness, expansion of modeling to include the entire cardiac cycle (valve opening and closure), and accounting for tissue–blood interaction, as their model was purely structural. Future models capable of incorporating varying leaflet thickness into their algorithm may provide more information on valve dynamics. Another method of modeling takes into account the complex interaction of soft tissues with a fluid environment, known as fluid–structure interaction analysis. This form of modeling analyzes structural stress in response to environmental forces and fluid dynamics [61]. Kunzelman et al. were one of the first groups to present such a mathematical model that couples the Lagrangian domain of structure elements and Eulerian domain of fluid flow [62]. The importance of fluid–structure interaction analysis lies in its potential application to model surgical repair.

10.4 Hemodynamics and Loads of Mitral Valve Apparatus

Investigating blood flow through the heart is important to understand its normal function as well as to characterize abnormal hearts. Detailed analysis may even help predict the progression of disease. One of the difficulties in modeling blood flow is to create and incorporate an accurate valve model. The mitral valve serves as the inlet to the left ventricle and thus plays a significant role in blood flow dynamics. Su and colleagues used cardiac MRI of volunteers and created a mathematical model of blood flow through the left ventricle with the mitral valve incorporated [63]. They described vortex structures during diastolic flow that propagated throughout the left ventricle. Comparing a normal subject with the one with pulmonary hypertension, they found disruption of the vortex structure due to bulging of the ventricular septum; however, the significance of these vortex structures requires further investigation. In a more recent work, Gao et al. further described a coupled left ventricle and mitral valve model in diastole and systole in a healthy volunteer and created a mathematical model based on cardiac MRI [64]. In their analysis, maximum flow velocity across the mitral valve was linear in fashion, with a trajectory toward the apex of the left ventricle, at a rate of 210 mL/s. With valve closure, they noted a small regurgitation volume of 7.2 mL, equal to approximately 10% of the filling volume. Ejection across the aortic valve reached 468 mL/s, with an ejection fraction of 51%. They found a close correlation between their model and cardiac MRIs. Interestingly, they reported a negative central LV pressure during early diastole, corresponding to active myocardial relaxation, facilitating rapid filling. As filling slowed and the negative pressure dissipated, diastolic filling became more dependent on atrial contraction. Gao et al. were able to adjust the endocardial pressure (which creates a negative pressure in the left ventricle) in their model and found enhanced diastolic filling at pressure values 12 mmHg and more. Endocardial pressure values 12 mmHg and less resulted in a less efficient filling, smaller stroke volume, and worse ejection fraction, closely modeling the physiology of diastolic heart failure.

Many groups have attempted to describe functional anatomy by using both animal and simulated mathematical modeling. The heart is designed to promote unidirectional blood flow. Blood fills the left atrium during cardiac systole and empties into the left ventricle during diastole. Closure of the mitral valve is a complex orchestration of both mechanical and fluid dynamics. As previously described in this chapter, the valve is anchored on the ventricular surface by chordae tendinae, acting like a parachute. Toward the end of diastole, as the ventricle enters into isovolumetric contraction, the papillary muscles contract to exert a vertical force on the leaflets, drawing them together [65,66]. In addition, blood flows through the valve orifice and enters the ventricle, heading toward the apex and creating a fluid vortex. As blood reaches the apex, it disperses circumferentially toward the chamber walls and back up toward the ventricular surface of the valve [67]. Therefore, the cumulative effects of negative pressure from fluid flowing through the mitral valve during atrial contraction, fluid vortex, and forces from flow along the chamber walls are to bring together the mitral leaflets and sustain closure during systole [68–70]. Advancements in cardiac imaging have allowed for detailed investigation of the inner workings of the heart, which was once thought to be a simple fill-and-pump mechanism. The formation of vortices is believed to play a critical role in cardiac function; however, the consequences of not having vortex formation are not yet known. Left ventricular vortices form at the tips of the mitral leaflets and are believed to help in the efficiency of diastolic filling, to sustain filling, and to aid in atrioventricular valve closure [68–71]. Charonko et al. performed contrast MRI studies on 14 subjects (4 normal and 10 with filling disorders) [71]. At the end of systole in healthy subjects, there was elongation of the left ventricle and recoil of the mitral annulus, which increased the distance between the apex and mitral valve and produced a large pressure gradient. At the inflow from the atrium, a large vortex was identified to start at the tips of the mitral leaflets; this vortex persisted throughout the phase of filling. Toward end-diastole and with atrial contraction, a second vortex was produced, which increased the short axis measurement of the ventricle. In the 10 patients with cardiac disease, Charonko et al. noticed a weaker initial flow and smaller pressure gradient across the mitral valve. This resulted in a smaller vortex at the tip of the mitral leaflets during early diastolic filling and less elongation and more lateral expansion of the ventricle compared with normal subjects. Patients with filling disorders were found to be more dependent on atrial contraction for filling. The researchers concluded that vortices create a suction effect that drives ventricular filling by maintaining inflow; therefore, vortex formation was not just a by-product of flow but also facilitated flow. Similar findings have been described by other groups [72–74], and they pose interesting questions for the future study of heart disease. Can abnormal vortices induce remodeling? How does mitral valve surgery influence the formation of vortices? Akiyama et al. performed intraoperative flow-dynamic assessment in patients who underwent mitral valve surgery [75]. Fifteen patients underwent repair, and 17 patients underwent mitral replacement with a bioprosthetic valve. Thirteen (86.7%) of the 15 patients in the repair group had normal vortex patterns in comparison with only one (5.9%) of the 17 patients in the replacement group. Moreover, the replacement group had significantly higher energy loss per cardiac cycle due to more dissipation from abnormal flow patterns. In patients with aortic stenosis, energy loss across the valve has been found to be an independent predictor of aortic valve events and a negative prognostic indicator, leading some to suggest that measurement of energy loss was part of the standard evaluation of such patients [76].

Whether a similar principle applies to the mitral valve would require further investigation. A translational study by Witschey et al. looked at flow dynamics in ovine models with varying annuloplasty rings [77]. They found that as ring size decreased, there was an increase in disturbance of intraventricular flow patterns and vortex formation. This finding may be an important contributing factor to the evolution of functional stenosis in patients after mitral repair [26,27] and may potentially help guide surgical therapy.

The mitral valve is a complex structure that intimately connects to the left ventricle. Innovation and advancement in imagining have allowed for detailed analysis and modeling of its function. Although a seemingly simple structure with two leaflets acting as a guardian between the left atrium and ventricle, disease of this structure can drastically influence the patient's quality of life and survival. Thus far, preservation by repairing the mitral valve has become the mainstay treatment in many circumstances. Continued research into predicting the outcome with computational models has the potential to play a significant role before knife hits the skin.

References

1. Wenink AC, Gittenberger-de Groot AC. Embryology of the mitral valve. *Int J Cardiol* 1986;11(1):75–84.
2. Wenink AC, Gittenberger-de Groot AC. The role of atrioventricular endocardial cushions in the septation of the heart. *Int J Cardiol* 1985;8(1):25–44.
3. Armstrong EJ, Bischoff J. Heart valve development: Endothelial cell signaling and differentiation. *Circ Res* 2004;95(5):459–470.
4. Combs MD, Yutzey KE. Heart valve development: Regulatory networks in development and disease. *Circ Res* 2009;105(5):408–421.
5. Schroeder JA, Jackson LF, Lee DC, Camenisch TD. Form and function of developing heart valves: Coordination by extracellular matrix and growth factor signaling. *J Mol Med (Berl)* 2003;81(7):392–403.

6. Misfeld M, Sievers HH. Heart valve macro- and microstructure. *Philos Trans R Soc Lond B Biol Sci* 2007;362(1484):1421–1436.

7. Fornes P, Heudes D, Fuzellier JF, Tixier D, Bruneval P, Carpentier A. Correlation between clinical and histologic patterns of degenerative mitral valve insufficiency: A histomorphometric study of 130 excised segments. *Cardiovasc Pathol* 1999;8(2):81–92.

8. Ranganathan N, Lam JHC, Wigle ED, Silver MD. Morphology of the human mitral valve. *Circulation* 1970;41(3):459.

9. Benfari G, Rossetti L, Rossi A, Luciani GB. Quadricuspid mitral valve: Of clefts, scallops, and indentations. *J Thorac Cardiovasc Surg* 2016;152(2):e51–e53.

10. Anderson RH. How many leaflets in the mitral valve? *J Thorac Cardiovasc Surg* 2016;152(2):e53–e54.

11. Victor S, Nayak VM. Definition and function of commissures, slits and scallops of the mitral valve: Analysis in 100 hearts. *Asia Pacific J Thorac Cardiovasc Surg* 1994;3(1):10–16.

12. Lam JH, Ranganathan N, Wigle ED, Silver MD. Morphology of the human mitral valve. I. Chordae tendineae: A new classification. *Circulation* 1970;41(3):449–458.

13. Chiechi MA, Lees WM, Thompson R. Functional anatomy of the normal mitral valve. *J Thorac Surg* 1956;32(3):378–398.

14. Rusted IE, Scheifley CH, Edwards JE. Studies of the mitral valve. I. Anatomic features of the normal mitral valve and associated structures. *Circulation* 1952;6(6):825–831.

15. Kunzelman KS, Cochran RP, Verrier ED, Eberhart RC. Anatomic basis for mitral valve modelling. *J Heart Valve Dis* 1994;3(5):491–496.

16. Cole WG, Chan D, Hickey AJ, Wilcken DE. Collagen composition of normal and myxomatous human mitral heart valves. *Biochem J* 1984;219(2):451–460.

17. Gross L, Kugel MA. Topographic anatomy and histology of the valves in the human heart. *Am J Pathol* 1931;7(5):445–474.

18. Muresian H. The clinical anatomy of the mitral valve. *Clin Anat* 2009;22(1):85–98.

19. Ritchie J, Warnock JN, Yoganathan AP. Structural characterization of the chordae tendineae in native porcine mitral valves. *Ann Thorac Surg* 2005;80(1):189–197.

20. Ho SY. Anatomy of the mitral valve. *Heart* 2002;88(Suppl 4):iv5–iv10.

21. Nkomo VT, Gardin JM, Skelton TN, Gottdiener JS, Scott CG, Enriquez-Sarano M. Burden of valvular heart diseases: A population-based study. *Lancet* 2006;368(9540):1005–1011.

22. Carpentier A. Cardiac valve surgery—the French correction. *J Thorac Cardiovasc Surg* 1983;86(3):323–337.

23. Pellerin D, Brecker S, Veyrat C. Degenerative mitral valve disease with emphasis on mitral valve prolapse. *Heart* 2002;88(Suppl 4):iv20–iv28.

24. Anyanwu AC, Adams DH. Etiologic classification of degenerative mitral valve disease: Barlow's disease and fibroelastic deficiency. *Semin Thorac Cardiovasc Surg* 2007;19(2):90–96.

25. Levine RA, Hagege AA, Judge DP, Padala M, Dal-Bianco JP, Aikawa E et al. Mitral valve disease—morphology and mechanisms. *Nat Rev Cardiol* 2015;12(12):689–710.

26. Chan KL, Chen SY, Chan V, Hay K, Mesana T, Lam BK. Functional significance of elevated mitral gradients after repair for degenerative mitral regurgitation. *Circ Cardiovasc Imaging* 2013;6(6):1041–1047.

27. Mesana TG, Lam BK, Chan V, Chen K, Ruel M, Chan K. Clinical evaluation of functional mitral stenosis after mitral valve repair for degenerative disease: Potential affect on surgical strategy. *J Thorac Cardiovasc Surg* 2013;146(6):1418–1423; discussion 23–25.

28. Chan V, Chu MWA, Leong-Poi H, Latter DA, Hall J, Thorpe KE et al. Randomised trial of mitral valve repair with leaflet resection versus leaflet preservation on functional mitral stenosis (The CAMRA CardioLink-2 Trial). *BMJ Open* 2017;7(5):e015032.
29. Remenyi B, ElGuindy A, Smith SC, Jr., Yacoub M, Holmes DR, Jr. Valvular aspects of rheumatic heart disease. *Lancet* 2016;387(10025):1335–1346.
30. Marijon E, Mirabel M, Celermajer DS, Jouven X. Rheumatic heart disease. *Lancet* 2012;379(9819):953–964.
31. Chockalingam A, Gnanavelu G, Elangovan S, Chockalingam V. Clinical spectrum of chronic rheumatic heart disease in India. *J Heart Valve Dis* 2003;12(5):577–581.
32. Yanagawa B, Butany J, Verma S. Update on rheumatic heart disease. *Curr Opin Cardiol* 2016;31(2):162–168.
33. Roberts S, Kosanke S, Terrence Dunn S, Jankelow D, Duran CM, Cunningham MW. Pathogenic mechanisms in rheumatic carditis: Focus on valvular endothelium. *J Infect Dis* 2001;183(3):507–511.
34. Tandon R, Sharma M, Chandrashekhar Y, Kotb M, Yacoub MH, Narula J. Revisiting the pathogenesis of rheumatic fever and carditis. *Nat Rev Cardiol* 2013;10(3):171–177.
35. Chauvaud S, Fuzellier JF, Berrebi A, Deloche A, Fabiani JN, Carpentier A. Long-term (29 years) results of reconstructive surgery in rheumatic mitral valve insufficiency. *Circulation* 2001;104(12 Suppl 1):I12–I15.
36. Chotivatanapong T, Lerdsomboon P, Sungkahapong V. Rheumatic mitral valve repair: Experience of 221 cases from Central Chest Institute of Thailand. *J Med Assoc Thai* 2012;95(Suppl 8):S51–S57.
37. Yakub MA, Dillon J, Krishna Moorthy PS, Pau KK, Nordin MN. Is rheumatic aetiology a predictor of poor outcome in the current era of mitral valve repair? Contemporary long-term results of mitral valve repair in rheumatic heart disease. *Eur J Cardiothorac Surg* 2013;44(4):673–681.
38. Roberts WC, Perloff JK. Mitral valvular disease. A clinicopathologic survey of the conditions causing the mitral valve to function abnormally. *Ann Intern Med* 1972;77(6):939–975.
39. Waller BF, Howard J, Fess S. Pathology of mitral valve stenosis and pure mitral regurgitation—Part II. *Clin Cardiol* 1994;17(7):395–402.
40. Chandrashekhar Y, Westaby S, Narula J. Mitral stenosis. *Lancet* 2009;374(9697):1271–1283.
41. Carabello BA. Modern management of mitral stenosis. *Circulation* 2005;112(3):432–427.
42. Rahimtoola SH, Durairaj A, Mehra A, Nuno I. Current evaluation and management of patients with mitral stenosis. *Circulation* 2002;106(10):1183–1188.
43. Rowe JC, Bland EF, Sprague HB, White PD. The course of mitral stenosis without surgery: Ten- and twenty-year perspectives. *Ann Intern Med* 1960;52:741–749.
44. Bayliss R, Clarke C, Oakley CM, Somerville W, Whitfield AG, Young SE. The microbiology and pathogenesis of infective endocarditis. *Br Heart J* 1983;50(6):513–519.
45. Freedman LR. The pathogenesis of infective endocarditis. *J Antimicrob Chemother* 1987;20(Suppl A):1–6.
46. Pettersson GB, Hussain ST, Shrestha NK, Gordon S, Fraser TG, Ibrahim KS et al. Infective endocarditis: An atlas of disease progression for describing, staging, coding, and understanding the pathology. *J Thorac Cardiovasc Surg* 2014;147(4):1142–1149.e2.
47. Thiene G, Basso C. Pathology and pathogenesis of infective endocarditis in native heart valves. *Cardiovasc Pathol* 2006;15(5):256–263.
48. Gammie JS, O'Brien SM, Griffith BP, Peterson ED. Surgical treatment of mitral valve endocarditis in North America. *Ann Thorac Surg* 2005;80(6):2199–2204.

49. Anyanwu A, Rahmanian PB, Filsoufi F, Adams DH. The pathophysiology of isch-emic mitral regurgitation: Implications for surgical and percutaneous intervention. *J Intervent Cardiol* 2006;19:S78–S86.

50. Grande-Allen KJ, Barber JE, Klatka KM, Houghtaling PL, Vesely I, Moravec CS et al. Mitral valve stiffening in end-stage heart failure: Evidence of an organic contribution to functional mitral regurgitation. *J Thorac Cardiovasc Surg* 2005;130(3):783–790.

51. Otsuji Y, Levine RA, Takeuchi M, Sakata R, Tei C. Mechanism of ischemic mitral regur-gitation. *J Cardiol* 2008;51(3):145–156.

52. Zeng X, Nunes MC, Dent J, Gillam L, Mathew JP, Gammie JS et al. Asymmetric versus symmetric tethering patterns in ischemic mitral regurgitation: Geometric differences from three-dimensional transesophageal echocardiography. *J Am Soc Echocardiogr* 2014;27(4):367–375.

53. Goldstein D, Moskowitz AJ, Gelijns AC, Ailawadi G, Parides MK, Perrault LP et al. Two-year outcomes of surgical treatment of severe ischemic mitral regurgitation. *N Engl J Med* 2016;374(4):344–353.

54. Levine RA, Handschumacher MD, Sanfilippo AJ, Hagege AA, Harrigan P, Marshall JE et al. Three-dimensional echocardiographic reconstruction of the mitral valve, with implications for the diagnosis of mitral valve prolapse. *Circulation* 1989;80(3):589–598.

55. Delgado V, Tops LF, Schuijf JD, de Roos A, Brugada J, Schalij MJ et al. Assessment of mitral valve anatomy and geometry with multislice computed tomography. *JACC Cardiovasc Imaging* 2009;2(5):556–565.

56. Chandra S, Salgo IS, Sugeng L, Weinert L, Tsang W, Takeuchi M et al. Characterization of degenerative mitral valve disease using morphologic analysis of real-time three-dimensional echocardiographic images: Objective insight into complexity and plan-ning of mitral valve repair. *Circ Cardiovasc Imaging* 2011;4(1):24–32.

57. McCulloch A, Waldman L, Rogers J, Guccione J. Large-scale finite element analysis of the beating heart. *Crit Rev Biomed Eng* 1992;20(5–6):427–449.

58. Kunzelman KS, Cochran RP, Chuong C, Ring WS, Verrier ED, Eberhart RD. Finite ele-ment analysis of the mitral valve. *J Heart Valve Dis* 1993;2(3):326–340.

59. Prot V, Haaverstad R, Skallerud B. Finite element analysis of the mitral apparatus: Annulus shape effect and chordal force distribution. *Biomech Model Mechanobiol* 2009;8(1):43–55.

60. Votta E, Caiani E, Veronesi F, Soncini M, Montevecchi FM, Redaelli A. Mitral valve finite-element modelling from ultrasound data: A pilot study for a new approach to understand mitral function and clinical scenarios. *Philos Trans A Math Phys Eng Sci* 2008;366(1879):3411–3434.

61. Lau KD, Diaz V, Scambler P, Burriesci G. Mitral valve dynamics in structural and fluid-structure interaction models. *Med Eng Phys* 2010;32(9):1057–1064.

62. Kunzelman KS, Einstein DR, Cochran RP. Fluid-structure interaction models of the mitral valve: Function in normal and pathological states. *Philos Trans R Soc Lond B Biol Sci* 2007;362(1484):1393–1406.

63. Su B, Tan RS, Tan JL, Guo KWQ, Zhang JM, Leng S et al. Cardiac MRI based numerical modeling of left ventricular fluid dynamics with mitral valve incorporated. *J Biomech* 2016;49(7):1199–1205.

64. Gao H, Feng L, Qi N, Berry C, Griffith BE, Luo X. A coupled mitral valve-left ventricle model with fluid-structure interaction. *Med Eng Phys* 2017;47:128–136.

65. Perloff JK, Roberts WC. The mitral apparatus. Functional anatomy of mitral regurgita-tion. *Circulation* 1972;46(2):227–239.

66. Silverman ME, Hurst JW. The mitral complex. Interaction of the anatomy, physiology, and pathology of the mitral annulus, mitral valve leaflets, chordae tendineae, and papillary muscles. *Am Heart J* 1968;76(3):399–418.

67. Reul H, Talukder N, Muller EW. Fluid mechanics of the natural mitral valve. *J Biomech* 1981;14(5):361–372.

68. Pedrizzetti G, Domenichini F. Nature optimizes the swirling flow in the human left ventricle. *Phys Rev Lett* 2005;95(10):108101.

69. Bellhouse BJ. Fluid mechanics of a model mitral valve and left ventricle. *Cardiovasc Res* 1972;6(2):199–210.

70. Kilner PJ, Yang GZ, Wilkes AJ, Mohiaddin RH, Firmin DN, Yacoub MH. Asymmetric redirection of flow through the heart. *Nature* 2000;404(6779):759–761.

71. Charonko JJ, Kumar R, Stewart K, Little WC, Vlachos PP. Vortices formed on the mitral valve tips aid normal left ventricular filling. *Ann Biomed Eng* 2013;41(5):1049–1061.

72. Elbaz MS, Calkoen EE, Westenberg JJ, Lelieveldt BP, Roest AA, van der Geest RJ. Vortex flow during early and late left ventricular filling in normal subjects: Quantitative characterization using retrospectively-gated 4D flow cardiovascular magnetic resonance and three-dimensional vortex core analysis. *J Cardiovasc Magn Reson* 2014;16:78.

73. Arvidsson PM, Kovacs SJ, Toger J, Borgquist R, Heiberg E, Carlsson M et al. Vortex ring behavior provides the epigenetic blueprint for the human heart. *Sci Rep* 2016;6:22021.

74. Toger J, Kanski M, Carlsson M, Kovacs SJ, Soderlind G, Arheden H et al. Vortex ring formation in the left ventricle of the heart: Analysis by 4D flow MRI and Lagrangian coherent structures. *Ann Biomed Eng* 2012;40(12):2652–2662.

75. Akiyama K, Nakamura N, Itatani K, Naito Y, Kinoshita M, Shimizu M et al. Flow-dynamics assessment of mitral-valve surgery by intraoperative vector flow mapping. *Interact Cardiovasc Thorac Surg* 2017;24(6):869–875.

76. Bahlmann E, Gerdts E, Cramariuc D, Gohlke-Baerwolf C, Nienaber CA, Wachtell K et al. Prognostic value of energy loss index in asymptomatic aortic stenosis. *Circulation* 2013;127(10):1149–1156.

77. Witschey WR, Zhang D, Contijoch F, McGarvey JR, Lee M, Takebayashi S et al. The influence of mitral annuloplasty on left ventricular flow dynamics. *Ann Thorac Surg* 2015;100(1):114–121.

11

The Mechanical Changes Associated with Aging in the Cardiovascular System

L. Horný

Contents

There are many well-known risk factors correlating with the incidence of cardiovascular diseases. Sedentary lifestyle, dyslipidemia, diabetes, genetic predisposition, and smoking are some examples. However, epidemiological studies have shown that the greatest risk of all is advancing age (Lakatta and Levy, 2003a). The role of age may be understood from two different viewpoints. On the one hand, as commonly known, there are diseases that correlate with age in terms of their incidence and degree of severity. Such diseases include atherosclerosis, hypertension, heart failure, atrial fibrillation, and stenosis or insufficiency of the aortic and mitral valves. They can be defined by signs contributing to a clinical picture. However, these pathological changes, although associated with advancing age, should not be confused with cardiovascular aging. Indeed, other structural changes also accompany increasing age that cannot be defined as symptoms. To be correct, only these changes should be referred to as cardiovascular aging. In contrast to a disease, which is a pathological state, aging is a normal and unavoidable process.

In this context, aging is understood as a process of persistent decline in the age-specific fitness components of an organism, due to internal physiological deterioration (Rose, 1991). In the cardiovascular system, this process leads to a cascade of changes exhibited at the molecular, cellular, and tissue levels, which alter the substrate on which cardiovascular diseases are superimposed and thus alter the occurrence, presentation, and manifestation of cardiovascular diseases in older persons (Lakatta and Levy, 2003b). Aging creates conditions under which people become more susceptible to a disease; aging also reduces the threshold for disease manifestation and intensifies the impact of a disease (Lakatta and Levy, 2003a).

Typical signs of aging in the human heart include left ventricular hypertrophy (Levy et al., 1988), thickening of the left ventricle wall (Gerstenblith et al., 1977), and the decrease of the maximum heart rate achievable during exhaustive, dynamic exercise (Fleg et al., 1995; Lakatta and Levy, 2003b). These signs are found in otherwise-healthy individuals. Arteries, which conduct blood and interact mechanically with it by affecting its velocity and pressure, also show age-associated changes that should not be interpreted as pathological. In particular, intimomedial thickening and dilatation are prominent with aging in elastic arteries (Lakatta and Levy, 2003a; Greenwald 2007; O'Rourke and Hashimoto, 2007). However, as will be detailed in this chapter, the most significant change is arterial stiffening, which ultimately affects the heart through the reflected pressure pulse wave (PWV). This biomechanical change leads to further stiffening, thereby establishing a vicious cycle.

11.1 The Heart

The most prominent structural change that the human heart undergoes with aging consists of a significant increase in the myocardial thickness (Gerstenblith et al., 1977). Simultaneously, cardiomyocyte enlargement is observed, which appears to be a compensatory reaction to the decrease in the number of cardiac cells (Olivetti et al., 1991; Strait and Lakatta, 2012). Figure 11.1 shows the relationship between the thickness of the left ventricle (TLV) and age as well as the relationship between the heart weight (HW) and age. The data presented are based on 610 autopsy measurements conducted by the author's colleagues (Horný et al., 2012, 2014a, 2017). The correlation coefficients are R (HW, age) $= 0.362$, with $p < 0.001$, and R (TLV, age) $= 0.221$, with $p < 0.001$. The symbols used in the figure highlight the increasing severity of the atherosclerotic lesions found in the aorta.

Although the correlation between age and HW is clear (Figure 11.1), it has to be noted that the increase in HW is not only due to aging. Studies that present data adjusted for hypertension and coronary artery disease and corrected for body surface area have suggested that there is no aging-induced change in HW in women, and data collected from men have even suggested a decrease in cardiac mass (Strait and Lakatta, 2012). This has been confirmed by echocardiographic measurements (Khouri et al., 2005) and magnetic resonance imaging examinations of healthy persons involved in the Baltimore Longitudinal Study of Aging (Hees et al., 2002). Thus, the apparent age-related changes in HW presented in Figure 11.1 are more likely the result of the mechanobiological adaptation of the heart to cardiovascular diseases such as hypertension and atherosclerosis rather than the result of aging (Chen et al., 1998).

The systolic function of the heart, expressed by means of the ejection fraction metric, is preserved during normal aging (Lakatta and Levy, 2003b; Strait and Lakatta, 2012). This finding does not apply to individuals suffering from, for example, dilated or ischemic cardiomyopathy; they do not satisfy the condition of normal aging anyway. However, the preservation of the systolic function is observed only at rest. During physical exercise, aging-related changes are much more evident. The maximum ejection fraction of the left ventricle decreases with age in healthy persons (Fleg et al., 1995) and so does the maximum heart rate during dynamic exercise (Fleg et al., 1995). With regard to diastolic function, early diastolic filling of the left ventricle progressively slows down after the age of 20 years (Schulman et al., 1992; Lakatta and

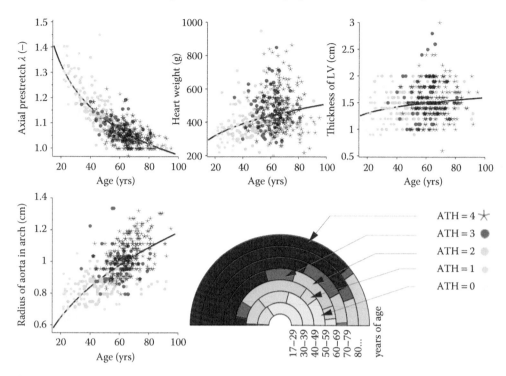

Figure 11.1   Selected age-associated changes in cardiovascular system. Upper left panel: axial prestretch in infrarenal aorta significantly decreases with age; $R(ln(\text{Age}),ln(\lambda)) = -0.865$, $p < 0.001$; equation of regression curve $y = 2.372x^{-0.1934}$. Upper mid panel: heart weight (HW) significantly increases with age; $R(ln(\text{Age}),ln(\text{HW})) = 0.409$, $p < 0.001$; equation of regression curve $y = 133.1x^{0.2916}$. Upper right panel: thickness of left ventricle (TLV) increases with age; $R(ln(\text{Age}),ln(\text{TLV})) = 0.227$, $p < 0.001$; equation of regression curve $y = 0.8929x^{0.1258}$. Lower left panel: aorta significantly dilates with age; $R(ln(\text{Age}),ln(\text{HW})) = 0.837$, $p < 0.001$; equation of regression curve $y = 0.2099x^{0.3756}$. Lower right panel: pie graph showing decades of age and distribution of atherosclerosis severity in decades. The severity of atherosclerosis (ATH) correlates positively with age (see Table 11.1 for characterization of severity). The graphs were created from merged data published by the author and his coworkers (Horný et al., 2012, 2014a, 2017). The total number of autopsy measurements is 610.

Levy 2003b). However, this is compensated in late diastole by augmented atrial contraction. Thus, the end diastolic volume is not compromised in healthy older individuals, but this is achieved at the cost of atrial hypertrophy (Lakatta and Levy 2003b).

The findings discussed earlier apply to normal aging, that is, aging in healthy subjects. However, aging creates a substrate for the development of pathological phenomena that impair all cardiovascular functions. Figure 11.2 summarizes age-related changes in the prevalence of selected cardiovascular diseases (arterial hypertension, heart failure, myocardial infarction, and total cardiovascular diseases) in the US and Canadian populations. The prevalence of heart failure clearly shows that the mechanical function of the heart worsens with age in the general population. By comparing the prevalence of cardiovascular disease and that of myocardial infarction and heart

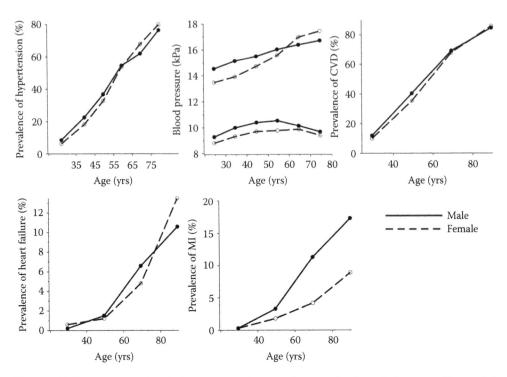

Figure 11.2 Age-associated changes in the prevalence of selected diseases. Upper left panel: prevalence of hypertension in US adults aged 20 years and older. Upper mid panel: age-related changes in systolic (upper solid and dashed curve) and diastolic (lower solid and dashed curve) pressures in the population aged 20–79 years in Canada. Upper right panel: total prevalence of cardiovascular disease (CVD) in US adults aged 20 years and older (hypertension, heart failure, coronary heart disease, and stroke are included). The lower panels show the prevalence of heart failure and myocardial infarction (MI) in US adults aged 20 years and older. Prevalence is expressed as a percentage of the population suffering from a disease with respect to the total population. Data for hypertension, CVD, heart failure, and MI were collected during the National Health and Nutrition Survey 2007–2012 and reported by the American Heart Association in Mozaffarian et al. (2016). Data for age-related changes in blood pressure were collected during the Canadian Health Measures Survey 2007–2009. (Adapted from Wilkins, K. et al., Blood pressure in Canadian adults. *Health Reports/Statistics Canada, Canadian Centre for Health Information*, 21, 37–46, 2010.)

failure in Figure 11.2, it appears that the dominant cardiovascular pathological condition is systemic hypertension. Statistics published by the American Heart Association showed that, in 2015, 102.7 million of US citizens had at least one cardiovascular disease and 96.1 million of them had hypertension (American Heart Association, 2017). In addition, 16.8 people suffered from coronary heart disease, 7.5 million had experienced a stroke, 5.8 million had congestive heart failure, and 5.2 million were diagnosed with atrial fibrillation (American Heart Association, 2017).

Systemic hypertension is a synonym for high arterial blood pressure; an individual is said to be hypertensive if a systolic pressure equal to or higher than 140 mmHg or a diastolic pressure equal to or higher than 90 mmHg is found during repeated measurements. Hypertension may be essential or primary, that is, idiopathic, with no clear and univocal cause, or it may be secondary, that is, with a clear cause, such as stenosis of the renal arteries. Although hypertension is an arterial disease, it has a crucial effect on the heart in that the heart has to adapt to be able to eject blood under changed pressure conditions in conduit arteries.

In contrast to the elastic properties of arteries, for which many experimental results obtained from uniaxial and biaxial tests document how arteries stiffen with age, the changes in the elastic properties of the heart muscle with age have not been well studied in the literature. Based on a recent study carried out by Sommer et al. (2015), age-related changes in the passive elasticity and viscoelasticity of the cardiac muscle do not seem to be as significant during normal aging as they are, for example, in the aorta and in the coronary arteries. Indeed, Sommer et al. (2015) reported that the results of planar biaxial tensile tests, shear tests, and relaxation tests on specimens obtained from the left ventricle wall did not demonstrate any significant correlation with age in 28 subjects aged 61 ± 15 years (range 31–93 years). However, although passive elastic properties may not significantly correlate with age, active mechanical properties, such as myocardial contractility, contractile reserve, and regulatory mechanisms, decline with age (Lakatta and Levy, 2003b).

11.2 Systemic Circulation

As mentioned earlier, in contrast to the passive elastic properties of the heart muscle, those of arteries do change significantly with aging. Arteries progressively stiffen and dilate (Greenwald 2007; O'Rourke and Hashimoto, 2007). However, this is more so for elastic arteries, whose main function is not only to transmit blood but also to attenuate pressure pulsations. Simultaneous permanent dilatation and loss of elasticity are usually referred to as arteriosclerosis (Greenwald, 2007; O'Rourke and Hashimoto, 2007). Arteriosclerosis, which must be distinguished from atherosclerosis, is associated with general nonatherosclerotic intimomedial thickening and with gradual fragmentation and calcification of the medial elastic lamellae (Elliott and McGrath, 1994). This condition is also referred to as elastocalcinosis or, sometimes, Mönckeberg sclerosis (Persy and D'Haese, 2009).

Arteriosclerosis predominantly affects the medial layer of an artery, while, as discussed in more detail in Chapter 7, atherosclerosis is a focal disease of the intimal layer and manifests itself by lesions that accumulate lipids, inflammatory cells, and fibrous tissue (Figure 11.3a vs. b and c vs. d). The lesions develop to form calcified plaque, which obstructs blood flow and may result in clinically significant ischemia. However, the most dangerous situation occurs when the so-called vulnerable plaque ruptures. The mechanical failure of the thin fibrous cap of the plaque results in the formation of thrombus, which may suddenly block an artery. Myocardial infarction frequently arises from this mechanism.

Both atherosclerosis and arteriosclerosis significantly correlate with age. In the case of atherosclerosis, empty yellow circles in Figure 11.1, denoting an anatomically normal intima, are abundant up to 40 years, whereas almost everyone older than

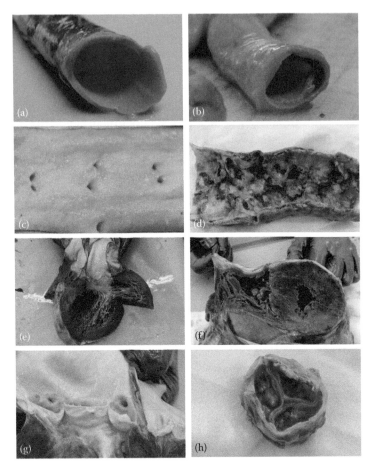

Figure 11.3 Age-associated changes in the heart and the aorta. (a) Intact intimal surface of the thoracic aorta versus (b) ruptured atherosclerotic lesion in the iliac artery. (c) Intact intimal surface of the thoracic aorta versus (d) calcified and ruptured atherosclerotic lesions in the thoracic aorta. (e) Cut left ventricle versus (f) hypertrophied wall of left ventricle. (g) Aortic valve leaflets with minimal calcification versus (h) highly calcified aortic valve. Pictures from the author's personal archive.

60 years of age shows a severity of atherosclerosis at least equal to 2, corresponding to the presence of advanced, calcified, or even ruptured plaques (see Table 11.1 for classification details). Since arteriosclerosis is characterized by the stiffening and dilatation of arteries, the lower left panel in Figure 11.1, showing the relationship between the aortic radius and age, documents how strong the correlation is between age and arteriosclerotic changes; the Pearson correlation coefficient computed for logarithms of age and radius is $R = 0.837$, with $p < 0.001$.

Another manifestation of age-related, arteriosclerotic, changes is the decrease in the axial prestretch of elastic arteries. At autopsy, when an arterial segment is excised from the body, one can observe that the in situ length is longer than the length measured after removal; this is because arteries retract when excised. The in vivo prestretch is believed to help the circulatory function by making arteries more distensible at physiological

TABLE 11.1   Classification of Atherosclerotic Lesions According to Kumar et al.

Characteristics	ATH
Intact artery and fatty streaks	0
Fibrofatty plaques	1
Advanced plaques	2
Calcified plaques	3
Ruptured plaques	4

Source: Kumar, V. et al., *Robbins and Cotran Pathologic Basis of Disease*, 8th ed., Elsevier Saunders, Philadelphia, PA, 2010.

pressures (Horný et al., 2014b; Horný and Netušil, 2016). However, as arteries stiffen and elastic fibers, which are assumed to bear the prestress (Horný et al., 2014a), fragment, the axial prestretch decreases (Kamenskiy et al., 2016). Some publications even reported axially precompressed, instead of prestretched, arteries in older individuals (Schulze-Bauer et al., 2003; Horný et al., 2017). Age-related changes in the prestretch are documented in Figure 11.1, where λ is defined as the ratio of in situ to ex situ lengths.

There are many studies documenting age-related stiffening in the human arteries. Roccabianca et al. (2014) recently sampled those that focused on the aorta under multiaxial loading and compared the components of the elasticity tensor to quantify regional differences in aging-induced changes with the mechanical behavior of the aorta. All papers included in the survey contained experimentally validated numerical parameters of constitutive models that reflected aging-induced changes in aortic biomechanics (Vorp et al., 2003; Vande Geest et al., 2004; Labrosse et al., 2009; Haskett et al., 2010; Martin et al., 2011; García-Herrera et al., 2012).

Figure 11.4 documents how age influences the stress–strain behavior of the human aorta. Panel (a) illustrates uniaxial testing responses, and Panel (b) shows the stress–strain curves computed at equibiaxial stretch of a planar sample, while pressure–deformation relationships for inflated cylindrical samples are demonstrated in Panel (c). As can be seen, the mechanical responses at increasing ages exhibit a leftward shift and a greater steepness of the curves in comparison with the biomechanical responses found in younger individuals. Although Figure 11.4 focuses only on the aorta, similar results have also been found for other elastic and muscular arteries (Valenta et al., 2002; Schulze-Bauer et al., 2003; Kamenskiy et al., 2016, 2017).

Age-related stiffening has been attributed, in part, to the calcification of the arterial wall (Elliott and McGrath, 1994; Atkinson, 2008). Other factors are thought to contribute as well, among which two are worth noting. One, very important, factor is the transfer of the load-bearing capacity from fragmented, thus mechanically inactive, elastin to significantly stiffer collagen. The other factor is the additional nonenzymatic crosslinking of collagen and elastin, which occurs in aging.

Although elastin contained in elastic fibers and membranes is a highly stable scleroprotein, studies focused on athero- and arteriosclerotic changes in arteries have found that enzymes degrading elastin, especially matrix metalloproteinases (MMP)-2 and

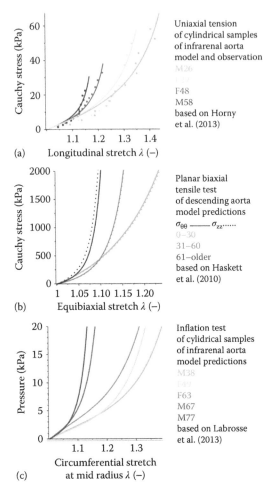

Figure 11.4 Age-related changes in the mechanical behavior of the human aorta. Aging is accompanied by a gradual left shift and an increased steepness of the stress–strain curves. Panel (a) shows stiffening of abdominal aorta observed in uniaxial tension of nonpressurized cylindrical samples (based on Horny et al., 2013). Panel (b) shows circumferential and axial stress at equibiaxial planar loading predicted by computational model, using average constitutive parameters found by Haskett et al. (2010) for three different age groups. Panel (c) shows examples of pressure–deformation relationships computed from data found by Labrosse et al. (2013) in experiments with human abdominal aorta. Age-related stiffening is exhibited as decreased circumferential distensibility. MXX = male, FYY = female, XX or YY = age in years.

MMP-9, occur in the surrounding of fragmented elastic fibers and exhibit increased serum levels (Stewart et al., 2003; Wang et al., 2003; Yasmin et al., 2005; Sherratt, 2009). Proteolysis damages elastic fibers by disrupting and fragmenting them. As a result, the load-bearing capacity of the arterial wall structure is transferred to collagen.

Collagen concentration in the arterial wall increases with age (Spina et al., 1983; Kohn et al., 2015). It is a consequence of medial fibrosis (Schlatmann and Becker, 1977), but collagen fibers are also synthetized by aged endothelial cells, which, during nonatherosclerotic intimal thickening, sustain morphological changes and acquire a phenotype resembling that of synthetic smooth muscle cells (Fleenor et al., 2012). Since collagen is much stiffer than elastin, the arterial wall stiffens. Additional crosslinking of collagen and elastin by advanced glycation end products further contributes to this stiffening (Bailey, 2001; Aronson, 2003; Sherratt, 2009).

Age-related changes in the elasticity of arteries have important consequences regarding fluid–structure interactions in the circulation. Mechanical interactions between arteries and blood are expressed via blood pressure. As discussed in Chapter 6, reduced elasticity in arteries contributes to an increased velocity of PWV. Noninvasive carotid–femoral in vivo measurement of PWV is well established and has been shown to provide a valuable and independent assessment of cardiovascular health (Greenwald, 2007; McEniery et al., 2007). A typical average value of PWV in young individuals is 5 m/s, whereas 12 m/s is expected for 80-year-old individuals (McEniery et al., 2007; O'Rourke and Hashimoto, 2007).

Increased PWV contributes to the systolic blood pressure through reflected pressure waves, which arise at every hydraulically nonsmooth site (i.e., arterial branching, resistant arteries, and sites of atherosclerotic plaques). Reflected waves travel back to the heart and, in the young elastic circulatory system, reach the heart when the ejection phase has been completed. Thus, reflected pressure waves contribute to the Windkessel function. This is also favorable to the blood supply of the heart muscle, which happens during diastole, when the heart is relaxed. However, this optimal tuning is lost in the aged, stiffened arterial tree. Reflected waves are transmitted more quickly and may reach the heart before the optimal systolic volume has been ejected. Yet, these reflected waves bear down on the aortic valve and increase the overall loading of the left ventricle. By this mechanism, reduced elasticity contributes to the development of hypertension and heart failure (Greenwald, 2007; O'Rourke and Hashimoto, 2007).

The situation is further compounded by the fact that remodeling mechanisms in arteries do not include effective elastin synthesis (Wagenseil and Mecham, 2009). The dominant component of extracellular matrix that is synthetized by fibroblasts and vascular smooth muscle cells in synthetic phenotype is collagen. However, as already mentioned, collagen is stiffer than elastin. In this vicious cycle, a stiff arterial wall, in reaction to elevated blood pressure, is remodeled to become stiffer.

11.3 Age-Related Changes in the Biomechanics of Heart Valves

Cardiac and arterial diseases are much more frequent than pathological changes in any other parts of the circulatory system. They also tend to have a more substantial impact on health and life expectancy. According to Mozaffarian et al. (2016), in the US population, the overall age-adjusted prevalence of any clinically diagnosed heart valve disease is 1.8%, which is in stark contrast to hypertension, whose age-adjusted prevalence is 32.6%. On the other hand, these numbers by no means suggest that age-related changes in heart valve biomechanics should be discounted: 1.8% of the US population represents a whopping 5,400,000 individuals, and the mortality directly related to valvular disease is 24,608 people a year (Mozaffarian et al., 2016).

Similar to cardiac and arterial functions, heart valve function shows significant age-related changes that are highlighted by the increasing prevalence of heart valve disease with age. According to the National Health and Nutrition Survey 2007–2012 reported by the American Heart Association in Mozaffarian et al. (2016), prevalence of heart valve disease is 0.3% from the age of 18 years to 44 years, 0.7% from 45 years to 54 years, 1.6% from 55 years to 64 years, 4.4% from 65 years to 74 years, and 11.7% in individuals older than 74 years (Mozaffarian et al., 2016).

Age-related degenerative disease (dysfunction) is a typical pathological change in heart valves. From a functional point of view, valvular stenosis and valvular insufficiency are distinguished. The condition wherein a valve inadequately opens and the hemodynamic resistance to blood ejection is consequently increased is referred to as valvular stenosis. On the other hand, valvular insufficiency refers to the imperfect closing of the heart valve leaflets, accompanied by a regurgitation of the blood into the upstream heart chamber. It is very frequent to observe both pathologies at the same time, because both are manifestations of valve sclerosis. Heart valve sclerosis, whereby a valve stiffens due to calcification, shares some characteristics with arterial atherosclerosis but differs from an etiological point of view (Butcher et al., 2011).

Both atherosclerosis and heart valve sclerosis are initiated by endothelial dysfunction and involve the differentiation of underlying medial cells (referred to as *interstitial cells* in the case of valvular anatomy). In addition, both atherosclerosis and valvular sclerosis create lipid-rich plaque with inflammatory infiltration and calcium deposits and are chronic self-propagating pathologies (Butcher et al., 2011). However, unlike atherosclerosis, valvular calcification can affect much younger and generally healthier patients. The changes in cell phenotype are also different. Moreover, plaque found in heart valve disease is characterized by large mineralized matrix nodules formed by osteoblast-like cells; this is in contrast to the small calcific nodules and large lipid and fibrous tissue accumulations found in atherosclerotic lesions (Persy and D'Haese, 2009; Butcher et al., 2011). This is illustrated in Figure 11.3d (atherosclerotic lesions) versus h (calcified nodules in aortic valve).

Contrary to atherosclerotic plaque, heart valve lesions usually do not rupture but enlarge to a state where the flexibility of the heart valve leaflets is significantly reduced. Besides calcification, heart valves show other age-related pathological changes in the extracellular matrix, such as the disruption of elastic laminae and disorganized matrix (especially collagen) deposition and remodeling (Butcher et al., 2011; Leopold, 2012), which, to some extent, may resemble arteriosclerosis rather than atherosclerosis. The development of heart valve dysfunction may also be linked to rheumatic fever (the most important cause of the heart valve diseases in the first half of the twentieth century) and infective endocarditis.

Overall, the age-related changes in heart valve biomechanics are determined by calcification (sclerosis), which leads to a gradual stiffening, manifested by an increased flexural rigidity. However, this stiffening depends on the anatomical location of the valves. Indeed, left heart (aortic and mitral) and right heart (pulmonary and tricuspid) valves differ in their mechanical properties because of the different pressure gradients that they sustain (Sacks et al., 2009; Pham et al., 2017). The age-related increase in the stiffness of the valves is accompanied by a simultaneous decrease in their extensibility (i.e., deformation at failure), a behavior similar to that known from arterial biomechanics (Pham et al., 2017). Qualitative changes associated with age in the stress–strain relationships of heart valve leaflets are the same as in arteries. The stress–strain curves exhibit a shift to the left and show greater steepness. It was also found that aging changes the degree of anisotropy of valvar tissues (Pham et al., 2017). Age-dependent numerical values of constitutive parameters suitable for the finite element modeling of human valves can be found, for example, in Oomen et al. (2016), who used an inverse finite element method for the regression analysis of microindentation tests. Age-specific values of constitutive parameters estimated from planar biaxial tests can be found in Pham et al. (2017).

References

American Heart Association. 2017. Cardiovascular disease: A costly burden for America – Projections through 2035. 1/17DS11775.

Aronson, D. 2003. Cross-linking of glycated collagen in the pathogenesis of arterial and myocardial stiffening of aging and diabetes. *Journal of Hypertension* 21 (1): 3–12.

Atkinson, J. 2008. Age-related medial elastocalcinosis in arteries: Mechanisms, animal models, and physiological consequences. *Journal of Applied Physiology* 105 (5): 1643–1651.

Bailey, A. J. 2001. Molecular mechanisms of ageing in connective tissues. *Mechanisms of Ageing and Development* 122 (7): 735–755.

Butcher, J. T., G. J. Mahler, and L. A. Hockaday. 2011. Aortic valve disease and treatment: The need for naturally engineered solutions. *Advanced Drug Delivery Reviews* 63 (4), 242–268.

Chen, C.-H., C.-T. Ting, S.-J. Lin, T.-L. Hsu, S.-J. Ho, P. Chou, M.-S. Chang et al. 1998. Which arterial and cardiac parameters best predict left ventricular mass? *Circulation* 98 (5): 422–428.

Elliott, R. J. and L. T. McGrath. 1994. Calcification of the human thoracic aorta during aging. *Calcified Tissue International* 54 (4): 268–273.

Fleenor, B. S., K. D. Marshall, C. Rippe, and D. R. Seals. 2012. Replicative aging induces endothelial to mesenchymal transition in human aortic endothelial cells: Potential role of inflammation. *Journal of Vascular Research* 49 (1): 59–64.

Fleg, J. L., F. O'Connor, G. Gerstenblith, L. C. Becker, J. Clulow, S. P. Schulman, and E. G. Lakatta. 1995. Impact of age on the cardiovascular response to dynamic upright exercise in healthy men and women. *Journal of Applied Physiology* 78 (3): 890–900.

García-Herrera, C. M., D. J. Celentano, M. A. Cruchaga, F. J. Rojo, J. M. Atienza, G. V. Guinea, and J. M. Goicolea. 2012. Mechanical characterisation of the human thoracic descending aorta: Experiments and modelling. *Computer Methods in Biomechanics and Biomedical Engineering* 15 (2): 185–193.

Gerstenblith, G., J. Frederiksen, F. C. P. Yin, N. J. Fortuin, E. G. Lakatta, and M. L. Weisfeldt. 1977. Echocardiographic assessment of a normal adult aging population. *Circulation* 56 (2): 273–278.

Greenwald, S. E. 2007. Ageing of the conduit arteries. *Journal of Pathology* 211 (2): 157–172.

Haskett, D., G. Johnson, A. Zhou, U. Utzinger, and J. Vande Geest. 2010. Microstructural and biomechanical alterations of the human aorta as a function of age and location. *Biomechanics and Modeling in Mechanobiology* 9 (6): 725–736.

Hees, P. S., J. L. Fleg, E. G. Lakatta, and E. P. Shapiro. 2002. Left ventricular remodeling with age in normal men versus women: Novel insights using three-dimensional magnetic resonance imaging. *American Journal of Cardiology* 90 (11): 1231–1236.

Horny, L., T. Adamek, and M. Kulvajtova. 2014a. Analysis of axial prestretch in the abdominal aorta with reference to post mortem interval and degree of atherosclerosis. *Journal of the Mechanical Behavior of Biomedical Materials* 33 (1): 93–98.

Horný, L., T. Adámek, and M. Kulvajtová. 2017. A comparison of age-related changes in axial prestretch in human carotid arteries and in human abdominal aorta. *Biomechanics and Modeling in Mechanobiology* 16 (1): 375–383.

Horny, L., T. Adamek, J. Vesely, H. Chlup, R. Zitny, and S. Konvickova. 2012. Age-related distribution of longitudinal pre-strain in abdominal aorta with emphasis on forensic application. *Forensic Science International* 214 (1–3): 18–22.

Horny, L., T. Adamek, and R. Zitny. 2013. Age-related changes in longitudinal prestress in human abdominal aorta. *Archive of Applied Mechanics* 83 (6): 875–888.

Horný, L. and M. Netušil. 2016. How does axial prestretching change the mechanical response of nonlinearly elastic incompressible thin-walled tubes. *International Journal of Mechanical Sciences* 106: 95–106.

Horný, L., M. Netušil, and T. Voňavková. 2014b. Axial prestretch and circumferential distensibility in biomechanics of abdominal aorta. *Biomechanics and Modeling in Mechanobiology* 13 (4): 783–799.

Kamenskiy, A., A. Seas, G. Bowen, P. Deegan, A. Desyatova, N. Bohlim, W. Poulson, and J. Mactaggart. 2016. In situ longitudinal pre-stretch in the human femoropopliteal Artery. *Acta Biomaterialia* 32: 231–237.

Kamenskiy, A., A. Seas, P. Deegan, W. Poulson, E. Anttila, S. Sim, A. Desyatova, and J. MacTaggart. 2017. Constitutive description of human femoropopliteal artery aging. *Biomechanics and Modeling in Mechanobiology* 16 (2): 681–692.

Khouri, M. G., M. S. Maurer, and L. El-Khoury Rumbarger. 2005. Assessment of age-related changes in left ventricular structure and function by freehand three-dimensional echocardiography. *The American Journal of Geriatric Cardiology* 14 (3): 118–125.

Kohn, J. C., M. C. Lampi, and C. A. Reinhart-King. 2015. Age-related vascular stiffening: Causes and consequences. *Frontiers in Genetics* 6. doi:10.3389/fgene.2015.00112.

Kumar, V., A. K. Abbas, N. Fausto, and J. C. Aster. 2010. *Robbins and Cotran Pathologic Basis of Disease*, 8th ed. Elsevier Saunders, Philadelphia, PA.

Labrosse, M. R., C. J. Beller, T. Mesana, and J. P. Veinot. 2009. Mechanical behavior of human aortas: Experiments, material constants and 3-D finite element modeling including residual stress. *Journal of Biomechanics* 42 (8): 996–1004.

Labrosse, M. R., E. R. Gerson, J. P. Veinot, and C. J. Beller. 2013. Mechanical characterization of human aortas from pressurization testing and a paradigm shift for circumferential residual stress. *Journal of the Mechanical Behavior of Biomedical Materials* 17: 44–55.

Lakatta, E. G. and D. Levy. 2003a. Arterial and cardiac aging: Major shareholders in cardiovascular disease enterprises: Part I: Aging arteries: A "set up" for vascular disease. *Circulation* 107 (1): 139–146.

Lakatta, E. G. and D. Levy. 2003b. Arterial and cardiac aging: Major shareholders in cardiovascular disease enterprises: Part II: The aging heart in health: Links to heart Disease. *Circulation* 107 (2): 346–354.

Leopold, J. A. 2012. Cellular mechanisms of aortic valve calcification. *Circulation: Cardiovascular Interventions* 5 (4): 605–614.

Levy, D., K. M. Anderson, D. D. Savage, W. B. Kannel, J. C. Christiansen, and W. P. Castelli. 1988. Echocardiographically detected left ventricular hypertrophy: Prevalence and risk factors. The Framingham heart study. *Annals of Internal Medicine* 108 (1): 7–13.

Martin, C., T. Pham, and W. Sun. 2011. Significant differences in the material properties between aged human and porcine aortic tissues. *European Journal of Cardio-Thoracic Surgery* 40 (1): 28–34.

McEniery, C. M., I. B. Wilkinson, and A. P. Avolio. 2007. Age, hypertension and arterial Function. *Clinical and Experimental Pharmacology and Physiology* 34 (7): 665–671.

Mozaffarian, D., E. J. Benjamin, A. S. Go, D. K. Arnett, M. J. Blaha, M. Cushman, S. R. Das et al. 2016. Heart disease and stroke statistics-2016 update a report from the American Heart Association. *Circulation* 133 (4): e1–e324.

Olivetti, G., M. Melissari, J. M. Capasso, and P. Anversa. 1991. Cardiomyopathy of the aging human heart. Myocyte loss and reactive cellular hypertrophy. *Circulation Research* 68 (6): 1560–1568.

Oomen, P. J. A., S. Loerakker, D. Van Geemen, J. Neggers, M.-J. T. H. Goumans, A. J. Van Den Bogaerdt, A. J. J. C. Bogers, C. V. C. Bouten, and F. P. T. Baaijens. 2016. Age-dependent changes of stress and strain in the human heart valve and their relation with collagen remodeling. *Acta Biomaterialia* 29: 161–169.

O'Rourke, M. F. and J. Hashimoto. 2007. Mechanical factors in arterial aging. A clinical perspective. *Journal of the American College of Cardiology* 50 (1): 1–13.

Persy, V. and P. D'Haese. 2009. Vascular calcification and bone disease: The calcification paradox. *Trends in Molecular Medicine* 15 (9): 405–416.

Pham, T., F. Sulejmani, E. Shin, D. Wang, and W. Sun. 2017. Quantification and comparison of the mechanical properties of four human cardiac valves. *Acta Biomaterialia* 54: 345–355.

Roccabianca, S., C. A. Figueroa, G. Tellides, and J. D. Humphrey. 2014. Quantification of regional differences in aortic stiffness in the aging human. *Journal of the Mechanical Behavior of Biomedical Materials* 29: 618–634.

Rose, M. R. 1991. *Evolutionary Biology of Aging.* Oxford University Press, New York.

Sacks, M. S., W. David Merryman, and D. E. Schmidt. 2009. On the biomechanics of heart valve function. *Journal of Biomechanics* 42 (12): 1804–1824.

Schlatmann, T. J. M. and A. E. Becker. 1977. Histologic changes in the normal aging aorta: Implications for dissecting aortic aneurysm. *The American Journal of Cardiology* 39 (1): 13–20.

Schulman, S. P., E. G. Lakatta, J. L. Fleg, L. Lakatta, L. C. Becker, and G. Gerstenblith. 1992. Age-related decline in left ventricular filling at rest and exercise. *American Journal of Physiology - Heart and Circulatory Physiology* 263 (6 32-6): H1932–H1938.

Schulze-Bauer, C. A. J., C. Mörth, and G. A. Holzapfel. 2003. Passive biaxial mechanical response of aged human iliac arteries. *Journal of Biomechanical Engineering* 125 (3): 395–406.

Sherratt, M. J. 2009. Tissue elasticity and the ageing elastic fibre. *Age* 31 (4): 305–325.

Sommer, G., A. J. Schriefl, M. Andrä, M. Sacherer, C. Viertler, H. Wolinski, and G. A. Holzapfel. 2015. Biomechanical properties and microstructure of human ventricular myocardium. *Acta Biomaterialia* 24: 172–192.

Spina, M., S. Garbisa, J. Hinnie, J. C. Hunter, and A. Serafini-Fracassini. 1983. Age-related changes in composition and mechanical properties of the tunica media of the upper thoracic human aorta. *Arteriosclerosis* 3 (1): 64–76.

Stewart, A. D., S. C. Millasseau, M. T. Kearney, J. M. Ritter, and P. J. Chowienczyk. 2003. Effects of inhibition of basal nitric oxide synthesis on carotid-femoral pulse wave velocity and augmentation index in humans. *Hypertension* 42 (5): 915–918.

Strait, J. B. and E. G. Lakatta. 2012. Aging-associated cardiovascular changes and their relationship to heart failure. *Heart Failure Clinics* 8 (1): 143–164.

Valenta, J., K. Vitek, R. Cihak, S. Konvickova, M. Sochor, and L. Horny. 2002. Age related constitutive laws and stress distribution in human main coronary arteries with reference to residual strain. *Bio-Medical Materials and Engineering* 12 (2): 121–134.

Vande Geest, J. P., M. S. Sacks, and D. A. Vorp. 2004. Age dependency of the biaxial biomechanical behavior of human abdominal aorta. *Journal of Biomechanical Engineering* 126 (6): 815–822.

Vorp, D. A., B. J. Schiro, M. P. Ehrlich, T. S. Juvonen, M. A. Ergin, and B. P. Griffith. 2003. Effect of aneurysm on the tensile strength and biomechanical behavior of the ascending thoracic aorta. *Annals of Thoracic Surgery* 75 (4): 1210–1214.

Wagenseil, J. E. and R. P. Mecham. 2009. Vascular extracellular matrix and arterial mechanics. *Physiological Reviews* 89 (3): 957–989.

Wang, M., G. Takagi, K. Asai, R. G. Resuello, F. F. Natividad, D. E. Vatner, S. F. Vatner, and E. G. Lakatta. 2003. Aging increases aortic MMP-2 activity and Angiotensin II in non-human primates. *Hypertension* 41 (6): 1308–1316.

Wilkins, K., N. R. Campbell, M. R. Joffres, F. A. McAlister, M. Nichol, S. Quach, H. L. Johansen, and M. S. Tremblay. 2010. Blood pressure in Canadian adults. *Health Reports/ Statistics Canada, Canadian Centre for Health Information = Rapports Sur La Santé/ Statistique Canada, Centre Canadien d'Information Sur La Santé* 21 (1): 37–46.

Yasmin, S. Wallace, C. M. McEniery, Z. Dakham, P. Pusalkar, K. Maki-Petaja, M. J. Ashby, J. R. Cockcroft, and I. B. Wilkinson. 2005. Matrix metalloproteinase-9 (MMP-9), MMP-2, and serum elastase activity are associated with systolic hypertension and arterial stiffness. *Arteriosclerosis, Thrombosis, and Vascular Biology* 25 (2): 372–378.

12

Mechanical Effects of Cardiovascular Drugs and Devices

K. May-Newman

Contents

12.1 Introduction

There are a number of medical conditions that alter the mechanics of the cardiovascular system and are ameliorated by drugs or devices, which restore some aspect of native structure or function. Both blood and tissue are each sensitive to altered biomechanics in different, sometimes counteracting, ways that complicate device design, integration, and long-term performance. In this chapter, an overview of the native mechanobiology of the cardiovascular system is presented in the context of medical devices and drugs, followed by detailed reviews of specific devices that include both engineering and regulatory requirements. Cardiovascular drugs and devices operate via intentional alterations in the biomechanics that result in unintentional clinical consequences. Two main considerations of mechanobiology are pertinent for the cardiovascular system: the response of the soft tissue and the response of the blood.

12.2 Response of Cardiovascular Soft Tissue to Altered Mechanics

We begin by a review of the soft tissue, which inherently applies the theories of solid mechanics. Two basic principles govern soft tissue mechanobiology: (1) the tissue is sensitive to changes in stress and strain, and (2) surgery and device placement produce an injury response, either short term or long term, which directly relates to the long-term success. Cardiovascular tissues are distensible viscoelastic composites of muscle and extracellular matrix (ECM), with a thin endothelial lining. Blood vessels are tubular structures with a laminar microstructure consisting of smooth muscle and ECM layers. Cardiac tissue is primarily muscle, with a small amount of ECM that organizes the muscle fiber structure within and throughout the heart wall. Both these tissues have endothelial linings, which are highly sensitive to mechanical and chemical cues.

The heart is the source of energy in the cardiovascular system, acting as a two-sided volume displacement pump to power systemic blood flow. Pressures inside the pumping chamber, the left ventricle, range from 0 to 120 mmHg during each cardiac cycle. The aorta, the blood vessel immediately distal to the heart, is the major outflow vessel that acts as an elastic reservoir to buffer the pressure pulse delivered by the heart, reducing the pressure range to 60–120 mmHg. The systemic circulation acts as a variable resistor, damping the pulsatility in the distal circulation, such that flow in capillaries is nonpulsatile. Smooth muscle in the blood vessel walls contracts and dilates to alter the distribution of blood flow to different tissues and organs based on oxygen demand.

A simple mechanical formula is used to relate a clinically important and measurable quantity, blood pressure, to the underlying wall stress, which governs vessel mechanobiology. The law of Laplace, shown in Equation 12.1, is derived from a force balance of pressure acting over the inner surface (lumen) of the vessel and the stress integrated across the wall thickness (Figure 12.1).

$$\sigma = (P \times R)/h \qquad (12.1)$$

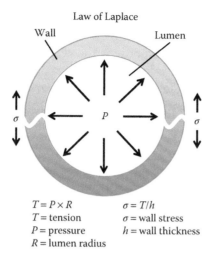

Figure 12.1 The Law of Laplace relates the blood pressure to the stress in the wall of an inflated vessel through a force balance.

Conditions, drugs, and devices that alter pressure or the natural response to pressure can be related through this relation. Hypertension, or high blood pressure, is a clinical problem that affects 16%–37% globally and is the biggest single contributor to the global burden of cardiovascular disease. Risk factors for hypertension are primarily environmental and include high-salt diet and smoking. The condition often goes undetected, as it is initially asymptomatic, but it places individuals at a high risk for extreme cardiac events such as heart attack and atherosclerosis. Treatments are aimed at reducing blood pressure and consist of calcium channel blockers, angiotensin-converting enzyme (ACE) inhibitors, and angiotensin receptor blockers. From the law of Laplace, we observe that increased pressure results in an increase in vessel wall stress, which triggers a remodeling response within the tissue. The response may alter the material properties, such as in fibrous tissue formation and aneurysmal weakening, or geometry, such as in intimal hyperplasia. Without addressing the driving stimulus, the hypertension, the chronically altered boundary conditions provide positive feedback and, ultimately, result in the need for medical intervention. Often, the function of a component, such as blood vessel and heart valve, is significantly affected, necessitating replacement.

The introduction of a blood-contacting medical device is a major insult to the body. Catheter-based devices require a percutaneous incision and have the potential to inflict damage to the blood vessel at any point along their tortuous path. Endothelium is damaged by any devices that come in contact with the vessel wall, and stress may be produced in deeper layers. In addition, all the materials are in contact with the bloodstream and must minimize thrombogenicity during use. Surgery to place an implant causes an injury to the affected tissue, and thus, a wound healing response is to be expected and managed, including systemic immune responses and local tissue remodeling. In general, a synthetic material placed in contact with body tissue will induce a foreign body response. A mild response will mimic normal wound healing, with restitution of tissue geometry and material properties. A severe response is associated with chronic inflammation, poor healing, and, ultimately, failure of the implant.

The classic soft tissue injury response is the acute inflammation phase, which is relatively brief (minutes to a few days). Capillary constriction produces hemostasis, which is followed by fluid leakage and neutrophil migration into the tissue. The neutrophils remove the injury debris by phagocytosis of microorganisms and small foreign particles. The classic symptoms of redness, swelling, heat, and pain accompany this phase of normal wound healing. This initial response usually resolves during the formation of granulation tissue, which replaces the injured native tissue with a provisional matrix consisting of a fibrin scaffold. Fibroblasts migrate to the injured site and use the scaffold as a framework for collagen deposition. Angiogenesis aids the progression of this process, during which the fibrin scaffold is degraded and the remaining collagen is organized and crosslinked to form a fibrous capsule. The capsule surrounds and isolates the implant from the immune system and, if no inflammation persists at the site, provides a stable tissue–biomaterial interaction. However, if chronic inflammation is present, tissue macrophages frustrated by the inability to phagocytose the foreign material, coalesce into large, multinucleated foreign body giant cells, which may persist at the tissue–implant interface for the implant's lifetime. The resultant response to tissue injury depends on both the regenerative capacity of the cells and the degree of preservation of the stroma framework (i.e., it is the part of a tissue that has connective and structural roles but does not carry out the specific functions of an organ) at the injury site. Tissue cells can be labile (continually proliferating), stable (can but do not normally replicate), and permanent (cannot reproduce after differentiation). Preservation of stroma framework leads to better restitution of tissue structure, whereas its destruction leads to fibrosis. These factors are also affected by local blood supply, and systemic conditions such as nutrition and disease. In general, an implant is a hindrance to healing and tissue regeneration and should be designed to best mitigate the body's natural healing responses.

One common example of a mechanically induced pathology is intimal hyperplasia, which occurs in the native circulation but also occurs much more rapidly following endovascular treatments such as percutaneous balloon angioplasty and stent placement. Intimal hyperplasia is usually initiated by an endothelial disruption, which occurs naturally during atherosclerotic plaque rupture or during a treatment of the blood vessel. During balloon angioplasty, the vessel wall is stretched, which results in an increase in smooth muscle cell proliferation. These cells migrate from the media to the intima, where they thicken the intimal layer and reduce the luminal opening of the blood vessel, restricting blood flow to downstream tissues.

12.3 Response of Blood to Altered Mechanics

The response of blood to altered mechanics are triggered by flow abnormalities and foreign surfaces that activate the coagulation system. As discussed in more detail in Chapter 8, blood is sensitive to changes in flow. The coagulation or clotting system of blood system is designed for localized hemostasis or for stoppage of blood flow following injury. This response is designed to protect the host from injury and consists of a cascade of chemical reactions in which the signal is amplified at each step. There are two entries into this system, the intrinsic and extrinsic systems, both of which collapse to a common pathway, with the conversion of prothrombin to thrombin. The concept of the coagulation cascade has evolved to reflect the multiple roles that thrombin plays in both coagulation and platelet activation. Thrombin is the most potent physiological activator of platelets and also activates leukocytes and endothelial cells, which can aggregate and occlude vessels downstream.

Platelet activation is initiated by mechanical disruption of the vessel wall that exposes tissue factor, which leads to the production of small amounts of thrombin. Platelets also respond, by adhering at the injury site. This initial signal is amplified, as thrombin activates and recruits more platelets and coagulation factors, setting the stage for large-scale thrombin production, which occurs on the surface of activated platelets. More thrombin converts fibrinogen monomers to fibrin, leading to a clot formation. Thrombin bound to fibrin remains active, and thus, the clot becomes a reservoir of active thrombin, which continues to activate platelets and promote its own generation. The burst of thrombin further fuels thrombosis, by activating cells and proteins involved in inflammatory and thrombotic responses. A thrombus attached to a surface can obstruct passage of blood flow or interfere with device function. If the clot detaches and becomes an embolus and floats downstream, it can become lodged in a small artery, obstructing blood flow to tissues. If the blocked artery is in the brain, the tissue dies and a loss of neurological function, either motor or cognitive, may occur. This type of stroke is ischemic, but hemorrhage strokes may also occur due to vessels that burst and bleed.

Three factors that affect coagulation are blood chemistry, activating surfaces, and extreme flow patterns, including stasis and high shear, classically articulated by Virchow's triad. Flow affects the local concentrations of coagulation cascade factors, which impact the activation, aggregation, and deposition of platelets that initiate a thrombus. Flow determines where a thrombus will form, its size, and composition, as well as whether or not it will remain attached or embolize. Under low-flow conditions, early platelet adhesion depends on diffusion of platelets to the surface (diffusion controlled), but under higher-flow conditions, adhesion also depends on surface properties (reaction controlled). Flow fields impart mechanical shear (see Chapter 3), which is the main mechanical signal for platelet activation; thus, the importance of flow patterns in thrombosis is well recognized but not well understood.

Often, in medical devices, anticoagulants, antithrombic, or antiplatelet agents are given to patients to reduce risk. Heparin and warfarin are the most common anticoagulants. Heparin hinders the formation of fibrin, and warfarin is a vitamin K antagonist. Antiplatelet agents include aspirin, which decreases platelet aggregation and release, dipyridamole, which decreases platelet adhesion, and agents that interfere with calcium such as ethylenediaminetetraacetic acid (EDTA) and citrate. Blood flow affects thrombogenicity, because it controls the rate of transport to artificial surfaces. Studies have shown that early platelet attachment to surfaces increases with increasing wall shear rate.

Undesirable blood–material interactions include chronic platelet activation, formation of thrombus, shedding or nucleation of emboli, destruction or damage of circulating blood components, and activation of the complement system or other immunological pathways. Thus, the design of a blood contacting medical device must consider the thrombogenic propensity of the device. This includes designs that allow regional accumulation of blood elements, such as thrombin, as well as areas of disturbed flow that lead to the formation of clots. Both local and systemic effects work together in order to determine the overall device thrombogenicity. An elegant example of a quantitative approach to device design for minimizing thrombogenicity is detailed in a series of papers; the reader is referred to the original publications for detail.[1-4]

The performance of medical devices is intertwined with the system of governmental regulation, which, in the United States, is overseen by the Food and Drug Administration (FDA). Federal law gives the FDA authority to grant permission for a device company to commercialize its device. The FDA is overseen by a commissioner and has five offices, one of which is the Office of Medical Devices and Tobacco. Within this office, there are four centers, one of which is the Center for Devices and Radiological Health, which oversees the regulation of medical devices.[5] Title 21 of the Code of Federal Regulations (CFR) spells out the definitions and requirements for submission and approval. Part 870 specifies the categorization and review of cardiovascular devices and is divided into six subparts, A–F (see Table 12.1). Part 870 device submissions are reviewed by the Circulatory System Devices Medical Device Advisory Committee (MDAC), 1 of 18 MDACs in the FDA review process.

Part 870 of CFR provides a detailed device classification system for the medical devices that specifies the level of regulatory control necessary for reasonable assurance of the safety and efficacy of each device, based on the level of risk. As device class increases from Class I to Class II and Class III, the level of regulatory controls also increases, with Class I subject to the least regulatory control and Class III subject to the most regulatory control. Class I devices are considered low to moderate risk and require general controls, as specified in Part 870 of CFR. General controls are regulatory requirements that apply to all medical devices, unless specifically exempted. Class II includes moderate- to high-risk devices, for which general controls alone are insufficient to provide reasonable assurance of safety and efficacy. Class II is further divided into subclasses related to the level of special control; these classes are specified based on input from industry and clinicians. Special controls are established for each product classification and may include performance controls, FDA guidance, consensus standards, patient registries, postmarket surveillance, and other requirements.

Many different options are available for categorizing medical devices, some of which have been listed earlier: Class I, II, or III; short- versus long-term exposure to body tissues; devices that treat the same condition; vascular versus cardiac devices; passive versus active (powered) devices; and delivery method (Table 12.1).

TABLE 12.1   The Food and Drug Administration Reference Information for Selected Cardiovascular Devices

Regulation Number	Product Code	Device Name	Device Class	Delivery Method	Anatomical Site	Passive/Active
870.5150	DXE	Embolectomy catheter	II (P)	Catheter	Peripheral vessel	Passive
870.3375	DTK	Cardiovascular intravascular filter	II (S)	Catheter	Inferior vena cava	Passive
870.3450	DSY	Vascular graft >6 mm	II (S)	Surgery	Vessel	Passive
	DYF	Vascular graft <6 mm	II (S)			
870.5100	LOX	PCI	II (S)	Catheter	Vessel	Passive
870.4075	DWZ	Endomyocardial bioptome	II (P)	Catheter	Heart	Passive
870.3535	DSP	Intra-aortic balloon pump	II (S)/III		Aorta	Active
870.4210	DWF	CPB—circuit	II (P)	Surgery	Heart	Active
870.4350	DTZ	Oxygenator	II (S)			
870.4260	DTM	Arterial filter	II (S)			
870.4100	BYS	ECMO—circuit	II (S)	Surgery	Heart or vessel	Active
		Oxygenator	II (S)			
	MAF	Stent	III	Catheter		Passive
	NIQ	Coronary				
	PNY	Drug-eluting Absorbable DE				
	MLV	Septal occluder	III	Catheter	Heart	Passive
	OZG	Atrial				
	OZH	Ventricular				
870.3800	KRH	Annuloplasty ring	II (S)	Surgery	Heart	Passive
	NKM	Mitral valve repair devices	III	Catheter	Heart	Passive
870.3925	DYE	Replacement heart valve	III	Surgery Catheter	Heart	Passive
870.3545	OKR	Ventricular assist device	III	Surgery	Heart and aorta	Active
870.3680	PMA	Cardiovascular permanent pacemaker electrode	III	Catheter	Heart	Active

The following review of cardiovascular devices generally follows the FDA device classification scheme, with some clustering of devices that impart similar mechanical interactions with the native tissue structures. Devices used for short-term treatments or procedures are presented first, followed by implants with longer-term exposure to the host physiology. Short-term vascular procedures conducted with devices can be divided into two types of exposure: (1) devices that pass through the bloodstream, and (2) bloodstream passes through the device. Devices in the first category include catheter-based therapies delivered via intravascular catheter, such as those used to treat vessel narrowing or blockage.

12.4 Device-Based Vascular Disease Treatment

One of the most prevalent diseases of the cardiovascular system is atherosclerosis, which has been reviewed in Chapter 7. Atherosclerosis is the buildup of cholesterol plaque in the walls of the arteries. The initial lesion usually occurs decades before clinically significant effects are observed; thus, treatment of lesions has evolved as the primary remedy for vessel narrowing due to atherosclerosis. The lesion is marked by intracellular lipid accumulation, forming a fatty streak in the vessel wall. Further lipid accumulation expands to an extracellular lipid pool, which provides a site for calcification. This is followed by increased proliferation of smooth muscle and collagen deposition. When the lesion is severe, it erupts through the vessel wall, attracting platelets and forming a thrombus at the site. Atherosclerosis occurs all over the body but is most problematic in the peripheral, coronary, and cerebral arteries, which feed important capillary beds.

If a peripheral vessel in the arms or legs is affected, the risk of a surface thrombus releasing from the surface is high. Embolization of a blood clot leads to a vessel blockage and reduces blood flow downstream, which deprives the tissue of oxygen and leads to necrosis and limb amputation. Embolectomy balloon catheters are part of the market for clot management devices (CMDs), which was valued at US $1.26 billion in 2015 and is projected to grow at an annual rate of 4.6% through 2024.[6] Clot management devices include percutaneous thrombectomy devices, used to aspirate blood clots, and catheter-directed thrombolysis devices, which dispense clot-dissolving medication at the thrombus site. Both the increase in atherosclerosis and venous thromboembolism rates and the demonstrated effectiveness of catheter-based therapies contribute to the anticipated growth of the CMD market.

12.4.1 Embolectomy Catheter

For large blood clots lodged in peripheral arteries, such as those of the arms and legs, the device developed to remove the clot is the embolectomy balloon catheter.[5] An embolectomy catheter is a balloon-tipped catheter used to remove blood clots, which have detached from the site of origin and migrated to another site in the vascular tree, where they become lodged in an artery. The catheter is inserted into a major artery and guided to the treatment site by using fluoroscopy and/or ultrasound imaging. The catheter tip is pushed through the clot, the balloon is inflated, and the device retracted, pulling the clot out through the insertion site. This procedure replaced a painful and risk surgery, decreasing the time of surgery to 1 hour and greatly reducing limb loss and the amount of pain during recovery. The most common mechanical injuries produced during an embolectomy procedure are relatively minor, consisting of the percutaneous insertion site and the disruption of the vessel endothelium where the balloon is applied. The embolectomy catheter is regulated as a Class II device under Subpart F: Cardiovascular Therapeutic Devices and must demonstrate conformance to performance controls, including dimensional verification, tensile strength of connections, balloon inflation/deflation time, fatigue and leakage tests, kink resistance, and torque strength of the device, as well as biocompatibility standards, to receive regulatory approval. The catheter must also demonstrate effective adherent clot removal, usually evaluated in animal studies. Previous studies have shown that while embolectomy produces partial injury to the endothelium (noted as partial denudation of the surface) in intact vessels, no apparent change in smooth muscle function results.[7]

12.4.2 Percutaneous Coronary Intervention

Percutaneous coronary intervention (PCI) is a well-established treatment for atherosclerosis and has expanded from balloon angioplasty to stent, vascular graft, and heart valve delivery. The short-term mechanical interactions consist mainly of the catheter advancing through the vascular system and the balloon inflating inside of the vessel lumen. Percutaneous coronary intervention utilizes a balloon-tipped catheter, similar to the embolectomy procedure, but the treatment involves higher risk, and thus, PCI devices are considered Class II, which require special controls for regulatory approval.[8] Percutaneous coronary intervention replaces the previous term percutaneous transluminal coronary angioplasty (PTCA).

A PTCA catheter is intended for balloon dilatation of a hemodynamically significant coronary artery or bypass graft stenosis in patients evidencing coronary ischemia, for the purpose of improving myocardial perfusion. A PCI catheter may also be intended for the treatment of acute myocardial infarction, as well as for the treatment of in-stent restenosis or postdeployment stent expansion. Percutaneous coronary intervention procedures use a system of components that work together and include a guidewire, a guide catheter, and a balloon catheter. The guide catheter is inserted through the femoral artery into the aorta, through which it is advanced around the aortic arch and positioned at the entrance of one of the main coronary arteries. Radiopaque contrast and fluoroscopy are used to identify the lesion sites and to position a thin guidewire that is advanced through the guide catheter and into the coronary branch to the lesion. The guidewire marks the lesion site for delivery of other devices, including balloon dilatation catheters (BDCs) and stents.

A PCI catheter operates on the principle of hydraulic pressure applied via an inflatable balloon attached to the distal end. A PCI balloon catheter has a single or double lumen shaft, depending on the chassis design. The catheter features a balloon of appropriate compliance for the clinical application, constructed from a polymer. The balloon is designed to uniformly expand to a specified diameter and length at a specific pressure, as labeled, with well characterized rates of inflation and deflation and a defined burst pressure. The device generally features a type of radiographic marker to facilitate fluoroscopic visualization of the balloon during use.

12.4.2.1 Clinical Complications
Early successes with PCI were rapidly challenged by the biological response to vessel injury, which resulted in rapid restenosis of the vessel. Approximately 57% of patients have a reoccurrence of stenosis within 6 months of PTCA. Some of the stenosis is due

to elastic recoil of artery, which occurs shortly after treatment. In the longer term, intimal hyperplasia and scar formation at the injured site reduce the lumen back to pre-PCI levels. This complication greatly diminished the success of PCI and spurred innovations to address restenosis, including stents, which are discussed later in this chapter. While the deployment of PCI is anticipated to produce some vessel injury, design focuses on minimizing this injury and the subsequent response, primarily by improving the accurate targeting of lesion treatment.

12.4.2.1.1 Percutaneous Coronary Intervention Catheter Design.   Generally, the design of dilatation catheters is divided into two construction types, over-the-wire (OTW) and rapid exchange (RX), and two balloon types, predilatation and postdilatation.

12.4.2.2 Chassis Construction
The worldwide dilatation market is approximately \$800 million, with little growth over the last years.[9] Europe and the United States make up more than 70% of this market. The OTW type is the original PCI chassis design, for which the entire catheter tracks over a 300-cm long coaxial guide wire. The OTW catheter shaft consists of two concentric tubes, an inner member for the guidewire, and an outer membrane that bounds the balloon inflation lumen, all connected at the proximal Luer hub and the distal tip. The force to insert the catheter is immediately distributed to the outer and inner members and then carried along the length of the shaft to the balloon. The OTW PCI requires two operators, one to operate the proximal catheter and one to manage the distal guidewire. The OTW system offers easy guidewire exchange, without compromising catheter position in the vessel. This is beneficial when treating chronically stenosed lesions; however, equipment changes can be time-consuming. For these reasons, the OTW systems are used in approximately 25% of cases; however, approximately 75% of laboratories stock the OTW catheters.

The RX chassis design was developed to reduce the PCI procedure to a single operator and a shorter 190-cm guidewire. Only the distal 25–30 cm of the RX catheter tracks over the guidewire, reducing the dual-lumen distance to the distal region. The RX catheters comprise 75% of systems used in the United States, and usage rates continue to increase because of reduced procedure time, x-ray exposure, and contrast usage. The RX catheter provides ease of base wire lesion access and rapid catheter exchange.

12.4.2.3 Catheter Shaft
Distal lesions in tortuous anatomy demand catheters with greater flexibility and deliverability than proximal lesions. Flexibility is driven by materials, tip design, and how the catheter is constructed. Profiles, including, tip, crossing, and balloon, influence the catheter's ability to cross the lesion. Smaller tip and crossing profiles lend to the catheter accessing tight calcific lesions easier than larger profiles. The RX shaft is composed of a stiffer hypotube that carries the applied force from the user to the RX notch and then joins a distal shaft consisting of an inner member, with an exit site for the guidewire and an outer membrane attached to the balloon. The outer member is coated beyond the guide wire notch to help maintain lubricity and durability during long cases. A well-designed

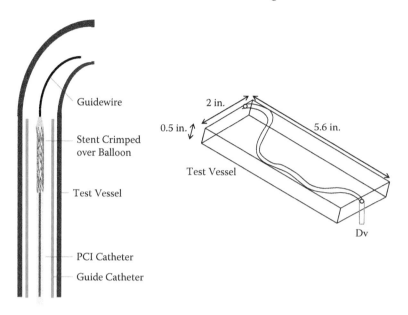

Figure 12.2 Tracking testing for stent delivery systems. The crimped stent on the uninflated balloon (left panel) is pulled through a tortuous vessel pattern (right pattern) of the appropriate diameter (Dv) to evaluate stent delivery. A small shim is used to test securement of the stent to the catheter shaft while the stent detatchment force is measured (see ASTM 2394 for more details).

balloon catheter should smoothly track over the guidewire, without interference from stent struts or calcified tissue (Figure 12.2). Track is driven by inner member and tip design. Push transmission is important for the device to reach distal lesions in tortuous anatomy, which requires maximizing stiffness at the proximal (user) end while maintaining a soft distal tip to avoid vessel damage. The RX shaft design typically consists of three sections, the proximal shaft, the midshaft, and the distal shaft. Generally speaking, each section has different design specifications, in order to optimize its role in the system. The proximal shaft requires stiffness for good pushability but does not require the large bending needed to track around the aortic arch. The distal shaft must be flexible to optimize access and deliverability and minimize tissue damage. The distal shaft is often a multilayer material extrusion, with an inner layer of low-friction, high-density polyethylene and an outer layer of nylon or Pebax®. The guidewire lumen must accommodate the 0.009-in-diameter guidewire, and the remainder of the cross-section must be utilized for the balloon inflation lumen. Low-profile shafts enable better distal access and are therefore considered more deliverable, but profiles that are too low may result in slow inflation/deflation times and experience mechanical interaction with the guidewire. In the midshaft, material stiffness should be transitioned from supportive proximal section to the flexible distal section. The midshaft connects the distal and proximal catheter shaft components and must accommodate a guidewire notch, which produces the largest diameter along the catheter length. The outer diameter is approximately (0.035–0.040 in). Both inner and outer membranes can be coated to provide lubricity for enhanced deliverability and to track through tortuous anatomy. Inner-membrane coatings minimize guidewire interactions in challenging cases. Dual-layer coatings are more durable than single-layer coating for lubricity in long cases but may contribute to "watermelon seeding," as will be defined in section 12.4.2.3.1.11.

12.4.2.3.1 Balloon Design

12.4.2.3.1.1 Balloon Material. Early-generation dilatation balloons were composed of linear low-density polyethylene (LLDPE), characterized as very flexible, large profile, and with a low pressure range. Polyethylene materials emerged later and produced less compliant balloons that can withstand higher pressures with minimal diameter change. Nylon and Pebax (polyamides) are commonly used in current clinical practice, especially for stent deployment PCI. The development of multilayer balloons resulted in more flexible, lower-profile balloons capable of dilating lesions at very high pressures. These characteristics are especially useful for dilating calcified/resistant lesions. Each company designs multilayer BDC differently and for different applications. Multilayer balloons can include one balloon inside another, as well as coextruded balloon material, where different polymers are combined in a molten state to create a single layer of material. The multiple layers serve several purposes: one is to offer lower profiles and enhanced performance, without compromising rupture strength, and another is to minimize the risk of pinholes and reduce material rupture.

12.4.2.3.1.2 Crossing a Lesion with an Uninflated Balloon. Percutaneous coronary intervention devices need to be able to cross the vascular lesion, regardless of how challenging it may be. Low profiles, flexible balloon and catheter materials, and good track and push, all help a dilatation catheter cross the lesion. Radiopaque markers aid in determining the length of the lesion when predilating and ensuring that the postdilatation balloon is positioned to minimize injury outside the treatment area.

12.4.2.3.1.3 Recrossing a Lesion with a Deflated Balloon. A PCI catheter's ability to recross a stent or lesion is important for minimizing the number of balloons used during a case, reducing overall procedural time, x-ray exposure, and use of contrast. A balloon's refold influences its ability to recross a lesion or access new lesions. Refold is influenced by balloon material, how the balloon is folded, the pressure to which the balloon is inflated, and how well the balloon refolds itself post expansion and deflation. Softer balloon materials are more flexible and tend to refold tighter than stiffer materials. Balloons inflated to higher pressures stretch more, causing the material properties to change, resulting in a flatter refold.

12.4.2.3.1.4 Balloon Inflation Targets. The nominal pressure is the pressure at which the balloon reaches its target diameter, which is one point on the compliance curve. Increasing or decreasing the pressure from this value will result in a change in diameter that is predicted by the compliance relation. This information allows a physician to vary the diameter slightly around the target value, in order to best match the native vessel diameter. The term "quarter size" refers to the pressure at which the diameter increases to ¼ mm above the target diameter. Another important point on the compliance curve is the rated burst pressure (RBP), which is the pressure at which 99.9%

of balloons will not rupture with 95% confidence, which is an industry-wide definition. Knowing this pressure gives the physician an idea of the safe range of inflation pressures for a particular balloon and is provided on the compliance chart included with each device.

12.4.2.3.1.5 Balloon Compliance.   Compliance is defined as the growth in balloon diameter per atmosphere of inflation pressure. The diameter corresponding to each 0.5-1 atmosphere of inflation pressure up to the RBP must be tabulated and reported as the compliance curve.

12.4.2.3.1.6 Clinical Applications: Predilatation and Postdilatation.   Balloon compliance describes the inflation behavior as the balloon diameter as a function of pressure. A compliant balloon continues to grow as pressure increases, while a noncompliant balloon grows very little with pressure increase. Most balloons are semicompliant, typically more compliant at lower pressures and more noncompliant at higher pressures. On the more compliant end of the spectrum are predilatation balloons, which expand as pressure increases. As with most medical treatments, reports in the scientific literature vary in their support of predilatation. Potential benefits that have been cited include evaluation of the lesion before stent implantation, based on assessment of balloon inflation within the lesion, and the ability to size the stent to be placed more effectively. Predilatation catheters need to be able to access tight lesions and track through tortuous anatomy. To achieve this, they have thinner, sleeker tips and smaller-diameter shafts, designed for good push transmission and support. Predilatation increases the success of device delivery by creating a "path" for easier stent deployment and maintaining the integrity of drug coating. Predilitation results in decreased complications and lumen loss related to inadequate stent expansion and apposition.

Toward the more noncompliant are high-pressure balloons, used primarily for postdilatation. This type of catheter has a broad working range and can also be used for predilatation. Postdilatation PCI catheters are designed to open up highly resistant lesions or postdilate a stent to ensure good stent expansion/apposition. To achieve this goal, they tend to have a more robust tip and slightly larger profiles. Accurate working length and alignment between balloon shoulder and markers are important to ensure that treatment is limited to the treatment area, to minimize injury to healthy tissue. The shaft is larger to offer rapid balloon deflation and restore flow. The balloon material tends to be stronger, stiffer, and more noncompliant, with a higher RBP to ensure complete stent expansion and apposition. The type of balloon material used impacts rewrap, flexibility, and deliverability, with stiffer materials being more difficult to advance and track through tortuous anatomy. The clinical benefits of postdilatation are directly related to achieving full stent expansion and include reduction in restenosis, avoidance of thrombosis, decreased target vessel revascularization (TVR), and uniform drug delivery. Clinical studies have shown that postdilatation significantly optimizes long-term outcomes.[10,11] However, each vessel's dilatation cycle increases mechanical loading and may result in stent overexpansion and additional vessel injury, especially at the outer edges of the stent.

12.4.2.3.1.7 Dimensional Accuracy/Longitudinal Shortening. The distal and proximal balloon tapers can be long or short, with short tapers designed for precise focal dilatation and long tapers designed for flexibility. Working balloon length is a balloon's stated size and the distance between the two markers. The center of markers should be aligned with the balloon shoulders to accurately indicate working length. Physicians desire balloons that stay true to their stated size, to reduce the risk of unnecessary injury to the vessel. Some balloons experience longitudinal growth, when the balloon grows longer than its stated size. This distance is undesirable in a noncompliant balloon, as physicians want to minimize injury to healthy tissue, outside of the stented area.

12.4.2.3.1.8 Dilating Force. Lastly, dilating force is the force or pressure exerted on the lesion and vessel wall by a balloon.

12.4.2.3.1.9 Inflation Time. Inflation time is the time required to achieve maximum stretch.

12.4.2.3.1.10 Dog Boning. Dog boning is stretching of a dilatation balloon along the path of least resistance, outside the lesion or stent margins.

12.4.2.3.1.11 Watermelon Seeding. Watermelon seeding is the retrograde movement of a dilatation balloon when inflated within a lesion, common in resistant lesions and in-stent restenosis.

12.4.2.3.1.12 Catheter Tip. Catheter tip diameter (0.43-0.51 mm) and length (3–5 mm) should be small for better access and cross, but the material and shape are also important. The material should be soft and flexible as well as durable, so that it does not stretch around curves; it is known as a "fishmouth." Tips can be straight or tapered. Straight tips are more uniform in diameter along the length of the tip, whereas tapered tips gradually increase in diameter as you move proximally and are designed to hug the guidewire. A blunt tip does not track as well as a tapered tip, which impacts the delivery to challenging anatomy or calcified lesions. Tip length is a critical factor in determining catheter flexibility, as it impacts how close the tip, inner member, and balloon seal are located. The greater the distance between these three points, the more flexible the balloon tip and the more deliverable the catheter. Tip seals can be gradual, meaning the bond between the tip and the inner member and between the balloon and the tip are spread out, enabling increased flexibility and deliverability compared with abrupt seal, where all three bonds occur in one location, resulting in a single point of high stiffness that translates to reduced catheter flexibility and deliverability. Tip designs vary between pre- and postdilatation catheters, as predilatation tips are designed to be low profile and to access or cross tight lesions. Tip material used on predilatation BDCs tends to be soft and flexible, allowing it to hug the guidewire around tight curves and through tortuous anatomy. The material needs to be strong and durable to ensure that no damage occurs when crossing calcium or previously deployed stent struts. Tip design in postdilatation catheters is also important, as stent struts may be malapposed to the vessel wall, necessitating the tip to deflect off stent struts to gain access to the lesion.

12.4.2.3.1.13 Balloon Taper.   Balloon tapers are another important design element of BDCs. Balloon tapers can be short, for focal dilatation and minimal vessel injury within the treatment area, especially when treating a lesion on a bend. Long tapers are typically considered more deliverable.

12.4.2.3.1.14 Regulatory Guidance.   Nonbinding recommendations from the FDA for dilatation catheters are detailed in Class II Special Controls Guidance Document for Certain PTCA.[8] Biocompatibility testing is suggested following ASTM F748.[12] Bench testing comprises dimensional measurements, including catheter diameter and deflated balloon profile, which determine compatibility with guidewires and guide catheters. Accuracy and radiopacity of the balloon markers are also recommended. Balloon rupture can result in device failure or vessel damage. The balloon compliance curve should be measured over the range of inflation pressure and provided on each package. The nominal pressure, at which the balloon reaches the target diameter, and the RBP must also be noted on the compliance curve. Inflation of the balloon temporarily obstructs blood flow, and excessively slow deflation can lead to prolonged ischemia and tissue damage. Thus, measurement of balloon inflation and deflation times is recommended. Balloon fatigue should also be measured, as balloons are often inflated multiple times during a procedure. Failure of the balloon to withstand at least 20 inflations can lead to vessel damage and device failure. Pull strength of the catheter shaft the tip should be measured, as well as testing at a bend radius that is appropriate for the intended anatomy to demonstrate that the catheter will not kink under compressive or torsional forces. Any coatings should be tested for delamination or degradation, which may form embolized particulates that cause clinical complications.

12.4.3 Endomyocardial Bioptome

Another catheter-based device is the bioptome for performing an endocardial biopsy. These devices consist of small stainless-steel cutting jaws on the end of a catheter controlled with an actuator at the handle; these devices are inserted through the jugular or femoral veins to remove samples of tissue from the inner wall of the right heart, primarily for surveillance of heart transplant rejection. These devices are regulated as Class II, requiring performance of sampling ability and safety for intravascular use. The devices are associated with a low serious complication rate (<1%), but risks of injury to the sample site include hematoma, disruption of the conduction system, and perforations. Site selection and sampling should be performed under fluoroscopic guidance.

12.5 Short-Term Device Systems to Support
Blood Circulation and/or Oxygenation

The devices described previously are considered passive devices, meaning that they do not require power to perform their intended function. For device systems in which the blood is routed through the device, power is required, and thus, these devices are considered active.

12.5.1 Intra-aortic Balloon Pump

Intra-aortic counterpulsation provides a minimally invasive method of support for failing left ventricular (LV) function by reducing afterload and improving myocardial oxygen supply–demand balance. However, the efficacy of counterpulsation depends on several factors, including intrinsic ventricular function. Counterpulsation therapy is produced by an intra-aortic balloon (IAB) and control system. The IABP consists of an inflatable balloon, which is placed in the aorta to improve cardiovascular functioning during certain life-threatening emergencies, and a control system for regulating the inflation and deflation of the balloon. The control system, which monitors and is synchronized with the electrocardiogram, provides a means for setting the inflation and deflation of the balloon with the cardiac cycle. The IABP provides counterpulsation therapy to adult patients with impaired LV function. The IAB is inserted via catheter into the femoral artery and positioned in the descending thoracic aorta 1–2 cm distal to the left subclavian artery. It provides hemodynamic support of blood pressure and reduced cardiac work through volume displacement principles.

The IABP delivers helium into the IAB during diastole to displace blood above and below the IAB, increasing blood pressure and perfusion to organs. In systole, the balloon rapidly deflates, reducing aortic pressure and LV afterload during ejection and improving forward flow from the heart. The net effect is to decrease systolic aortic pressure by as much as 20% and increase diastolic pressure by 20–30 mmHg. The IABPs are often controlled to assist every other (2:1) or every third (3:1) cardiac cycle. An appropriately timed IABP will effectively lower impedance to LV ejection and augment diastolic pressure. The net effect on myocardial mechanics is to decrease myocardial oxygen consumption, increase cardiac output, and lower peak LV wall stress.[13] The magnitude of counterpulsation hemodynamic effect depends on several factors, including the relation of balloon volume to aorta size, heart rate and rhythm, and aortic compliance.[14,15] Selection of balloon size is determined by the height of the patient. For patients shorter than 5 ft, a 25-cm^3 balloon is recommended, while, for patients taller than 6 ft, a 50-cm^3 balloon is available, with three to four balloon sizes in the range from 25-50 cm^3.

The IABPs are classified differently for different pathological conditions. For deterioration of cardiac function predicted to be short term, such as in acute coronary syndrome, cardiac and noncardiac surgery, and complications of heart failure (HF), these devices are classified as Class II with special controls. These special controls recommend testing of nonimplantable components, including the IABP control system, to ensure electrical safety and compatibility with other hospital equipment, as well as software verification and validation. The IAB must demonstrate biocompatibility, mechanical integrity, durability, and reliability to support its intended purpose. Rate limit testing should be conducted to verify that the IABP can successfully inflate and deflate the available range of IAB balloons (30–50 mL) connected to the IABP system. Electrocardiography (ECG) trigger validation testing can be conducted using recordings of real ECG waveforms from the American Heart Association database. Reliability testing is recommended to confirm that the IABP system could run continuously for 9 days and perform as intended. If the IABP is to be used for septic shock and pulsatile flow generation, these devices require Class III approval.[5]

12.5.2 Cardiopulmonary Bypass

The second category of short-term blood-contacting devices is external circuits through which blood is pumped and oxygenated. These include cardiopulmonary bypass (CPB), used during open heart surgery, and extracorporeal membrane oxygenation (ECMO), which provides longer-term support when evaluating treatment options for cardiopulmonary dysfunction. Cardiopulmonary bypass was developed in 1953 by Dr. John Gibbons at the Mayo Clinic to support the open-heart surgery needed for heart transplantation. In CPB, the patient's heart is arrested and blood is diverted through an external circuit for gas exchange before being returned to the body. This provides a static bloodless field for the surgeon to repair the heart chamber or valves, replace valves or blood vessels, implant a left ventricular assist device (LVAD), remove clots from the pulmonary artery, and transplant a heart. The circuit is connected to the circulation under general anesthesia, with aortic cannulation for return of oxygenated blood and right atrial cannulation for gravity-assisted drainage of deoxygenated blood into the circuit. A perfusionist monitors and regulates blood flow and blood oxygenation to optimize tissue perfusion and protection. Most procedures strive to limit the time on CPB to 1 hour or less.

The CPB circuit consists of several devices, connected by tubing, that support the pumping and gas exchange of blood during cardiac surgery. The circuit components typically include a roller pump; an oxygenator with a built-in heat exchanger; an arterial filter, connected with sterile tubing; reservoirs for managing fluid volumes; and cannulae for attachment to the native vessels. The blood volume needed to fill the circuit requires expansion of the native blood with a priming solution, which dilutes hematocrit. All the CPB circuit components are Class II, with most needing only performance controls for regulatory approval. Exceptions are devices that perform critical functions, such as the oxygenator and arterial line filter. These two components require special controls, as described in the FDA guidance documents "Guidance for Cardiopulmonary Bypass Oxygenators 510(k) Submissions"[16] and "Guidance for Cardiopulmonary Bypass Arterial Line Blood Filter 510(k) Submissions."[17]

12.5.2.1 Cardiopulmonary Bypass Oxygenator

Oxygenators provide exchange of oxygen and carbon dioxide between the blood and a source from respiratory gases. Bubble oxygenators enable direct transfer by mixing gases directly with the blood. Membrane or hollow-fiber designs separate blood and gas with a semipermeable membrane. In the hollow-fiber design, gas flows inside the fibers and blood on the outside, filling the chamber surrounding the fibers. Blood and gas flows are countercurrent, and gas is usually carbogen (95% oxygen/5% carbon dioxide). This design reduces the gradient between blood and gas, the membrane fiber area, as well as the trauma produced by passage of blood inside of the fibers. The major resistance to gas exchange in these devices is on the blood side, as fluid boundary layers limit transport at the fiber surface. Carbon dioxide transport occurs more rapidly than oxygen transport; thus, materials with good permeability to oxygen and resistance to plasma leakage are selected. Commonly used fiber materials include silicone and microporous polypropylene. Blood damage to abnormal shear exposure within the oxygenator can produce significant hemolysis of blood. High doses of anticoagulants are needed to reduce clot formation within the circuit, which can plug tubing and the hollow fibers of the oxygenator. Arterial filters are important to prevent nonbiological particles and emboli from being infused back into the patient.

Bench testing of CPB components requires a mock circulatory loop of bovine blood that uses a large venous reservoir and a second oxygenator for the simulated patient. The second oxygenator uses a mixture of nitrogen and carbon dioxide as the gas to deoxygenate the blood. Following the recommendations in the guidance document, the oxygenator must be investigated for leaks, toxicity, loss of gas transfer efficiency, gas embolism, thromboembolism, and blood damage. The circuit components should be tested at a blood flow rate of 5 L/min for 6 hours. Operating specifications for CPB oxygenators include an inflow oxygen transfer requirement of 250 mL/min and an outflow carbon dioxide elimination of 200 mL/min at a blood flow rate of 5 L/min.[18] Most oxygenators also serve as heat exchangers and must be characterized for safety and performance. The heat-exchange performance factor is calculated from the difference in blood temperature across the oxygenator, divided by the difference between water and blood temperature at the oxygenator inlet. The water side pressure difference should be monitored. The arterial line filter must be evaluated for hemolysis separately from the oxygenator, and platelet functionality must be characterized. Excessive pressure drop across the filter over the time of use may result in inadequate blood flow and should be measured. The filtration efficiency measures the ability of the device to remove solid and gaseous emboli by using a bubble generator and detector in the circuit. Standard hemocompatibility and sterility testing are also expected.

12.5.3 Extracorporeal Membrane Oxygenation

Extracorporeal membrane oxygenation, or extracorporeal life support (ECLS), as it is currently known, is essentially a long-term version of CPB that provides circulatory and respiratory support for hours to days. The standard CPB provides temporary cardiopulmonary support during various types of cardiac surgical procedures, while the purpose of ECMO is to allow time for intrinsic recovery of the lungs and heart. Extracorporeal life support is almost always "partial" bypass, as opposed to "total" bypass, which is required for cardiac operations. The amount of blood flow is based on the degree of support required, which is based on a series of physiological monitors in the circuit and on the patient. Many days may be required for the native heart or lungs to regain adequate function, and continuous anticoagulation is required. In general, ECLS is indicated in acute severe reversible cardiac or respiratory failure, when the risk of dying from the primary disease despite optimal conventional treatment is high (50%–100%). Usually, a patient on ECMO will also be on a ventilator, to give the lungs a chance to heal. The current survival rate is 80% for neonatal respiratory failure, 60% for pediatric respiratory failure, 50% for adult respiratory failure, 45% for pediatric cardiac failure, and 40% for adult cardiac failure.[19]

An ECMO circuit is a system of devices and accessories that provides assisted extracorporeal circulation and physiological gas exchange of the patient's blood in patients with acute respiratory failure or acute cardiopulmonary failure, where other available treatment options have failed and continued clinical deterioration is expected or the risk of death is imminent. The main devices and accessories of the system include, but are not limited to, the console (hardware), software, and disposables, including, but not limited to, an oxygenator, blood pump, heat exchanger, cannulae, tubing, filters, and other accessories (e.g., monitors, detectors, sensors, and connectors). In contrast to CPB, ECMO in adults is often performed by utilizing vessels closer to the surface (femoral and jugular). Cannulation can be performed under local anesthesia, and the ECMO circuit is more compact and controlled by a console. Two types of cannulation are as follows: V-A ECMO routes blood from the internal jugular or femoral vein through the circuit and into the femoral artery, providing almost total cardiopulmonary support. Blood passing through the native lungs dilutes downstream oxygenation, and thrombotic complications are a major source of morbidity. V-V ECMO oxygenates venous blood by connecting one or both internal jugular veins to the circuit, enabling 100% of the blood to pass through the heart. Extracorporeal membrane oxygenation is extensively used in neonates with severe respiratory failure, refractory to maximal medical management, with potentially reversible etiology. It serves as a bridge-to-decision device and provides temporary assistance for patients with single ventricle or other congenitally complex cardiovascular anatomies undergoing cardiac repair surgeries.[20] Similar to CPB, ECMO components are bundled into circuits selected by each hospital. Thus, many of the components are shared, except for the ECLS oxygenators, which are designed for longer-term use than CPB oxygenators, as they are designed with smaller priming volumes (150 mL, adult) and membrane surface area ($1.2 m^2$, adult), as well as with better materials for plasma leak resistance.

12.6 Implantable Vascular Devices

This section addresses devices with long-term exposure to blood and cardiovascular tissue. These are divided into vascular implants and cardiac implants. Long-term complications resulting from implanted devices include those mentioned previously from vessel wall damage and thrombosis, as well as complications from surgical attachment. Dehiscence is the failure of the wounds inflicted during surgery to heal, usually at the sutured connection of the device to the native tissue. During surgery, the sutures can be tied too tightly, causing necrosis or ischemia, especially when postoperative edema expands the tissue volume. Conversely, sutures that are tied too loosely can become untied, allowing the wound to open before it is healed. This can result in a separation of the implant from the native tissue at the attachment site. When this occurs in vascular implants, there can be leakage into the tissue, outside of the vascular space. When dehiscence occurs in the heart, as with heart valves or annuloplasty rings, it results in a paravalvular orifice that allows for regurgitation, ultimately causing implant failure and a need for reoperation. Dehiscence is often accompanied by infection, either from the initial implant surgery or developing later from some other source of endocarditis.[21]

12.6.1 Intravascular Blood Filter

Vascular implants include devices delivered by catheter, as well as traditional surgery. One of the least invasive of the catheter-delivered devices is the intravascular blood filter. A cardiovascular intravascular filter is an implant that is placed in the inferior vena cava (IVC), primarily for preventing thromboemboli from flowing into the right side of the heart and pulmonary circulation. These devices are usually deployed in patients with documented deep vein thrombosis (DVT), a blood clot in the legs that is formed mostly by immobility. Parts of this thrombus can break off and travel up the IVC, the main vessel that drains blood from the legs to the heart. The blood clot will travel through the IVC and into the heart. If the clot reaches the heart, it will pass into and lodge in a branch of the pulmonary artery, the main vessel that supplies blood to the lungs. If this happens, the lung tissue begins to die, which can result in death. The IVC filters are also placed in patients who exhibit other complications with the normal anticoagulation-based approach to DVT and for patients with a high risk of DVT, leading to pulmonary embolism (PE), including trauma and surgical procedures of the lower abdomen.

To prevent PE, an IVC filter can be placed.[22] The IVC filters consist of collapsible cages made from nitinol wires that are delivered via catheter through the femoral vein and released into the IVC. The filter is a nonobstructive cage that can trap blood clots before they reach the heart. To insert the device, a small catheter is introduced into a vein in the leg and advanced into the IVC under image guidance, until it reaches the target location, where it is deployed. As the filter is pushed out of the catheter, it begins to expand, filling the IVC. Hooks on the filter attach to the wall of the IVC, holding it securely in place. As blood clots break off, they are trapped by the filter and slowly dissolved by the body's natural agents. Once the risk for PE has ceased, the filter can be removed. Removal of the filter is similar to the placement. A catheter is advanced up to the location of the filter. A snare is place inside the catheter and advanced to the filter, where it is looped around a hook. As the snare pulls on the filter, the hooks detach from the wall of the vessel, collapsing easily back into the catheter. The filter and catheter are then removed.

Although retrievable IVC filter are approved for temporary and permanent use, only 14%–75% of temporary filters are retrieved, leaving the potential for long-term complications. Although mortality related to IVC filter is very low, significant complications occur in up to 27% of cases.[23] One of the most prevalent is migration of the IVC filter from the deployment site, either at the initial procedure or subsequently. Minor local migration is commonly reported and does not appear to be associated with clinically significant events. The walls of the IVC move with respiration, and changes in intra-abdominal pressure occur, which induce flexion on the filter struts. Regional migration of several centimeters may result in occlusion of the renal arteries or the IVC itself, especially if flow disturbances are created during the migration, and contribute to thrombus growth within the IVC filter. Distal migration has been reported in 2%–5% of cases and involves the filter detachment from the IVC and entry into the right atrium of the heart. Misalignment, including tilting, angulation, and incomplete opening of the IVC filter, may also result in thrombotic complications and damage to the vessel wall. Filter fracture can occur at several stages during deployment and presents a serious risk of emboli for the patient.

Owing to the high risk of complications from IVC filter, special controls are required for FDA approval of this Class II device.[24] Submissions are recommended to demonstrate that the filter is nonthrombogenic; possesses a high filter efficiency, without impeding the blood flow; is securely fixed within the IVC during its use; exhibits a low rate of associated morbidity; is magnetic resonance (MR) compatible; and can be inserted safely and rapidly by using a percutaneous procedure. In addition to biocompatibility testing, bench testing must be performed to demonstrate clot-trapping ability without significant reduction in overall blood flow. Fatigue and corrosion resistance of the filter must also be evaluated, as well as the forces of the hooks on the IVC wall, the limits of detachment and caval perforation; and thrombogenicity. Appropriate labeling of warnings must accompany the results of testing for regulatory consideration.

12.6.2 Stents

An intravascular stent is a synthetic tubular structure intended for permanent implant in native or graft vasculature. The stent is designed to provide radial mechanical support after deployment, which is meant to enhance vessel patency over the life of the device. The stent is delivered with a catheter inserted into an arterial vessel, in the same type of procedure used for vascular dilatation. Once the stent reaches the target location under image guidance, it is expanded by a balloon or self-expanding mechanism. Stents were developed to address the growing problem with restenosis following balloon angioplasty treatment. As mentioned previously, restenosis rates of 25%–50% within 6 months are common, which diminishes the cost-effectiveness of PCI.

The majority of peripheral stents are bare-metal stents, made from stainless steel, Co–Cr alloy, or Nitinol. The first two are plastically deformed into place by using a balloon, inflated as described during PCI. Nitinol, otherwise known as shape-memory alloy, is delivered from a cooled catheter into the heated bloodstream; it springs into position by assuming superelastic properties in that temperature range. When the stent is placed in the vessel, it produces both a surface injury to the endothelium and a stretch injury to the underlying vascular tissue. As detailed earlier in this chapter, the vessel wall injury exposes underlying collagen and plaque; this presents an early risk of thrombosis, which is reduced by anticoagulant therapy for the first month. The stretch injury causes inflammation and cell proliferation, resulting in intimal hyperplasia and restenosis or a reoccurrence of narrowing of the vessel lumen. Stents are manufactured in a range of diameter and lengths to accommodate most lesions. When crimped onto the balloon, the largest diameter is the crossing profile, which limits the size of the lesion that can be traversed without puncture, typically around 1 mm. The stent is positioned within the target artery by using radiopaque markers. Optimal selection and deployment of the stent include achieving maximal vessel lumen diameter and minimal vessel wall injury. Both undersized and oversized stents are associated with higher restenosis rates.[25]

A coronary stent is a metal scaffold placed via a delivery catheter into the coronary artery or a saphenous vein graft to maintain the lumen open for blood flow. In the short term, the device increases blood flow through the vessel. Over the long term, the device must heal into the surrounding tissue while maintaining the open lumen of the blood vessel. Stents are typically made of a metal mesh that covers only 7%–20% of the solid vessel wall beneath it. The mesh is constructed of wires that can be open- or closed-cell, coiled, laser-cut, or multilinked. The stent should be flexible enough to conform to tissue anatomy but stiff enough to provide vascular support. As observed with PCI, intimal hyperplasia results from treatment-induced injury and causes rapid restenosis of bare-metal stents in the coronary circulation in approximately 30% of patients within 12 months. Although a significant improvement over unstented PCI, this complication diminished the cost-effectiveness of the procedure. In 2003, the first drug-eluting stent (DES) was approved. The DES is a bare-metal stent that is coated with a drug-imbedded polymer that slowly releases anti-inflammatory agents into the tissue to reduce restenosis.[26] Clinical results demonstrated a 90% reduction in restenosis within 12 months, a dramatic improvement in treatment longevity. Some studies have indicated that the DES presents an increased risk of late-stage thrombosis, possibly related to the depletion of the drug coating, accompanied by cessation or reduction of anticoagulant therapy. Many speculated that this complication was not observed in bare-metal stents, because they were coated with a protective layer of endothelial cells and the stent struts were "embedded" into the wall of the artery, thereby becoming an "inside the wall" support. Recommendations for the DES and late-stage thrombosis include extending antiplatelet use to 1 year and improving deployment practices to reduce malapposition. A recent innovation is the resorbable stent, which functions as a DES for the first year but gradually resorbs over time, leaving the vessel free to heal. The device is an absorbable scaffold polylactide with a drug-eluting coating; it is placed via a delivery catheter into the coronary artery or saphenous vein graft to maintain the lumen. The drug coating is intended to inhibit restenosis. The absorbable stent provides mechanical support to the treated artery and a drug agent to prevent restenosis of the treated artery. It then gradually dissolves and is absorbed by the body within approximately 3 years.

12.6.2.1 Stent Design

All intravascular stents are Class III devices, which are governed by extensive ASTM standards and a FDA guidance document.[27] An extensive battery of nonclinical engineering testing on material characterization, stent dimensional and functional attributes, delivery system dimensional and functional attributes, shelf life, and biocompatibility is recommended. Many of these fall within standard engineering metrology and quality testing, but some are related to the mechanical interaction of diseased blood vessels and stents. The design and functionality of the stent delivery system design have essentially the same requirements as PCI: the catheter must safely and reliably deliver the stent to the intended location, without damage to the tissue or stent. Tip and balloon properties are critical to stent deployment and should follow the principles described in Section 12.4.2.

12.6.2.1.1 Foreshortening/Recoil.
Foreshortening is a dimensional change that may occur when deploying a stent, influencing the final stent length. Foreshortening is calculated as the change in length during loading, normalized by the loaded length; it is reported as a percentage and included in the labeling. Typical values of foreshortening range from 0% to 20%. Recoil is reported as the measured change in stent diameter between the postballoon expansion state during loading and after unloading, when the balloon is deflated. It is reported as a percentage, normalized by the expanded diameter.

12.6.2.1.2 Radial Stiffness, Strength, and Force.
The ability of the stent to resist collapse in compliant vessels under short-term or long-term external loads is critical. Radial stiffness is measured as the change in stent diameter as a function of uniformly applied external radial pressure and radial strength, with notation of the pressure at which the stent experiences irrecoverable deformation, which may differ with stent diameter and length. The outward force imposed by the stent is balanced by radial and hoop stresses in the tissue, as described by the law of Laplace. These stresses should be minimized to reduce the mechanobiological response that leads to intimal hyperplasia.

12.6.2.1.3 Mechanical Properties, Stress/Strain, and Fatigue.
Finite element analysis (FEA) can be used to model the stent, loading surfaces, and boundary conditions. The details of the analysis, including vessel compliance, loading conditions, contact elements, and mesh geometry must be rationalized, and the results must be validated with appropriate bench testing. Loading conditions should include radial dilation, torsion, bending, axial tension/compression, and crushing (peripheral applications).

Although stents add to the cost of PCI procedures, they are used in 75% of PCI treatments, constituting a $8 billion market.

12.6.3 Vascular Graft Prosthesis

A vascular graft prosthesis is an implanted device intended to repair, replace, or bypass sections of native or artificial vessels and to provide vascular access. It is commonly constructed of materials such as polyethylene terephthalate and polytetrafluoroethylene (PTFE), and it may be coated with a biological coating, such as albumin and collagen, or a synthetic coating, such as silicone. The graft structure is not made of materials of animal origin, including human umbilical cords.

12.6.3.1 Large Grafts (Diameter Greater than 6 mm)

Vascular prostheses for large vessels are designed to treat patient with occlusive or aneurysmal diseases and trauma patients that require vascular replacement and to provide dialysis access. The simplest of these prostheses are woven conduits that rely on controlled thrombosis of the graft surface, which is then encapsulated by fibrous tissue, forming a neointimal surface that is thromboresistant. These conduits often replace the native vessel, which is removed. Catheter- delivered vascular grafts have been very successful in treating abdominal aneurysms, with less mortality and morbidity risks for the patient. Abdominal aortic aneurysm results from weakening of the abdominal aortic wall, which causes bulging, further thinning the wall, and increased risk of rupture. These devices consist of a vascular graft mounted within a stent, which is expanded into the vessel with a dual-catheter procedure. The stent graft covers the native vessel, creating a new flow path with a normal aortic diameter.

12.6.3.2 Small Grafts (Diameter Less than 6 mm)

Small-diameter vascular grafts are needed to replace or bypass sections of the coronary arteries for patients with severe multivessel coronary artery disease or HF. Thus far, the patency of synthetic small-caliber grafts has been poor, and they have not been practical for coronary artery bypass grafting (CABG). The major causes of graft failure have been thrombosis and intimal hyperplasia of the graft. Satisfactory synthetic materials have not been successful for CABG so far because of their poor long-term patency rates. Although polyester and expanded PTFE (ePTFE) grafts have been used successfully in peripheral revascularization cases, these small-caliber vascular grafts have failed for coronary replacement. Polyester grafts suffer from thrombosis and neointimal proliferation. ePTFE grafts also have had poor patency rates because of surface thrombogenicity. In general, patency rates have varied widely between 60% at 1 year and 14% at approximately 3 years. For this reason, autologous vessels such as the internal mammary artery and saphenous vein are preferred for coronary artery bypass grafts.

The risks and complications associated with large- and small-diameter grafts are generally similar, include a variety of blood and tissue responses, and must be assessed and mitigated to ensure success of the device design.[28] Thromboembolic complications can arise from material biocompatibility or property mismatch at the anastomosis to the native vessel. Depending on the strength and distribution of stress along the sutured connection, property mismatch may lead to dehiscence or failure of the graft at the suture line. Appropriate testing to ensure suture retention strength is recommended. As with all blood-contacting devices, if the surgical integration produces flow alterations such as stasis, then thrombus risk is increased. The woven materials comprising vascular grafts are often porous and somewhat permeable to water and blood seepage. A false aneurysm can occur if leakage of fluid into the space between the graft and the native vessel wall or soft tissue encapsulation takes place. For this reason, extensive special controls are suggested for Class II regulatory approval, as recommended in the FDA guidance document.[28] This includes a study of biostability or the degradation of properties following implantation, porosity, permeability, strength, and suture retention strength. Assurance that the graft will not kink or collapse under physiological pressures must be provided.

12.7 Cardiac Implantable Devices

12.7.1 Septal Occluder

Atrial and ventricular septal defects are common congenital heart defects. These arterial–venous shunts cause oxygenated blood to mix with deoxygenated blood and reduce[29] systemic tissue oxygenation. Although it produces serious symptoms in some patients, it goes undetected until adulthood in 25%.[30] Traditionally, these defects required open heart surgery for repair, but in 2009, a catheter-based treatment, known as the septal occlude, was developed, which is used widely today. The device is a permanent implant placed in septum for the closure of atrial or ventricular septal defects. The septal occluder consists of loops of metal wire (Nitinol), supporting a microporous polyurethane patch that is delivered via a venous catheter system. Two patches are used in the procedure, one on either side of the hole, and cinched together. Fibrous encapsulation integrates the devices into the tissue, providing permanent septal closure. These are regulated as two different products, one for atrial septal defect and the other for ventricular septal defect; both are Class III devices. Each product must demonstrate safety and efficacy for long-term implantation to obtain regulatory approval.

12.7.2 Annuloplasty Ring

An annuloplasty ring is a rigid or flexible ring implanted around the mitral or tricuspid heart valve for reconstructive treatment of valvular insufficiency. The ring is sutured to the annular tissue to reshape, reinforce, and tighten the valve; this enables more complete leaflet closure. The stiff ring alters annular biomechanics, reducing the ability of the annulus to change size, which can lead to lower cardiac outputs. Valve repair with annuloplasty rings does not usually require long-term anticoagulant therapy, but short-term complications common with all cardiac surgery occur; therefore, it requires careful monitoring and appropriate physician training.

Annuloplasty rings are usually constructed of a PTFE core covered with polyester fabric, which can be a source of thromboembolism. Some materials cause blood damage and must be verified for hemocompatibility and hemolysis. Excessive stress resulting from heart dilation or overload may cause ring fracture. Material defects, including corrosion, may weaken material, resulting in failure. Dehiscence at the suture line is observed in some patients, which allows a paravalvular orifice for regurgitant flow. Clinical complications from annuloplasty result from a variety of sources, including progression of native cardiovascular disease. Although regurgitation is greatly reduced following proper repair, some of it may still be present and worsen with time. Reoperation for additional repair or valve replacement should be done before a decline in ventricular function occurs. Valvular stenosis may progress following annuloplasty, resulting in blood flow abnormalities and ultimately leading to fibrosis and calcification of the valve.

The device was reclassified from Class III to Class II special controls in 1999' recommendations are provided in a FDA guidance document.[31] The special controls for annuloplasty rings include biocompatibility, sterility, packaging, performance testing, and labeling recommendations. Performance testing includes computational structural analysis, mechanical testing, sterilization, and shelf life validation. Computational analysis, such as FEA, is used to evaluate the structural integrity of a new annuloplasty ring design with a solid core. The results must be validated by in vivo comparisons. Tensile testing is used to measure the strength of the annuloplasty ring to ensure that structure failure will occur at loads far greater than those experienced in vivo. Tensile testing serves as a special control to address ring fracture and the failure of the sewing ring fabric. Suture pull-out testing is used to determine the strength of the fabric component and to ensure that the sewing cuff can retain the suture in the heart annulus. This test is used to verify that the fabric can withstand forces experienced in vivo. Suture pull-out tests are recommended as a special control to help prevent ring dehiscence.

12.7.3 Mitral Valve Repair

The rapidly growing area of mitral valve repair devices has expanded from annuloplasty rings to a variety of catheter-based devices tailored to address specific valve dysfunctions. Only one, the MitraClip®, has gained regulatory approval at this time. It is designed to reduce mitral regurgitation by performing the edge-to-edge procedure, also known as the Alfieri stitch, using a cloth-covered metal clip that crimps over the edges of both leaflets together.[32] Blood flows through two smaller valve orifices on either side of the clip. Over time, the device is covered by a fibrous encapsulation, becoming integrated with the valve tissue. This device is regulated as a Class III device, as well as the catheter delivery system that performs the crimp.

12.7.4 Heart Valve Replacement

A replacement heart valve is a device intended to perform the function of any of the heart's natural valves. Heart valve prostheses fall into two categories, mechanical and bioprosthetic. Mechanical heart valves (MHVs) are made with all synthetic materials, usually rigid, attached to a flexible cloth-covered sewing ring for suturing to the native tissue. Both single-leaflet MHV designs, also known as tilting disk, and bileaflet MHV designs are available, but bileaflet MHV is preferred towing to fewer complications. All MHVs require anticoagulant therapy for the lifetime of the valve in the patient. Bioprosthetic valves are trileaflet valves that resemble the native aortic valve geometry and are made from porcine aortic or bovine pericardium treated with glutaraldehyde and chemicals to remove immunogenic material; however, they retain the native tissue properties. These valves are also mounted on a cloth-covered sewing ring for attachment. The design of these valves emulates the natural valve, with a central orifice that opens to allow forward flow. Anticoagulant therapy is not required for bioprosthetic valves, reducing associated bleeding complications. Bioprosthetic valves are vulnerable to calcification over time and degenerate more rapidly than MHVs, often lasting no more than 10 years, before requiring replacement. Traditionally implanted with an open-chest procedure, heart valve replacements are now also delivered transcutaneously via catheter.

Heart valves are made in a range of sizes to match the native geometry, based on the annulus diameter. Selection is based on imaging of patient geometry, as well as metal sizers that can be placed in the valve space during surgery and manually oriented. Each heart valve design accomplishes the job of a check valve in different ways, which require a detailed explanation and rationale for the design choices, in addition to bench testing. Thus, the valve locations, annulus positions, and suture technique must all be specified, along with the number and articulation of leaflets and how they occlude flow, including the fully open and closed angles, and travel arc in between. In addition, the fabrication of the support framework, including the sewing ring and stent for the leaflets, how it is attached, and how alignment is ensured during placement, must be indicated.

All heart valve replacements are Class III devices and require extensive testing for regulatory approval.[33] The goal of valve replacements is to improve cardiac function by maximizing forward flow and reducing regurgitant flow. Clinically, valve function is assessed with Doppler echocardiography to measure flow velocity during the cardiac cycle. Effective orifice area, EOA, is a global index that estimates the equivalent area for valvular flow from the continuity equation. The EOA is measured using the continuity equation:

$$EOA = A_{LVOT} * VTI_{LVOT} / VTI \tag{12.2}$$

where A_{LVOT} is the cross-sectional area of the left ventricular outflow tract (LVOT) and VTI_{LVOT} and VTI are the velocity time integrals measured by Doppler echocardiography for the LVOT and native valves, respectively. The VTIs can be calculated using the echo machine software or with the following equation:

$$VTI = Mean\ velocity \times ejection\ time \tag{12.3}$$

This relationship can be applied to either the mitral or aortic valve, as long as no regurgitation is present. If aortic regurgitation is present, then the continuity equation applied to the mitral valve will overestimate the EOA. In this condition, the pulmonic valve values should be used for A_{LVOT} and VTI_{LVOT}. If significant mitral regurgitation is present, the continuity method will underestimate mitral valve EOA and the pressure half-time (PHT) approach is recommended:

$$EOA = 220/PHT \qquad PHT = 0.29 \times \text{deceleration time} \qquad (12.4)$$

The performance index is obtained from the EOA divided by the preimplant measured orifice area of the replacement valve.

Transvalvular flow is also an important index for both aortic and mitral valves, calculated using the echo software or from the following equation:

$$\text{Flow} = \text{Valve cross-sectional area} \times VTI/\text{ejection time} \qquad (12.5)$$

Doppler velocity can be converted into pressure gradients by using the Bernoulli equation to assess the clinical hemodynamic performance:

$$\Delta P = K\left(V_d^2 - V_p^2\right) \qquad (12.6)$$

where K is a constant and depends on valve type, ΔP is the pressure gradient, V_d is the distal velocity measured by continuous wave Doppler, and V_p is the proximal velocity measured by pulsed Doppler. K has a theoretical value of 4, which can be compared with the experimentally measured value. Large deviations may affect clinical measurements of pressure gradients, for diagnosis and prognosis.[34]

Materials of MHVs must exhibit excellent corrosion and fatigue resistance. Cavitation testing is recommended, as cavitation erosion has been observed in failed valves. Bioprosthetic valve tissue must demonstrate appropriate failure strength and resistance to fatigue damage, as evaluated by histology and stress–strain testing. Accelerated wear testing for durability is recommended to ensure a 600 million cycle lifetime for MHVs and 200 million cycle lifetime for bioprosthetic valves under pulsatile flow and physiological loading. Valves should be tested at 120 mmHg peak LV pressure at a maximum flow rate of 7 L/m, increasing the LVP up to 200 mmHg. The systolic ratio should be set at 35%.

12.7.5 Mechanical Circulatory Support

Heart failure is a debilitating condition that is responsible for more than 300,000 deaths each year and costs the US healthcare system more than $39 billion annually.[35] Advanced HF is an end-stage disease in which the heart is unable to pump blood sufficiently to meet tissue oxygen demand. Both the conditions that contribute most to the development HF are mechanical: hypertension, or high blood pressure, and coronary artery disease, which reduces blood flow to the heart tissue. Incidence of HF is currently at 20% and growing. The condition has a high mortality rate, with a 1-year mortality of

20% and a 5-year mortality of 50%.[36] Consequences of HF include dilation of the LV chamber and thinning of the myocardial wall, both of which contribute to decreased cardiac efficiency. The traditional treatment for advanced HF is heart transplantation, considered the gold standard in terms of survival, but it suffers from limited availability and concomitant immunosuppressive therapy, which compromises quality of life.

Over the past decade, a treatment for HF by using long-term mechanical circulatory support (MCS) has been developed and is growing rapidly. Implantation of an LVAD, a mechanical pump that is surgically connected to the heart and aorta, boosts systemic blood flow and improves tissue oxygenation. The current generations of LVADs are rotary flow pumps, consisting of a metal impeller and housing, through which blood flows from the heart. Power for the LVAD is received from an external source through a transcutaneous cable. The pumps are valveless, and the flow rate is highly dependent on the pressure gradient across the LVAD, the pump pressure–flow (H–Q) curve, and the LVAD pump speed.

The LVADs provide tremendous benefits for patients by reducing the symptoms of HF; however, 17%–20% of LVAD patients have a stroke within the first year of implantation[37] and 25% have a major bleeding event requiring hospitalization.[38-40] Thrombus development is often a consequence of altered blood flow dynamics, which can produce areas of flow stasis or turbulence that promote coagulation.[3,41] The long-term success of LVADs depends on optimizing the host response to the device, which changes with time and is patient-specific.[42,43] Implantation of the LVAD creates one of the most thrombogenic situations in cardiovascular medicine owing to the simultaneous combination of (1) a proinflammatory state after the surgery, (2) the presence of the device, and (3) alterations of the normal flow.

Implantation of the LVAD abruptly changes the natural blood flow path through the heart, introducing alterations in the normal pattern that are associated with thromboembolic events (TE).[2,44,45] The LVAD inlet is typically located at the LV apex and the outlet anastomoses to the ascending aorta, bypassing the aortic valve. Implantation of the LVAD provides an immediate increase in systemic blood flow and end-organ perfusion, providing an alternate pathway for blood to flow from the heart to the arterial system. The LVAD support unloads the heart, decreasing the magnitude and pulsatility of LV pressure, which can fall below the level needed to fully open the aortic valve during myocardial contraction. As identified in previous studies,[45,46] the abnormal flow pattern creates a region of flow stasis adjacent to the aortic valve, which creates a high risk for TE that could be embolized by a sudden strong contraction of the native heart. The risk of flow-mediated thrombus formation during LVAD support has been the subject of considerable study.[47] Platelets are activated by high shear stress, such as that experienced in the housing gaps of the LVAD, and the level of activation is proportionally related to the time exposure, accumulating with repeated exposures.[1,4] Flow-induced shear platelet activation causes both platelet aggregation and thrombin generation, with high potential for TE.[48] Thus, the benefit of anticoagulation therapies in LVAD recipients needs to be balanced against their associated increase in bleeding risk. Despite significant evidence indicating that anticoagulants reduce thrombosis in patients with MCS, the lack of suitable markers of thrombogenesis makes it difficult to manage anticoagulation regimens.

The LVADs are currently the most available and effective treatment for advanced HF. Although biological solutions such as stem cells and bioactive injectibles are in clinical trials, years remain before their widespread adoption. Until then, LVADs will play an increasing role in health care, as evidenced by the recent acquisitions of two small LVAD companies by large medical device institutions. A plethora of other MCS devices is available or in development, which will fill the treatment gap for patients with short-term or intermediate-stage HF.

12.7.6 Implantable Leads for Rhythm Management

An implantable pacemaker pulse generator is a device that has a power supply and electronic circuits that produce a periodic electrical pulse to stimulate the heart. An implantable lead is used to sense electrical signals and apply pacing according to thresholds set by a clinician. This device is used as a substitute for the heart's intrinsic pacing system to correct both intermittent and continuous cardiac rhythm disorders. This device may include triggered, inhibited, and asynchronous modes and is implanted in the thoracic cavity. A pacemaker electrode consists of flexible insulated electrical conductors, with one end connected to a pacemaker pulse generator and the other end applied to the heart. The device is used to transmit a pacing electrical stimulus from the pulse generator to the heart and/or to transmit the electrical signal of the heart to the pulse generator. Temporary electrodes are used for mapping cardiac conduction before permanent electrode placement. All implanted components of the ECG system are Class III devices.

12.8 Conclusion

Cardiovascular medical devices pose significant challenges to the human system, and their integration must strike a balance between preventing and harnessing the body's natural responses. A wide range of short- and long-term functions is enabled by device-based therapies, which range in materials, form, and their mechanical effect. Devices placed in direct contact with endothelium, such as stents, vascular grafts, and septal occluders, must manage both the initial injury response and the chronic presence of a foreign body. In contrast, devices that extend into the bloodstream must manage the activation and destruction of blood components, which manifest clinically as hemolysis, thrombosis, bleeding, and stroke. For catheters, heart valves, blood filters, CPB components, and mechanical circulatory assist devices, the success largely depends on repelling protein adsorption and platelet activation. Active implants such as pacemaker electrodes, extracorporeal membrane oxygenators, and LVADs must also maintain long-term performance, without degradation of function.

References

1. Xenos M, Girdhar G, Alemu Y et al. Device thrombogenicity emulator (DTE) – Design optimization methodology for cardiovascular devices: A study in two bileaflet MHV designs. *J Biomech* 2010;43(12):2400–2409. doi:10.1016/j.jbiomech.2010.04.020.

2. Girdhar G, Xenos M, Alemu Y et al. Device thrombogenicity emulation: A novel method for optimizing mechanical circulatory support device thromboresistance. *PLoS One* 2012;7(3):e32463. doi:10.1371/journal.pone.0032463.

3. Bluestein D. Research approaches for studying flow-induced thromboembolic complications in blood recirculating devices. *Exp Rev Med Dev* 2004;1(1):65–80. doi:10.1586/17434440.1.1.65.

4. Bluestein D, Chandran KB, Manning KB, Luestein DB, Handran KBC, Anning KBM. Towards non-thrombogenic performance of blood recirculating devices. *Ann Biomed Eng* 2010;38:1236–1256. doi:10.1007/s10439-010-9905-9.

5. U.S. Food and Drug Administration. Center for Devices and Radiological Health. https://www.fda.gov/MedicalDevices/default.htm.

6. Grand View Research. *Clot Management Devices Market Analysis By Product (Neurovascular Embolectomy Devices, Embolectomy Balloon Catheters, Percutaneous Thrombectomy Devices, Catheter-Directed Thrombolysis Devices), By End User, And Segment Forecasts 2013–2024.* Pune, India: Grand View Research, 2016.

7. Jerius H, Bagwell D, Beall A, Brophy C. The impact of balloon embolectomy on the function and morphology of the endothelium. *J Surg Res* 1997;67(1):9–13. doi:10.1006/jsre.1996.4908.

8. Food and Drug Administration. *Class II Special Controls Guidance Document for Certain Percutaneous Transluminal Coronary Angioplasty (PTCA) Catheters.* Silver Spring, MD: U.S. Food and Drug Administration, 2015.

9. Angioplasty Balloons Market Analysis By Type (Normal Balloons, Drug Eluting Balloons, Cutting Balloons, Scoring Balloons), By Application (Peripheral Vascular Disease, Coronary Artery Disease), By End Use, By Region, And Segment Forecasts, 2018–2024, Grand View Research, Report GVR-1-68038-356-0, 2017.

10. Brodie BR. Adjunctive balloon postdilatation after stent deployment: Is it still necessary with drug-eluting stents? *J Interv Cardiol* 2006;19(1):43–50. doi:10.1111/j.1540-8183.2006.00103.x.

11. Fujii K, Carlier SG, Mintz GS et al. Stent underexpansion and residual reference segment stenosis are related to stent thrombosis after sirolimus-eluting stent implantation: An intravascular ultrasound study. *J Am Coll Cardiol* 2005;45(7):995–998. doi:10.1016/j.jacc.2004.12.066.

12. ASTM. *ASTM F748-06 Standard Practice for Selecting Generic Biological Test Methods for Materials and Devices.* West Conshohocken, PA: ASTM International, 1999.

13. Urschel CW, Eber L, Forrester J, Matloff J, Carpenter R, Sonnenblick E. Alteration of mechanical performance of the ventricle by intraaortic balloon counterpulsation. *Am J Cardiol* 1970;25(5):546–551.

14. Weber KT, Janicki JS. Intraaortic balloon counterpulsation. A review of physiological principles, clinical results, and device safety. *Ann Thorac Surg* 1974;17(6):602–636.

15. Kern MJ. Intra-aortic balloon counterpulsation. *Coronary Artery Dis* 1991:649–660.

16. U.S. Food and Drug Administration. *Guidance for Cardiopulmonary Bypass Oxygenators 510(k) Submissions. Guidance for Industry and FDA Staff*, 2000. http://www.fda.gov/downloads/MedicalDevices/DeviceRegulationandGuidance/GuidanceDocuments/ucm073670.pdf.

17. FDA. *Guidance for Cardiopulmonary Bypass Arterial Line Blood Filter 510 (K) Submissions*. 2000.

18. Cooney DO. *Biomedical Engineering Principles* (Bekey GA, Reneau DD, Eds.). New York: Marcel Dekker, 1976.

19. Lequier L, Horton S, McMullan D, Bartlett RH. Extracorporeal membrane oxygenation circuitry. *Pediatr Crit Care* 2013;14:1–10. doi:10.1097/PCC.0b013e318292dd10.Extracorporeal.

20. ELSO. *Extracorporeal Life Support Organization (ELSO) Guidelines for Neonatal Respiratory Failure*. Ann Arbor, MI: ELSO, 2013, pp. 1–5.

21. Brown MR, Javorsky G, Platts DG. Accuracy of 3-dimensional transoesophageal echocardiography in assessment of prosthetic mitral valve dehiscence with comparison to anatomical specimens. *Cardiol Res Pract* 2010;2010:2–3. doi:10.4061/2010/750874.

22. Deyoung E, Minocha J. Inferior vena cava filters: Guidelines, best practice, and expanding indications. *Semin Intervent Radiol* 2016;33(2):65–70. http://www.embase.com/search/results?subaction=viewrecord&from=export&id=L610282085%0Ahttp://dx.doi.org/10.1055/s-0036-1581088.

23. Cipolla J, Weger NS, Sharma R et al. Complications of vena cava filters: A comprehensive clinical review. *OPUS 12 Sci* 2008;2(2):11–24.

24. United States Food and Drug Administration. *Guidance for Cardiovascular Intravascular Filter 510(k) Submissions*. Rockville, MD: Center for Devices and Radiological Help, Interventional Cardiology Devices Branch, 1999.

25. Lui HK. The perfect fit: Getting the most out of your coronary stent. *Cath Lab Dig* 2005;13(10):20–26.

26. U.S. Food and Drug Administration. *Guidance for Industry: Coronary Drug-Eluting Stents—Nonclinical and Clinical Studies*. Silver Spring, MD: U.S. Food and Drug Administration, 2008.

27. FDA. *Non-clinical Engineering Tests and Recommended Labeling for Intravascular Stents and Associated Delivery Systems*, 2010. http://www.fda.gov/medicaldevices/deviceregulationandguidance/guidancedocuments/ucm071863.htm.

28. FDA. *Guidance Document for Vascular Prostheses 510 (K) Submissions*. Rockville, MD: FDA, 2000.

29. Dee KC, Puleo DA, Bizios R. *An Introduction to Tissue-Biomaterial Interactions*. Hoboken, NJ: John Wiley & Sons, 2002.

30. Kim MS, Klein AJ, Carroll JD. Transcatheter closure of intracardiac defects in adults. *J Interv Cardiol* 2007;20(6):524–545. doi:10.1111/j.1540-8183.2007.00304.x.

31. FDA. *Guidance for Annuloplasty Rings 510 (K) Submissions*. Silver Spring, MD: U.S. Food and Drug Administration, 2001.

32. Fedak PWM, McCarthy PM, Bonow RO. Evolving concepts and technologies in mitral valve repair. *Circulation* 2008;117(7):963–974. doi:10.1161/CIRCULATIONAHA.107.702035.

33. U.S. Food and Drug Administration. *Draft Guidance for Heart Valves - Investigational Device Exemption (IDE) and Premarket Approval (PMA) Applications*, 2010. http://www.fda.gov/downloads/MedicalDevices/DeviceRegulationandGuidance/GuidanceDocuments/UCM198043.pdf.

34. Zoghbi W, Enriquez-Sarano M, Foster E et al. Recommendations for evaluation of the severity of native valvular regurgitation with two-dimensional and doppler echocardiography. *J Am Soc Echocardiogr* 2003;16:777–802.

35. Go AS, Mozaffarian D, Roger VL et al. Heart disease and stroke statistics-2013 update: A report from the American Heart Association. *Circulation* 2013;127(1):e6–e245. doi:10.1161/CIR.0b013e31828124ad.
36. Mozzafarian D, Benjamin EJ, Go AS et al. On behalf of the American heart association statistics committee and stroke statistics subcommittee. Heart disease and stroke statistics–2016 update: A report from the American heart association. *Circulation* 2016;133:e38–e360.
37. Petrucci RJ, Rogers JG, Blue L et al. Neurocognitive function in destination therapy patients receiving continuous-flow vs pulsatile-flow left ventricular assist device support. *J Heart Lung Transplant* 2012;31(1):27–36. doi:10.1016/j.healun.2011.10.012.
38. Harvey L, Holley CT, John R. Gastrointestinal bleed after left ventricular assist device implantation: Incidence, management, and prevention. *Ann Cardiothorac Surg* 2014;3(5):475–479. doi:10.3978/j.issn.2225-319X.2014.08.19.
39. Lopilato AC, Doligalski CT, Caldeira C. Incidence and risk factor analysis for gastrointestinal bleeding and pump thrombosis in left ventricular assist device recipients. *Artif Organs* 2015;39(11):939–944. doi:10.1111/aor.12471.
40. Whitson BA, Eckman P, Kamdar F et al. Hemolysis, pump thrombus, and neurologic events in continuous-flow left ventricular assist device recipients. *Ann Thorac Surg* 2014;97(6):2097–2103. doi:10.1016/j.athoracsur.2014.02.041.
41. Goswami KC, Yadav R, Bahl VK. Predictors of left atrial appendage clot: A transesophageal echocardiographic study of left atrial appendage function in patients with severe mitral stenosis. *Indian Heart J* 2004;56(6):628–635.
42. Adamson RM, Mangi AA, Kormos RL et al. Principles of heartMate II implantation to avoid pump malposition and migration. *J Card Surg* 2015;30:296–299. doi:10.1111/jocs.12478.
43. Taghavi S, Ward C, Jayarajan SN et al. Surgical technique influences HeartMate II left ventricular assist device thrombosis. *Ann Thorac Surg* 2013;96(4):1259–1265.
44. Fyrenius A, Wigström L, Ebbers T, Karlsson M, Engvall J, Bolger AF. Three dimensional flow in the human left atrium. *Heart* 2001;86(4):448–455. doi:10.1136/heart.86.4.448.
45. Wong K, Samaroo G, Ling I et al. Intraventricular flow patterns and stasis in the LVAD-assisted heart. *J Biomech* 2014;47(6):1485–1494. doi:10.1016/j.jbiomech.2013.12.031.
46. Reider C, Moon J, Ramesh V et al. Intraventricular thrombus formation in the LVAD-assisted heart studied in a mock circulatory loop. *Meccanica* 2017;52(3):515–528. doi:10.1007/s11012-016-0433-z.
47. Reider C, Moon J, Ramesh V et al. Intraventricular thrombus formation in the LVAD-assisted heart studied in a mock circulatory loop. *Meccanica* 2016. doi:10.1007/s11012-016-0433-z.
48. Hellums JD. 1993 Whitaker lecture: Biorheology in thrombosis research. *Ann Biomed Eng* 1994;22(5):445–455. doi:10.1007/BF02367081.

Index

Note: Page numbers in *italics* and **bold** refer to figures and tables, respectively.

Printed and bound by CPI Group (UK) Ltd, Croydon, CR0 4YY

17/10/2024

01775663-0006